Genetics and Medicine

Order this book online at www.trafford.com
or email orders@trafford.com

Most Trafford titles are also available at major online book retailers.

Note for Librarians: A cataloguing record for this book is available from Library
and Archives Canada at www.collectionscanada.ca/amicus/index-e.html

Printed in Victoria, BC, Canada.

ISBN: 9781-4269-0555-1 (soft cover)
ISBN: 9781-4269-0557-5 (eBook)

Our mission is to efficiently provide the world's finest, most comprehensive book publishing service, enabling every author to experience success. To find out how to publish your book, your way, and have it available worldwide, visit us online at www.trafford.com

Trafford rev. 08/10/09

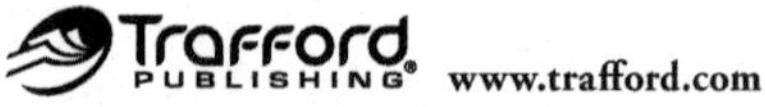

www.trafford.com

North America & international
toll-free: 1 888 232 4444 (USA & Canada)
phone: 250 383 6864 ♦ fax: 812 355 4082 ♦

Genetics and Medicine in Great Britain 1600 to 1939

Alan R. Rushton, M.D., Ph.D.

Trafford Publishing

To Nancy

Contents

Preface

The science of genetics is both old and new. It is old in the obvious sense that "like begets like." Such a statement is made evident for most of us in our day-to-day interactions with our own family members. Children often do resemble their parents in many respects. The new science of genetics is also young. The British biologist William Bateson coined the term "genetics" in 1905 to encompass both the fields of heredity and organ development beginning with the fusion of egg and sperm (Bateson, B., 1928). The new genetics aims to apply this scientific theory to the systematic understanding of transmission—how characters are passed from parent to child, and then of expression—how those inherited characters guide cellular growth and development throughout a lifetime.

Medical aspects of genetics have also been obvious for centuries. In daily practice, physicians often encountered characters—both normal and diseased—that appeared to "run in the family," being transmitted from parent to child. *Genetics and Medicine in Great Britain 1600 to 1939* has been written to provide a broad picture of how ideas on heredity evolved within the British medical community before World War II. The work is encyclopedic in its effort to touch upon the major areas within medicine that have found ideas on heredity and disease to be useful, not just theoretical. The book has utilized medical texts, journals and personal letters of scientists and physicians to illuminate the interaction between the science of heredity and the application of those concepts to medical practice.

Many sciences proceed at a steady pace over centuries of time, studying the chemical elements, rocks or insects. Only occasionally does a truly new science burst upon the intellectual landscape as "genetics" did in 1900. The study of heredity as practiced in animal and plant breeding had existed for centuries, of course. Breeding of parental types with specific characters often produced offspring with a similar constitution. Inbreeding then was utilized to maintain the desired traits in the flock or the field. In the 1860s, a monk living at the abbey in Brno, Czech Republic, began a series of plant breeding experiments that would revolutionize and define the modern science of genetics. Gregor Mendel was a science teacher and had extensive experience in mathematics and physics. He made thousands of crosses with garden peas and then tabulated the results of different physical characters. He concluded that the specific ratios of different traits that he obtained indicated the presence of some type of physical hereditary element that passed via egg from the mother, or via sperm from the father, to form a fertilized egg [zygote]. Knowing the pattern of segregation for each trait, it was then possible to accurately predict the outcome of any two parental crosses. In 1865, Mendel presented his findings at two meetings of the Naturforschenden Verein in Brno. The material was subsequently published in the *Verhandlungen des naturforschenden Vereines in Brunn*, which was then distributed to more than 120 libraries around the world (Zirkle, 1964).

Mendel's work was so radical in its application of statistical analysis to biological data that leading scientists of the day paid little attention to the monk's breeding studies. However, several botanists mentioned Mendel's paper in works published over the next three decades. W.O. Focke cited the work in his 1881 *Die Pflanzenmischlinge*, a book on plant breeding. Liberty Bailey also mentioned Mendel in his 1894 text *Plant Breeding*. And the ninth edition of the *Encyclopedia Britannica* also reported Mendel's studies (Zirkle, 1964).

Systematic plant breeding was taken up in the 1890s by several prominent botanists who were also interested in heredity. Pehr Bohlin from Sweden examined segregation of characters in peas and barley. He noted in 1897 that the outcomes of particular crosses "could be predicted with almost mathematical accuracy" (Von Tschermak-Seysenegg, 1951). Hugo de Vries was Professor of Botany at the University of Amsterdam. In 1894, he began a systematic study of heredity using poppies and *Oenothera* [evening primrose]. He believed that the characters segregated independently at fertilization. By the end of the decade, he had accumulated data on transmission of many traits from more than 30 different varieties of plants. He attempted to apply statistics to the analysis of his breeding results and noted cases of what would later be called dominant and recessive characters. In early 1900, de Vries prepared a summary of seven years work and submitted the manuscript to *Comptes Rendu de l'Academie des Sciences* on 14 March (de Vries, 1900a). Shortly thereafter, he received a copy of Mendel's 1865 paper from a friend, Professor Beijerinck from Delft, whose accompanying letter observed, "I know you are studying hybrids, so perhaps the enclosed report of the year 1865 by a certain Mendel which I happen to possess is still of some interest to you" (Muller-Wille, 2007). De Vries then revised a longer article on his data to include this material rediscovered 35 years later. He submitted the second paper to *Berichte der Deutschen Botanischen Gesselschaft.* In the text, he commented "...I conclude that the splitting law of hybrids as discovered by Mendel has a very general application to the plant world, and that it has a fundamental significance for the study of units of which the specific character is composed" (Stamhuis, Meijer and Zevenhuizen, 1999; Olby, 1987; de Vries, 1900b; Zirkle, 1964). In a very real sense, the analytical methods utilized by de Vries in his breeding studies paralleled those of Mendel. De Vries almost stumbled upon the same general principles for heredity outlined by Mendel in 1865 (Mayr, 1982a).

Another prominent plant breeder of this era was Carl Correns, Dozent in Botany at the University of Tubingen. He too had embarked on a study of plant heredity and likewise found characteristic ratios for the inheritance of particular traits. His notebook for 16 April 1896 mentions that he had read Mendel's 1865 paper after seeing the reference in Focke's book, but was not particularly impressed by the results. Three years later when he began to consolidate his own breeding data, Correns reread Mendel's report, and noted, "like a flash," Mendel's analysis of the breeding data made sense of his own experimental results (Rheinberger, 1995). He subsequently received a reprint of de Vries *Comptes* paper in April 1900. The next day, Correns mailed an article to the *Berichte* to report his own plant breeding studies (Correns, 1900; Von Tschermak-Seysenegg, 1951; Muller-Wille, 2007).

Erich von Tschermak was a young botanist who studied plant breeding at the Austrian Imperial Family Foundation Estate. He had also noted characteristic ratios of traits in successive generations of plants and published the results in his Habilitationschrift [dissertation] in January 1900. After reading the de Vries papers, von Tschermak realized that his own studies showed dominant and recessive patterns of inheritance, as outlined by Mendel. He then prepared a paper for the June 1900 *Berichte* to publicize his research findings (Von Tschermak, 1900; Dunn, 1991a; Von Tschermak-Seysenegg, 1951).

The English biologist William Bateson from Cambridge University had likewise been doing systematic breeding studies of both plants and animals during the 1890s. When he became aware of Mendel's work in 1900, Bateson immediately saw how these laws illuminated his own breeding data. He noted, "We are in the presence of a new principle of the highest importance." His enthusiasm knew no bounds because the "Mendel experiments [are] worthy to rank with those which laid the foundation of the atomic laws of chemistry" (Olby, 1985).

The fact that this group of plant breeders quickly understood the relevance and usefulness of Mendel's theory for heredity in understanding their own work suggests that the intellectual climate in 1900 was prepared to be impressed by the new theory. It was an event just waiting to happen. In fact, shortly before the rediscovery in 1900, Bateson had spoken on the topic of heredity before the Royal Horticultural Society. He recognized the meager knowledge then available on the details of hereditary mechanisms. He noted,

> We want to know the whole truth of the matter, we want to know the physical basis, the...essential nature, the causes...of heredity. We also want to know the laws which the outward and visible phenomena [of heredity] obey...Of the nature of the physical basis of heredity we have no conception at all.
>
> We do not know what is the essential agent in the transmission of parental elements, and whether it is a material agent or not (Bateson, W., 1900).

In fact, cytological research completed before 1900 had already convinced many biologists that there was a physical unit for heredity and that it resided in the cell nucleus.

As early as 1883, Wilhelm Roux had postulated a theoretical explanation for the elegant pattern of cell division seen in all plants and animals. He reasoned that the dark staining chromatin fibers in the nucleus were not all uniform, but qualitatively different. The accurate division of chromatin fibers and their segregation to the daughter cells in mitosis and meiosis thus separated and distributed qualitatively different material to the two daughter cells. If this were not the case, then he thought that the whole complicated process of cell division would be "superfluous" (Wilson, 1900a). The botanist Edouard Strasburger observed the fusion of one male and one female nucleus to form the fertilized egg. He argued that the "fibers" in the nuclei had to be the physical agents for heredity from one generation to the next.

> The nuclear filaments of all the following nuclear divisions will contain approximately similar pieces of the nuclear filaments from the father and the mother...The carrier of the hereditary elements is really the cell nucleus, and its structures as well as its complicated division process result from this function (Churchill, 1987).

Further substantiation for the notion that the chromatin carried unique pieces of hereditary information was provided by the work of Theodor Boveri, Professor at the University of Wurzberg. He began to examine the role that the hereditary elements played in embryonic development of the sea urchin. Adult sea urchins usually contained 36 chromosomes in each cell nucleus. After meiosis, both egg and sperm contained 18 chromosomes. Fertilization of one egg fusing with one sperm then returned the chromosome number to 36 once again. Boveri sought to demonstrate that each chromosome was qualitatively distinct. He devised a method to fuse 2 sperm with each egg cell. After such fertilization, abnormal cell division occurred, resulting in sea urchin embryos with variable numbers of chromosomes. If the chromosomes were all equivalent, such maldistribution should have little effect on embryonic development. What Boveri found was that only those embryos with exactly 36 chromosomes began normal development. Hence, embryogenesis required not just some chromosomes, but the right number as well (Baltzer, 1964, 1967; Mayr, 1982b).

The American biologist E.B. Wilson summarized the current understanding of heredity and cells in the 1890s:

> We reach the remarkable conclusion that inheritance may, perhaps, be affected by the physical transmission of a particular chemical compound from parent to offspring (Wilson, 1895).

The transmission of that substance, chromatin, had been observed in numerous plants and animals, and

> ...must have a deep significance...The contrast points unmistakably to the conclusion that the most essential material handed on by the mother-cell to its progeny is the chromatin, and that this substance therefore has a special significance in heredity (Wilson, 1900b).

The association between the physical elements of chromosome fibers and the segregation of the theoretical hereditary units was further substantiated by cytological studies shortly after the rediscovery of Mendel's work in 1900. In September 1902, William Bateson traveled to the United States and lectured on Mendelian heredity. A young student, Walter Sutton, who worked with E.B. Wilson at Columbia University in New York City, attended one of these talks. Bateson captivated Sutton's interest in heredity and planted the seed in his mind that meiotic segregation of chromosomes and of hereditary elements had to be connected. Sutton observed that same year,

> I may call attention to the probability that the association of the paternal and maternal chromosomes in pairs and their subsequent separation during the reduction division [meiosis]... may constitute the physical basis of the Mendelian law of heredity (Sutton, 1902).

Sutton then convinced his mentor of these facts. Wilson publicized the association of Mendelism and chromosome segregation the following year.

> In view of the great interest that has been aroused of late by the revival and extension of Mendel's principles of inheritance, it is remarkable that, as far as I am aware, no one has yet pointed out the clue to these principles, if it be not an explanation for them, that is given by the normal cytological phenomena of maturation [of germ cells in meiosis] (Wilson, 1902).

Boveri likewise agreed on the importance of unifying the two fields of cytology and inheritance.

> The more our insight grows, the more we perceive that 'morphological' in these matters is only the sub-structure of what we eventually want to know; what in fact these chromatin elements, which bear such remarkable destinies, possess in respect of physiological significance (Dunn, 1991b).

> We see here that two areas of study which developed quite independently of each other have yielded results which are so harmonious as if one had been derived theoretically from the other...The probability is extraordinarily high that the characters dealt with in Mendel's experiments are truly connected to specific chromosomes (Baltzer, 1964).

In this case, the whole appeared to be greater than the sum of the individual parts.

In such manner, the science of genetics rapidly evolved during the first decade of the twentieth century. *Genetics and Medicine* has begun a new inroad to study how ideas on inheritance and disease developed in the minds of practicing British physicians. Before 1900, there was no "genetics," only rather ill defined notions of heredity. With the rediscovery of Mendel's work in 1900, the application of the new theory to both biological and medical sciences quickly developed. The author hopes that the material presented here will form a basis for other historians to examine this area of medicine in greater detail. This work is an outgrowth of a twenty-five year project that has reviewed the development of ideas on heredity and medicine in both Britain and the United States. The work in America resulted in the 1994 publication of *Genetics and Medicine in the United States 1800-1922.*

Professionals at several libraries contributed to the acquisition of reference material for this project. Grateful thanks are given to the media staff of Firestone Library at Princeton University; New York Academy of Medicine Library; College of Physicians of Philadelphia Library; American Philosophical Society Library in Philadelphia; the British Library, Royal Society of Medicine Library and University College London Special Collections Library in London; and the John Innes Center Library at the Norwich Bioscience Institute in Norwich, England for their efforts in locating the many references utilized in this research. The medical librarian, Jeanne Dutka, at Hunterdon Medical Center in Flemington, New Jersey, assisted in obtaining copies of more recent articles.

My wife, Nancy Spencer Rushton, endured piles of index cards and a distracted husband for the years of this project with her usual good humor. Her insightful editorial comments were also greatly appreciated.

Permission to quote extracts from unpublished archival material has been graciously granted by the following institutions:

American Philosophical Society Philadelphia, PA	Letters of William Bateson Letters of Charles Darwin
Scientific Manuscripts Collection Syndics of Cambridge University Library Cambridge, England	Letters of William Bateson Letters of Charles Darwin
Special Collections Division University College Library London, England	Manuscripts of Karl Pearson
Bateson Archives John Innes Foundation Norwich Bioscience Institute Norwich, England	Manuscripts of William Bateson

Part I
Heredity and Medicine 1600 to 1800

One
The Origins of Modern Science and Medicine

In 1657, the English physician William Harvey wrote a letter to a colleague, Dr. Vlackweld of Haarlem in the Netherlands:

> Nature is nowhere accustomed more openly to display her recent mysteries than in cases where she shows traces of her workings apart from the beaten path; nor is there any better way to advance the proper practice of medicine than to give our mind to the discovery of the usual laws of nature by careful investigation of cases of rarer forms of disease. For it has been found in almost all things, that what they contain of useful or applicable nature is hardly perceived unless we are deprived of them, or they become deranged in some way (Willis, 1848).

This letter reflected observations made over a long and distinguished career in trying to gain a better understanding of the function of the human body in both health and disease. Harvey's experience at the anatomy dissection table and the patient's bedside had convinced him that observing variations from the norm was an important method for understanding the relationship between anatomy and human disease.

It may seem somewhat unfounded to mention William Harvey, the discoverer of the circulation of the blood, in the beginning of a book on the history of genetics in English medicine. In fact, Harvey serves as a paradigm of the "new science" of the seventeenth century that would revolutionize not only English medicine, but the other natural sciences as well. Harvey learned by direct observation of nature itself, not just from an ancient Greek or Roman text. He carried out experiments and quantified blood flow. His claim to fame is not so much in what he did, but how he did it. He formulated hypotheses, tested them by experiment, and produced quantitative data to support his ideas. These steps formed the basis of natural science and methods of scientific investigation, as we know them today (Wear, 1995a; Sloan, 1996).

Harvey was born in 1578 and attended King's School at Canterbury until enrolling in Caius College Cambridge at age sixteen. After receiving a classical education there, he began the study of medicine in 1597. Although human dissections were performed during the medical course, the method for learning human anatomy relied more on memorizing quotations from Galen rather than direct observation of the human body itself (Keynes, 1966). It was customary for English students to subsequently attend a continental medical school for more detailed study than was available in England at the time. Harvey enrolled at the Padua medical school in Italy early in 1600 and found himself in a whole new and exciting world of innovative medicine. The Renaissance, a rebirth of arts and learning, had begun after 1500 in Italy and eventually spread throughout Europe. The goal of many teachers of the period was to rediscover the ancient Greek and Roman sources of knowledge and to modify or discard the erroneous portions that had accumulated in the more recent past. In medicine, many physicians attempted to retranslate original Greek and Roman texts of Hippocrates and Galen. The

Arabic and Latin translations from the Middle Ages were felt to be corrupt and untrustworthy. The introduction of the printing press allowed wider dissemination of the new Latin translations of classic medical texts that were believed to reflect more accurately the spirit of the original works. In something approaching a religious fervor, medical faculty came to accept the newly available sources as icons. Sylvius of the Paris Faculty of Medicine noted that Galen and Hippocrates "had never written anything in physiology or other parts of medicine that is not entirely true" (Conrad, Neve, Nutton et al., 1995a).

The study of human anatomy at Italian medical schools, however, raised serious questions about the validity of such a blanket acceptance of the ancient wisdom. From early in the 1500s, anatomy professors such as Berengario de Capri at Bologna and Niccolo Massa at Venice had urged their students to use their own senses to observe carefully during human dissections. A close reading of Galen, in fact, revealed that most of his anatomical studies had been done on apes, not humans. The work of Andreus Vesalius epitomized the quest for knowledge which accepted the Greek anatomy as a starting point, but then expanded and modified these facts based upon direct observation of human cadavers. Vesalius was appointed lecturer in surgery and anatomy at Padua in 1537 and gradually became convinced of Galen's many errors. He taught that human anatomy could not be learned solely from the ancient texts, but rather from detailed dissection of the human body (Conrad, Neve, Nutton et al., 1995b).

Vesalius published *De Humani Corporis Fabricia* in 1543 as the first systematic work to compare Galen's anatomy with direct observations on human material. The text came to represent a cornerstone in Renaissance thinking, that knowledge should be gained empirically. The work had a profound effect on the method physicians then used to learn about the human body. Valverde of Spain observed, "Vesalius started to open the eyes of many, showing that faith must not be given to everything which is found in writing...The lazy should not try to defend their ignorance by means of the authority of this or that author and particularly in those things in which the contrary can be touched by hand" (Conrad, Neve, Nutton et al., 1995c).

The young Harvey studied medicine at Padua for only two years. Its university was the lone college in Italy that did not require a religious test for the medical degree. This freedom from religious authority allowed creative thought to flourish there unlike any other European school (Booth, 1979). Harvey became convinced that the method of direct observation was the only way to learn about nature. Years later, he noted that his own works were derived not from books, but from dissections; not from the tenets of philosophers but from "the fabric of nature" (Frank, 1980a). He received the M.D. degree from Cambridge in 1602 and then began medical practice in London. Harvey was elected Fellow of the Royal College of Physicians in 1607, and in 1615 became its Lumleian lecturer on anatomy, a post he held until 1656 (Willius and Keys, 1941). His most famous work, *De Motu Cordis*, was published in 1628 and recounted his anatomical and physiological studies on the circulation of the blood from the heart to the lungs and back to the heart before being transported to other parts of the body (Conrad, Neve, Nutton et al., 1995d).

Harvey devoted the latter portion his life trying to explain "the origin of life itself" (Guyton, 1989). He had been appointed physician to Charles I in 1639 and spent the next several years with the royal family as they campaigned throughout England during the Civil War. After the battle of Edgehill in October 1642, the royal retinue wintered at Oxford. Harvey was to remain there for the next four years. In addition to providing medical attention to the Royal court, he became involved in the activities of the University. Harvey was named Warden at Merton College and worked there on the study of embryology, the formation of individual structures during gestation (Frank, 1980b).

Girolamo Fabricius (b 1537) had been appointed Professor of Anatomy at Padua in 1562, and observed and recorded the features of embryonic development of avian eggs, giving embryology, as well as anatomy, of the day an "empirical habitus" (Bodemer, 1974). As early as 1604, in the text *On the Formation of the Fetus*, he examined the generation of both animals and man, investigating the origin and function of the egg and sperm, and the formation of embryos. Specific study of bird development appeared posthumously in *On the Formation of the Egg and the Chick* published in 1621. Harvey had studied with Fabricius during his tenure at Padua. He later decided to examine embryology himself after a 1625 visit with Joseph of Aromatori in Venice, who also had examined chick development. Joseph claimed that a miniature chick was present at the beginning of development and then enlarged, due to local heat, food in the yolk and vital spirits from the air (Meyer, 1936). Later in 1643, Harvey collaborated with several local Oxford physicians on the detailed study of embryonic development of the chicken. A Fellow of Trinity College, George Bathurst "had a hen to hatch eggs in his chamber, which they dayly opening to discerne the progress and way of generation" (Frank, 1980c). John Greaves of Merton College had traveled to Egypt and reported to Harvey how the local people incubated eggs in ovens. Harvey used this incubator method to ensure a steady supply of eggs to study.

Charles Scarburgh, who had originally been trained in mathematics, came to Oxford to join the King during the war. His friendship with Harvey encouraged him to study medicine, and the two collaborated on embryology as well. Anthony Wood of Merton College reported the men working together and eventually preparing observations for publication:

> While he [Scarburgh] abode in Merton College, he did help the said Dr. Harvey, then Warden of that house (in his chamber at the end of the said library there) in the writing of his book *De Generatione Animalium* which was afterwards published by the said Harvey (Frank, 1980d).

Although the final work did not appear until 1651, it contained Harvey's lifelong theme for seeking the truth based on personal experience. He urged the reader,

> to be sure to weigh all that I deliver in these Exercitationes, touching the Generation of Living Creatures, in the steady scale of experiment, and give no large credit to it, than thou perceivest it to be securely bottomed by the faithful testimony of thy own eyes (Harvey, 1651a).

In embryology as well as anatomy, he noted that opinions of the ancients were "erroneous and hasty conclusions" which "suddenly vanished before the light of anatomical inquiry" (Harvey, 1651b). His goal was always "diligent observations" (Harvey, 1651c). He made those observations using a hand magnifying lens examining the daily development of structures within the chick egg and concluded that the parts of the embryo "are not fashioned simultaneously, but emerged in their due succession and order" (Harvey, 1651d). And "the processes of growth and formation are carried out at the same time, and a separation and distinction of the parts takes place in a regularly observed order, so in this case there is no immediate pre-existing material present..." (Harvey, 1651e).

Harvey also believed that both the male and female parents contributed to the formation of the fertilized egg and developing embryo. He observed, "And first is manifest that an Egge cannot be made fertile without the help of the Cock and the Henne. For without a Cock it cannot be fruitful, and without a Henne it cannot be at all" (Harvey, 1651f). He noted hybrid offspring which clearly had features derived from both parents, suggesting to him that the contribution of the sexes was equal (Knobil, 1981). "...An egg is to be viewed as a conception proceeding from the male and female, equally endued with the virtue of either and constituting the unity from which a single animal is engendered" (Harvey, 1651g). Harvey concluded,

> ...the offspring is of a mixed nature, inasmuch as a mixture of both parents appears plainly in it, in the form and lineaments, and each particular part of its body, in its color, mother-marks, <u>disposition to diseases</u> and other accidents. In mental constitution, also, and its manifestations, such as manners, docility, voice, and gait, a similar temperament is discoverable. For as we say of a certain mixture, that is composed of elements, because their qualities or virtues, such as heat, cold, dryness, and moisture are there discovered the association of a certain similar compound body, so, in like manner, the work of the father and mother is to be discerned in the body and mental character of the offspring...[emphasis added] (Muller-Wille, 2007; Muller-Wille and Rheinberger, 2007).

Harvey's observations of both animal and human development suggested that each parent contributed "elements" to the formation of the offspring. Normal characters such as color and voice, as well as abnormal ones, such as liability to disease, clearly were inherited.

But the origin of the human embryo was problematic. Harvey observed no male semen or female eggs in the uterus after coition and concluded that the embryo could not be formed of these factors at all. Clearly,

> It is to the uterus that the business of conception is chiefly intrusted...but since it is certain that the semen of the male does not so much as reach the cavity of the uterus, ...and that it carries with it a fecundating power by a kind of contagious property, the woman after contact with the spermatic fluid in coition, seems to receive influence and to become fecundated without the cooperation of any sensible corporeal agent...When this virtue is once received, the woman exercises plastic power of generation and produces a being after her own image...(Harvey, 1651h).

Harvey concluded that the parents were solely instruments of the power of creation in nature which then seemed to initiate embryonic development:

> The male and female, therefore, will come to be regarded as merely the efficient instruments [of generation], subservient in all respects to the Supreme Creator or father of all things. In this sense, consequently, it is well said that the sun and moon engender man; because, with the advent and succession of the sun, come spring and autumn, seasons which mostly correspond with the degeneration and decay of animated beings.... (Muller-Wille, 2007).

The embryo then resulted from the activation of a vital principle, not from physical elements contributed by the parents. Heredity then was not an event, but rather a process of gestation, maturation and adaptation.

The question of physical elements first derived from the parents and then subsequently constituting the developing embryo had been raised in an earlier generation by the French writer Michel de Montaigne in his 1582 *Essais*. The observation of the same condition in a parent and his children was commonplace. Montaigne asked:

> What monster is it that this teare or drop of seed whereof we are ingendered brings with it, and in it the impressions, not only of corporal forme, but even of the very

> thoughts and inclinations of the fathers? Where doth this droppe of water contain or lodge this infinite number of formes? And how bear they these resemblances of so rash and unruly a progresse, that the childe's childe shall be answerable to his grandfather, and the nephew to his uncle? (Lopez-Beltran, 2007).

However, Harvey was reluctant to speculate when his observations failed to explain natural phenomena. He realized the limitations of conjectures: "In general, the first processes of nature lie hid, as it were, in the depths of night, and by reason of their subtlety escape the keenest reason no less than the most piercing eye" (Harvey, 1651d). Personal observation of natural phenomena and experiments, coupled with particular attention to unusual variations from the norm came to characterize Harvey's method for doing medical science.

Harvey's development as a medical scientist in the first half of the seventeenth century reflected significant changes in the intellectual climate that occurred in England during that era. The opinions on the state of science and its need for reform expressed earlier by Francis Bacon provided an outline for the evolution of modern empirical science. Bacon was born in 1561 and educated at Trinity College Cambridge. He was elected to the House of Commons in 1584 and served both Elizabeth I and Charles I as political adviser. He is best known for his works that attempted to change the way science was done. Bacon was not a scientist himself, but an "agent of reform" (Ravetz, 1972). He outlined the sad state of contemporary science, proposed a plan for changing the way men thought about science, and then gave reasons for making such changes at that time. In *Novum Organum* (1620) he observed:

> Those who have taken upon themselves to lay down the laws of nature as a thing already searched out and understood, whether they have spoken in simple assurances or professional affectations, have therein done philosophy and the sciences great injury. For as they have been unsuccessful in inducing belief, so they have been effective in quenching and stopping inquiry, and have done more harm by spoiling and putting an end to other men's efforts than good by their own (Warhaft, 1965a).

Those who study nature, "the mechanic, the mathematician, the physician, the alchemist and the magician...(as things are now)" have had "scanty success" for their efforts (Warhaft, 1965b). They may add something to the "sum of science," but they "little advance the science" (Warhaft, 1965c). Bacon concluded that the reason such meager understanding of nature existed resulted from incorrect methodology. "The logic now in use seems rather to fix and give stability to the errors which have their foundation in commonly received notions than to help the search after truth. So it does more harm than good" (Warhaft, 1965d). Bacon proposed nothing less than the "total reconstruction of sciences, arts and human knowledge, raised upon the proper foundations" (Warhaft, 1965e). He argued first that man should divest the mind of all prejudices ("idols"), which clouded clear thinking. He proposed a form of inductive logic to systematically collect data from nature and then analyze it in such a fashion as to discern principles that explained natural phenomena. He sought to find the "forms of simple natures" (Hesse, 1970; Gould, 2000).

> The induction which is to be available for the discovery and demonstration of sciences and arts must analyse nature by proper reflections and exclusions, and then, after sufficient number of negatives, come to a conclusion on the affirmative instances...(Warhaft, 1965f).

The posthumous *New Atlantis* (1627) outlined Bacon's notions of a state-supported college for scientific research. At this learned institution, the "House of Solomon" he called it, researchers would be provided laboratories in which to perform experiments to learn about nature. "Interpreters" then would analyze the data by induction and propose further "observations, axioms and aphorisms" (Hesse, 1970). Bacon never viewed discovery as an end in itself. Rather, it was to be a means for the greater good of society. The true goal was not to be "for the pleasure of the mind, or for contention, or for superiority to others, or for profit, or power, as any of these inferior things, but for the benefit and use of life, and that they perfect and govern it in clarity" (Warhaft, 1965g).

Bacon perceived the study of nature as nearly a religious duty. In his earliest works, he argued that knowledge was given by God to man for one purpose: "the benefit and relief of the state and society of man." The application of knowledge and philanthropy was thus designed to improve the human condition. Knowledge was not idly collected facts; it had to be useful (Harrison, 2001). He noted he was "labouring to lay the foundation not of any sect or doctrine, but of human utility and power" (Warhaft, 1965g). In summary, Bacon's aim was not to perform scientific work himself but rather to plead a course, to reform how science was, in fact, to be done (Ravetz, 1972).

In his earliest work *The Advancement of Learning* (1605), Bacon had encouraged detailed study of organisms both during life and after death. All available means of observation, such as the microscope, were to be used "for inspecting blood, urine and wounds" and to collect information about nature (Keele, 1974). Harvey later put into practice careful observation and experiments in anatomy, embryology and physiology in order to achieve those principles that better explained how nature worked. At the end of his career, he concluded in *De Generatione Animalium*,

> For whosoever they be that read the word of authors and do not by this aid of their own senses abstract therefore true representations of the things themselves as they are described in the author's works, they do not conceive in their own minds aught but deceitful eidola[1] and vein fancies and never true ideas. And so they forme certain ...chimeras and all their theory and contemplation, which nonetheless they count knowledge, represents nothing but working men's dreams and sick men's fancies (Wear, 1995b).

Careful personal observation of nature, reasoned experiments and particular attention to unusual variations from the norm would characterize Harvey's method for doing medical science. Although Harvey may not have perceived himself as a part of "the new science" in England that developed before 1660, he, like Bacon, was an agent of change. His method of research and writings set an example for the younger man who would revolutionize science and medicine, first in Oxford and later in London after the restoration of the monarchy.

Two

Oxford Science, Medicine and Heredity

The development of "science" in Oxford occurred during the 1640s and thereafter, because of a unique confluence of university structure and the interests of chemists and physicians that produced an interconnected and highly diverse learning community. The university campus itself had grown dramatically since 1600. The number of students enrolled grew six-fold in the century before 1620. The demand for facilities engendered construction of new colleges and the expansion of existing quadrangles. A "Physick Garden" was established to grow botanical specimens that were used for the preparation of medications. The faculty of sciences also expanded to seven endowed chairs by 1640 (compared to only two at Cambridge). The statesman Sir Thomas Bodley rebuilt the library collection to more than 40,000 books that included all the major scientific works of the day (Frank, 1980a). The Oxford medical community also expanded greatly during this time. The number of medical students tripled between 1600 and 1650. Teaching expanded in anatomy, botany, physiology and clinical medicine as new faculty with more scientific interests were appointed (Frank, 1980b; Sinclair, 1974).

Approximately 110 men were ultimately involved in this "Oxford Renaissance" from about 1640 to 1670. The historian Robert Frank has identified 13 major scientists who, along with William Harvey, led the way. Robert Boyle (b 1627) became the leading chemist of his day and gave the first precise definition of chemical elements and reactions (Wooley, 1998). Walter Charleton (b 1619) trained as a physician and studied human anatomy and physiology. His work helped bridge the transition from the ancient scholastic style of learning to the more modern one of observation based on experimental knowledge. Nathaniel Highmore (b 1613) also studied medicine and had broad interests in pathology and embryology. Thomas Willis (b 1621) was an Oxford physician who defined the circulation and nerve origins of the human brain. Robert Hooke (b 1635) worked with Willis on human anatomy and with Robert Boyle on the construction of an air pump used to study the physics of gases and respiration. Richard Lower (b 1631) completed his medical studies at Oxford and worked with Willis on the detailed anatomy of the human brain. John Mayow (b 1641) was another physician who collaborated with Willis and Lower. He was particularly interested in the anatomy and physiology of respiration. Walter Needham (b 1631) was a medical colleague who studied the anatomy of the human fetus and placenta. William Petty (b 1623) became the Professor of Anatomy at Oxford. The final member of this group was Christopher Wren (b 1623). As a student at Oxford, he assisted Charles Scarburgh in anatomical classes. He experimented with blood transfusions in animals, and later developed his career in astronomy and architecture. In sum, more than 75 percent of the men in this elite group had some medical training.

The second set of about 50 men was classified by Frank as "minor" scientists who were actively involved in the Oxford period. About 75 percent of these had also been trained in medicine. The final group of 50 was comprised of men who supported the local scientific effort, but did little original work themselves. About 35 percent of these men had also completed medical school (Frank, 1980c).

It is therefore safe to say that physicians were prime movers in the initiation and support of anatomical and physiological studies in Oxford during the Civil War and after the 1660 Restoration of Charles II as monarch. The younger men had been inspired by Harvey's experimental approach to learning about human anatomy, physiology and disease (Wooley, 1998). In 1648, Harvey summarized his philosophy to a friend, George Ent, as follows:

> No one indeed has ever rightly ascertained the use or function of a part who has not examined its structure, situation, connexion by means of vessels and other accidents in various animals, and carefully weighed and considered all he has seen (Keynes, 1966a).

Not only in disease, but in heredity, observation was the key to new understanding. For centuries it had been frequently noted that children resembled their parents in many physical attributes. The historian Nicholas Russell summarized this as "like engend'ring like" (Russell, 1986). It was also common knowledge that disease was often passed from one generation to the next. The explorer Robert Thorne (d. 1527) was quoted by Richard Hakluyt in *The Principal Navigations, Voyages and Discoveries of the English Nation* (1589) as observing that "some sicknesses are hereditarious, and comme from the father to the sonne" (Hakluyt, 1589). John Jones agreed in *A briefe Discourse of the Naturell Beginning of all Growing and Living Things* (1574) that such familial transmission occurred, "as not only hereditall sickness doth show, but also deformed persons doth prove" (Jones, 1574). Tobias Whitaker in *The Tree of Humaine Life, or the Blood of the Grape* (1638) gave the example of "children, which are hereditarily subject to the [bladder] stone" (Whitaker, 1638). Edmund Gayton in *Pleasant Notes upon Don Quixat* (1654) observed that the "dropsies, gouts...and most diseases are as hereditable from our Parents, as their estates" (Gayton, 1654). Robert Burton noted in *Anatomy of Melancholy* (1621) that a man who inherits his father's land, may also have the "inheritance of his infirmities...Where the complexion and constitution of the father is corrupt, the complexion and constitution of the son must needs be corrupt" (Zirkle, 1946). And the prognosis for such inherited disorders was not too hopeful. Thomas Morley found, "The fault which like unto a hereditable leprosy in a man's bodie is incurable" (*A Plaine and Easie Introduction to Practicall Musick*) (Morley, 1597).

Four prominent physicians of this Oxford era studied human heredity and made valuable contributions to an understanding of how traits were passed from parents to their children. Thomas Browne (b 1605) began his study of medicine at Oxford, and traveled to Montpelier, Padua and Leyden to further his studies, eventually receiving the Leyden M.D. in 1633. He settled in Norwich and developed a busy medical practice, but maintained an extensive interest in scientific developments. He agreed with Harvey's experimental approach to the study of nature and corresponded extensively throughout his life with members of the Oxford group (Sloan, 1996a; Keynes, 1965, 1972). He felt that most people were too willing to trust ancient authority. In 1646, he published *Pseudodoxia Epidemica* in which he proposed to test many accepted beliefs using reason and experience, rather than tradition alone. He did not reject the ancient authorities, but used them as a starting point for experimentation and observation of the real world (Grell and Cunningham, 1996a).

Browne first considered the origin of Negro skin color. The ancient authors generally accepted this as the result of "heat and scorch of the Sonne." While black people often lived in the tropics and were darkened by the sun, Browne observed, however, that other tropical animals did not uniformly exhibit dark skin colors. Migration from hot to cold climates also did not change human skin color. As long as they continued to breed among their own kind, the dark complexion was maintained. Other races exposed to the same degree of sunlight did not always develop black skin. Inhabitants of tropical Asia often had yellow skin color. And Negro children were noted to be dark at birth, even before they had been exposed to the sun. Browne argued instead that skin color was a racial characteristic just like facial features of different ethnic groups:

> However, therefore this complexion was first acquired, it is evidently maintained by generation and by the tincture of the skin as a spermaticall part transduced from father unto son, so that they which are strangers contract it not, and the Natives which transmigrate omit it not, without conmixture, and that after diverse generations (Browne, 1672).

He was not clear about how such variants, or "mutations" had occurred originally, but was convinced that they had been passed from one generation to the next.

Nathaniel Highmore (b 1613) completed the M.B. at Oxford in 1641. He met Harvey there and collaborated with him on the study of chick embryology. His 1651 book *History of Generation* summarized his daily observations of the developing chick embryo. He was the first English scientist to use a microscope to make such observations, and was able to discern the appearance of structures at an earlier time during development than had other investigators (Highmore, 1651a; Frank, 1980d; Gordon, 1972; Godon, 1966). Highmore concluded that all different parts of the parents contributed to the development of the embryo:

> The seminal atomes constituting the fetus, collected from the blood of the testicles, and joyned together in the womb or vitellary,[2] contract to them from the fecund blood that round body which serves afterwards for their nourishment, receives nourishment from the blood, until they come to their accomplisht bignesse (Highmore, 1651b).

He pictured the embryo as formed from the beginning of development:

> So in an Egg before incubation, where both seeds are conjoyned, by the conjuncture and regular disposure of these atomes; which while they were parts of the blood, served for the nourishment and increase of that body from whence they were taken but now serve to make up another individium of the same species (Highmore, 1651c).

The embryo thus began as the union of two seeds, bearing "atomes" from each parent. The female acted to "fix and cement the spiritual atomes together, that they might mutually cohere the one to the other," while the male seeds acted to "activate, enliven and to act for all the rest" (Highmore, 1651d). This explained the common observation that offspring generally resembled both parents (Frank, 1980a).

But Highmore's own observations indicated that this was not always the case. He recorded an example of breeding true for the character if both parents had the trait, and of the trait's segregation when breeding with normal individuals took place:

> Myself also have seene a kinde of Poultry without rumps; which breeding with their own kinde, still brought forth children wanting that part; If with others, sometimes they had rumps, sometimes but part of a rump" (Highmore, 1651e).

He also made observations on the supposed heredity of acquired characters:

> I saw a Mongrel Bitch, that had her tail cut close to her body almost, whose whelps were half without tails and half with tails. The next year following, she brought them forth all with long tails as she had before the cutting off...which doth it seems to favor...this opinion, it doth in no way confirm it, as may appear by the frequent perfect generations of mutilated creatures, which begat children or issue with two legs or arms though they had but one...We must therefore look at some other way, how this may be done without the parts themselves (Highmore, 1651f).

If the part was lacking, it would be difficult to explain the origin of the "atomes" needed in egg or sperm to produce the same structure in the offspring of the next generation.

The third friend of Harvey had quite a different life story. Kenelm Digby (b 1603) attended Oxford for only two years and left without a degree in 1620. He then toured Europe and became friendly with royalty from several different countries. In 1627 he sailed as a privateer to the Mediterranean to put down Venetian pirates, hoping to gain further favor at the English court by serving his country. He next spent two years (1633-1635) studying chemistry at Gresham College in London. Harvey and Digby shared a mutual interest in animal reproduction and both used artificial incubators to synchronize embryogenesis. Both concluded that the embryo's organs developed from the formless fertilized egg in specific sequence during generation. Digby's interest in biology and medicine continued to evolve. Although he was entirely self-taught, he served Charles II as his unofficial and unlicensed court physician for many years (Sloan, 1996b; Fulton, 1937; Frank, 1980e; Keynes, 1966b).

Digby reported his observations on heredity in his major work *Two Treatises in One of which the Nature of Bodies, in the Other, the Nature of Man's Soule* (1645). During his travels in the Mediterranean, he had encountered a family in which several women had peculiar thumbs in successive generations:

> And another particular that I saw when I was at Algiers...which was of a woman that having two thumbs upon the left-hand; four daughters that she had all resembled her in the same accident, and so did a little child, a girl of her eldest daughter, but none of her sonnes. While I was there I had a particular curiosity to see them, although it is not easily permitted unto a Christian to speak familiarly with Mohametan women; yet the condition I was in there and the civility of the Bassha, gave me the opportunity of full view and discourse with them; and the old woman told me that her mother and grandmother had been in the same manner (Digby, 1645).

Digby noted the occurrence of the defect in five successive generations, affecting only females. And he placed himself at some personal risk by seeking to personally interview the Islamic women. He also observed a case of supposed heredity of acquired characters. A cat had its tail cut off at a very young age. It went on to have kittens: half of the offspring had tails and half were born without tails, "as if nature could supply but one partner's side, not both" (Digby, 1645). Digby believed that the blood carried "severall parts" derived from all the organs of the parents which were then concentrated in the sexual organs. The embryo was eventually formed from these "severall parts" transmitted by both parents, because "generation is made of the blood." Defects in the offspring could therefore result from an imbalance of these hereditary factors:

> Whence it followeth, that if any part be wanting in the body whereof this seed is made, or be superabundant of it; whose virtue is not in the rest of the body, or whose superabundance is not allaid by the rest of the body; the virtue of that part, cannot be in the blood, or will be too strong in the blood, and by consequence, it cannot be at all, or it will be too much in the seed. And the effect proceeding from the seed, that is, the young animal will come into the world savouring of that origine; unless the mother's seed, do supply or temper what the fathers was defective or superabundant in; or contrariwise the fathers do correct the errours of the mothers (Digby, 1645).

Both Highmore and Digby subscribed to an early theory of pangenesis. Elements from different body parts circulated in the blood, eventually resting in the female egg and the male sperm. Mixture of egg and sperm resulted in the embryo. Defects could occur if there was an imbalance of either maternal or paternal elements.

Francis Glisson (b 1597) became one of the most distinguished physicians of the day. As a young physician, he was impressed by Harvey's work on circulation and subsequently began his own detailed anatomical and pathological studies (Munk, 1878). He completed the M.D. at Cambridge in 1634 and was appointed Regius Professor of Physic there two years later. His best-known work is *A Treatise of the Rickets* (1668) in which he defined the nature of a hereditary disease. The question to be determined was:

> ...Hereditary disease be distinguished into that properly and that improperly so-called. And indeed the hereditary disease properly so-called is even supposed to be pre-existent in both or one of the two Parents; and from thence to be derived to the Progeny. But a hereditary disease improperly so-called, is not supposed to be preexistent in the same kind, either in both or one of the Parents; yet the same fault must always necessarily precede (perhaps altogether in a different kind) at least in one of them, by vertue whereof a certain disposedness is imprinted in the children, whereby they are made obnoxious to fall into this improperly called hereditary disease.
>
> Moreover, a hereditary disease properly so-called is twofold; either in the confirmation, as when a lame person begets a lame; a deaf father a deaf son, or a blind a blind; or in the similarly constitution: as when a gouty father begets a gouty child. It is to be noted, that in the first kind there is an hereditary fault whereat in the first affected parts of the confirmation. But the latter, there is no necessity that a disease of the same kind with the disease of the parents, should be actually inherent in the Embryon, for the first formation. But such a disposition imprinted by one or both of the parents is sufficient, which as the life is lengthened may be actuated into the same, by the concourse of other intervening causes. Again, an hereditary disease improperly called, may be likewise twofold; namely either in the confirmation, or in the similar constitution. In the formation, as when neither of the Parents is blind, pore-blind, lame, etc., yet have begotten a Son blind, pore-blind, or lame, by the very fault of formation. For in these cases, that very fault which is sensible and conspicuous in the issue, flowed from the same fault in the Parents, although perhaps a different kind, and so it may be called, although improperly, an hereditary disease. And in like manner in the similar constitution of the issue, there may reside an hereditary disease, improperly so-called, as when a Melancholy, sedentary or an intemperate Parent begeteth a child subject to the gout or the cachexia, although perhaps the Parent was never troubled either with one or the other (Glisson, 1668).

Glisson thus attempted to clearly define what inherited disease actually was. The common use of the term "hereditary" to describe an alleged predisposition passed from parent to child that could explain diverse disease in successive generations was vague; this was his "improper" use of the word hereditary. True hereditary disease implied the direct transmission of the defect from parent to child. This could be either a structural defect or predisposition to disease that could produce symptoms if specific triggering life events occurred. This was his "properly" called hereditary disease.

Other physicians also attempted to define the nature of hereditary disease at this time. John Floyer (b 1649) completed his medical studies at Oxford in 1680 (Stephen, 1889). He suffered from asthma himself and described in excruciating detail the agonies associated with attacks during which he could barely breathe. Asthma often ran in families, but not always. Floyer noted, "As my asthma was not hereditary from my ancestors, so, I thank God, neither of my two sons are inclined to it, who are now passed the age in which it seized me" (Floyer, 1698). Floyer pointed out the fact that many hereditary diseases often became apparent at specific ages, some in childhood, others not until much later in life.

Thomas Willis observed that the predisposition to gout was also often hereditary, but sometimes acquired through an intemperate diet (Willis, 1685a). Migraine headaches could also be hereditary. The disease often passed from a parent to the children. Its predisposing cause was a "vicious or weak constitution of the affected parent" (Willis, 1685b).

Francis Bacon's notion of induction had encouraged William Harvey to study nature by direct observation and experiment before drawing conclusions to explain what he had observed. The young men who followed Harvey in the Oxford Renaissance continued the empirical approach to learning in science, in general, and medicine, in particular. But only a beginning had been made. Joseph Glanvill (b 1636) was a cleric who befriended many of the Oxford scientists of this era. He was impressed with the many new discoveries made during that exciting time, but was sober enough to know that "We have no such thing as natural philosophy; natural history is all we can pretend to; and that, too, as yet, is but in its rudiments" (Glanvill, 1676).

Others expected rapid progress in these new fields of endeavor. A long-time friend of Thomas Browne, Henry Power (b 1623) had completed the M.D. degree at Cambridge in 1655. He reported experiments on human anatomy and physiology, especially using the microscope to observe in great detail the physical changes produced by disease (Robb-Smith, 1974). He was hopeful for the future of science and noted in his *Experimental Philosophy* (1664):

> And this is the age wherein all mens Souls are in a kind of fermentation, and the spirit of Wisdom and Learning begins to mount and free itself from those drossie and terrene Impediments wherewith it hath been so long clogg'd and from the insipid phlegm and Caput Mortuum of useless Notions, in which it has endured so violent and long a fixation.
>
> This is the age wherein (methinks) Philosophy comes in with a springtide; and the Peripateticks (that is, the followers of Aristotle) may as well hope to stop the current of the tide, or (with Xerxes) to fetter the Ocean, as hinder the overflowing of free Philosophy: Methinks, I see how all the old rubbish must be thrown away, and the rotten buildings be overthrown, and carried away with so powerful an innundation.

> These are the days that must lay a new foundation of a more magnificent Philosophy, never to be overthrown: that will Empirically and Sensibly canvass the phenomena of Nature, deducing the Causes of things from such originals in Nature, as we observe are producible by Art, and infallible demonstration of Mechanicks: and certainly, this is the way, and no other, to build a true and permanent Philosophy (Grell and Cunningham, 1996a).

Many of the other men involved in the Oxford Revolution were also convinced that a cooperative effort could further enhance the sharing of observations necessary to produce such a "true and permanent Philosophy." They subsequently began to meet in social groups that would eventually result in the formation of the Royal Society.

Three

The Commerce of Ideas:
The Royal Society, Medicine and Heredity

During 1681, William Dampier (b 1652) led an expedition to the Moskito [*sic*] Indians living on the Caribbean coast of Central America, called Darien at that time. The subject of his investigation was a mixed population of Native Americans and descendents of runaway African slaves. Dampier had become a well-known cartographer for the British Admiralty. Published accounts described the Indians as "tall, well-made, raw-bon'd, lusty, strong and nimble of Foot, long-visaged, dark black Hair...and of dark Copper-colored Complexion" ("New World Voyages", 1999). The young surgeon on the voyage, Lionel Wafer (b ?1660) had learned his trade by working as a servant for another surgeon on previous sea voyages. He functioned as both naturalist and physician for the exploration, and actually lived among the Moskito Indians for several months. He treated their physical ills and was held in high esteem by them (Pearson, Nettleship and Usher, 1911). Wafer published his own account of the voyage in 1699 and recounted experiences with the "White Indians," an unusual group within the Moskito tribes. He noted:

> The natural complexion of the Indians is a Copper colour, and orange tauney, and their eyebrows are naturally black as jet.
>
> There is one complexion so singular, among a sort of people of this country, that I never saw nor heard of any like them in any part of the world.
>
> They are white, and there are of them of both sexes; yet there are but few of them in comparison of the copper-color'd, perhaps but one to two or three hundred. They differ from the other Indians chiefly in respect to colour, tho' not in that only. Their skins are not of such a white as those of fair people among Europeans with some tincture of a blush or sanguine complexion, neither yet is their complexion like that of our paler people, but 'tis rather a milk-white, lighter than the color of any European, and much like that of a white horse.
>
> For there is further remarkable in them, but their bodies are beset all over, more or less, with a fine short milk-white down, which adds to the milk-whiteness of their chins: for they are not so thick-set with their down, especially over the cheeks and forward, but that the skin appears distinct from it. The men would probably have white bristles for beards, did they not prevent them by their custom of plucking the young beard up by the roots continually. But for the down all over their bodies, they never tried to get rid of it. Their eyebrows are milk-white, also, and so is the hair of their heads, and very fine withal, about the length of six or seven inches.
>
> They are not so big as other Indians, and what is yet more strange, their eyelids bend and open in an oblong figure, pointing downward at the corners, and forming

> an arch or crescent with the points downward. From hence, and from their seeing so clear as they do in a moon-shining night, we us'd to call them moon-ey'd. For they see not very well in the sun, peering in the clear state, their eyes being but weak, and running with water if the sun shine towards them; so that in daytime they care not to go abroad, unless it be a cloudy dark day. Besides they are but a weak people in comparison of the other, and not very fit for hunting or other laborious exercise ...When moon-shining night come, they are all life and activity running abroad and into the woods, skipping about like wild-bucks, and running as fast by moon-light...as other Indians by day. They are not a distinct race by themselves, but now and then one is bred of a copper-color'd father and mother; and I have seen a child of less than a year old of this sort. Some would be apt to suspect they might be the offspring of some European father. But besides that the Europeans come little here, and have little commerce with the Indian-women when they do come, these white people are so different from the Europeans in some respects, as from the copper color'd Indians in others. And besides, when a European lives with an Indian-women, the child is always a...Tauney, as is well-known to all who have been in the West Indies...but neither is a child of a man and woman of these White Indians, white like the parents, but copper-coloured as their parents were.
> For so Laurento told me, and gave me this as his conjecture how these came to be white, that 'twas through the force of the mother's imagination, looking on the moon at the time of conception; but this I leave to others to judge of...
> (Wafer, 1699).

Wafer's 1699 book describing these unusual white Indians was one of many works published in London during this era of exploration, recounting unusual people, plants and animals from all over the world. The white Moskito Indians were the offspring of tawny colored parents, and had characteristic facial features and photosensitivity that made it difficult for them to function in the bright tropical sun. But the trait did not breed true, as matings between affected men and women produced tawny colored children, as the grandparents had been. Although the cause of the unusual pigmentation could have been maternal impression, i.e., the woman looking toward the moon at the moment of conception, and then transmitting that effect to the developing embryo, Wafer was not certain of that notion and decided not to speculate on the matter.

Another explanation for the existence of the white Indians came from a fictional account of the historical Scottish expedition that attempted to establish a trading colony on the Isthmus of Panama (Darien) at the same time. A member of the crew, one Rev. Mackay, had studied more than twenty of the world's languages and was struck by evidence that Gaelic was "the closest descendant of the original tongue," the language spoken by all people before the Tower of Babel dispersion described in the Bible. Some groups had clung closely to the original tongue and had settled in Scotland, or so he claimed. The local language, Gaelic, then had to be the "purest relic of the original tongue." The Reverend was convinced that these so-called white Indians were, in fact, descendents of the first Scots, able seamen who crossed the Atlantic Ocean long before "that mountebank, that thief Columbus." In one sense, the Scottish expedition was not going abroad, but rather actually coming home (Galbraith, 2001).

FOUNDING OF THE ROYAL SOCIETY

William Harvey had urged physicians of the 1600s to pay attention to just such unusual cases as a means for understanding the functioning of the normal human body. The attitude of modern science proposed by Francis Bacon in the previous generation was to "understand and control nature for the benefit of mankind" (Sloan, 1996). Scientists of the early 1700s were generally optimistic, believing that the scientific method of testing hypotheses by observation and experiment was the way to social progress. The Royal Society in London became the institution that centralized and fostered this attitude. Sir John Hoskins, a lawyer and friend of Christopher Wren, was one of the early presidents of the Royal Society. He noted in 1661 that the members distrusted "lengthy discussions and elaborate theories...being convinced that the close study of the realities of nature was the only sound way of advancing philosophy" (Lyons, 1944a). The mathematician Isaac Newton agreed: "Nothing on principle should be assumed that is not proved by phenomena" (Hunter, M., 1981a).

The turbulent years of the Cromwellian Revolution (1642-1660) upset the universities, and traditional medical and scientific teaching at Oxford in particular. Several men who were interested in "experimental philosophy" happened to meet in London about 1645 and began to regularly discuss new developments in medicine and science in general. Most of the early members of this group had been friends of William Harvey at Oxford. The mathematician John Wallis (b 1616) recounted the establishment of what has been called the "1645 Club." He remembered years later that he "had the opportunity of being acquainted with diverse worthy persons, inquisitive into natural philosophy, and other parts of human learning" (Wallis, 1700). Five of the earliest participants in the group were physicians who had been colleagues of Harvey. Jonathan Goddard (b ?1617) was a Cambridge M.D. and was appointed Gulstonian lecturer in anatomy at the Royal College of Physicians in 1648. Charles Scarburgh (b 1616) received his M.D. from Oxford in 1646, lectured on anatomy at the Royal College of Physicians and the Barber-Surgeons Company, eventually becoming physician to Charles II. Christopher Merret (b 1614) was another Oxford M.D. and became actively involved in the Royal College of Physicians as well. George Ent (b 1604) was also an Oxford M.D. and eventually became president of the Royal College of Physicians. Francis Glisson (b 1597) earned the Cambridge M.D. and became Regius Professor of Physic there in 1636. He was also involved in administration of the Royal College of Physicians and served as its president (Munk, 1878). Although Wallis had studied mathematics, he too had assisted Glisson on human anatomical investigations while a student at Cambridge. The members of the group defined their business "to discourse and consider of Philosophical Enquiries, and such as related thereunto: as physics, anatomy, geometry, astronomy, navigation, statics, magnetics, chemics, mechanics and natural experiments" (Wallis, 1700). The group met regularly at different London locations, and avoided "all discourses of divinity and state affairs." They focused on attempting to understand "the New Philosophy," espoused by Francis Bacon (Wallis, 1700; Stimson, 1948a).

In 1649, Wallis was appointed Savilian Professor of Geometry at Oxford. John Wilkins, another mathematician and member of the London group, was appointed warden of Wadham College at the same time (Stimson, 1948a). Jonathan Goddard also moved to Oxford, and the nucleus for an Oxford scientific group developed. Regular meetings for discussion were held, as in London, and the group was formally organized as the Philosophical Society in1651. Proceedings were recorded until the company finally ceased meeting in 1690 (Stimson, 1948b). Notable participants here included Robert Boyle who developed an extensive chemical laboratory (Frank, 1980a). The Sedleian Professor, Thomas Willis (b 1621), studied human brain anatomy. Christopher Wren was actively involved in experiments on blood transfusion in conjunction with local physicians (Frank, 1980a). The organization grew in size until typical meetings numbered 25-30 members. Approximately half of these were physicians (Frank, 1980a; Laslett, 1960). Discussions at the meeting were characterized by intellectual freedom and vigor. Friendships and professional interests fostered extensive collaboration between the "scientists" such as Boyle and Wren and the "physicians." Each group learned from the other as they examined joint topics such as human anatomy and physiology (Frank, 1980a).

With the restoration of Charles II to the throne in 1660, the locus for scientific meetings again shifted to London, the center of both political and commercial England. The population of the metropolis had increased dramatically in the previous century, going from 93,000 in 1563 to more than 500,000 in 1660. The next largest cities such as Newcastle, Norwich and Bristol had only 25,000 inhabitants each. By this time, London had more people than the next 50 British cities combined (Braudel, 1981; Morgan, 1997a). It was evolving into the cultural and intellectual center of the country as well.

Gresham College became the London establishment in which those interested in the New Philosophy began to meet. Sir Thomas Gresham (b ?1519) was a wealthy financier and ambassador to the Netherlands and had established the college in 1597. The Corporation of London provided land for a building, and Queen Elizabeth I awarded it the royal appellation ("Gresham College," 2000; Kenyon, 1992). Seven professorships were endowed by rents paid on commercial businesses in London. The Professor of Physic was supposed to lecture on modern theories of physiology, pathology and therapeutics, in English, not Latin (Sinclair, 1974). Christopher Wren was appointed Professor of Astronomy at Gresham in 1657. His rooms provided the meeting site for the developing London group of philosophers. After 1660, they agreed to meet weekly to continue their experiments and discourse. Five physicians were among the early members of the discussion group. Jonathan Goddard had been appointed Professor of Physic at the College in 1655, and encouraged its use for the meetings. George Ent, Francis Glisson, Christopher Merret and Ralph Bathurst (b 1620), another Oxford M.D. who had worked with Thomas Willis there, had removed to London by this time. They were all distinguished for "zeal and energy in promoting natural knowledge" (Lyons, 1944b).

The original dozen members then compiled a list of 40 leading men who were invited to join this "Philosophers Society." Fifteen of the proposed members were physicians (Lyons, 1944a). By December 1660, the list had grown to 115 men who agreed to meet weekly to debate and develop ideas on "Experimental learning". King Charles II was intensely interested in promoting the society's aims and granted its Royal Charter on 15 July 1662 (Stimson, 1948b; "Royal Society," 2000). The charter described the society's aims as "advancing the knowledge of nature and useful arts by experiments to the glory of God The Creator and application to the good of mankind" (Prest, 1998). Physicians comprised about half of the original members, a fact that would continue well into the nineteenth-century (Lyons, 1944c).

During the same era, the center for medical learning in England shifted dramatically from the College of Physicians to the newly established Royal Society. The College of

Physicians remained bound to tradition, while the Royal Society fostered discussion, experimentation, and observation relating to physiology, anatomy and medicine. Members were open-minded, and claimed to embrace the inductive method of Bacon which they believed would eventually produce new understanding of the natural world (Wear, 1995; Hesse, 1970). The early historian of the Society, Thomas Sprat, observed that the members came together to share observations on "the Constitution of Men's Bodies." They focused on the human body as "the Natural Engine," utilizing experiments based on "Touch and Sight" (Keele, 1974).

However, in the two decades before the establishment of the Royal Society, the Royal College of Physicians had, in fact, been very active in fostering research in clinical medicine. Harvey himself had funded the construction of a new library and meeting rooms. Lectures on pathology were regularly given, and committees met to study chemistry, pharmacology and underlying causes of diseases. Numerous anatomical studies were also completed under the auspices of the College which had the Royal Charter for human dissection. Glisson studied the liver in great detail, while Scarburgh focused on the spleen. George Joyliffe examined the lymphatic system, and Thomas Wharton investigated the glands of the body. In 1656, Harvey endowed an annual lecture—The Harveian Oration—which was supposed to encourage the Fellows to "search and studdy out the secrett of Nature by way of Experiment" (Frank, 1980b).

Another friend of Harvey, Walter Charleton, published a report on activity at the College of Physicians in 1657. He had acted as physician to the King and was exiled after Cromwell came to power. He subsequently returned to England and eventually practiced in London. His assessment of the situation was that "...in the College of Physicians, I may pronounce it to be the most eminent Society of men, for Learning, Judgment and Industry, that is now or any time has been in the Whole World. You may behold 'Solomon's House' in reality" (Webster, 1967). He cited examples of research in comparative anatomy on all types of animals, circulation of the blood, especially as it related to disease pathology, the mechanics of animal motion, the collection of plants for medicinal use, brewing, metals and minerals, and medicinal chemistry. The College established a laboratory in 1648, and revised the *Pharmacopoeia Londinensis* in 1650. Charleton reported that both physicians and other researchers cooperated "for the Common design, the erecting an active and durable Fabrick of Solid Sciences..." (Webster, 1967).

But public confidence in the Fellows of the Royal College of Physicians dwindled during the Great Plague of 1655 as most physicians left London, and those remaining could do little to help the suffering public. Harvey subsequently died in 1657. The Royal College of Physicians was later destroyed in the Great Fire of London in 1666, and the College as an organization went into a rapid decline. One historian of the College, George Clark, observed, "In matters relating to medical thought and science little activity can be traced after 1666" (Hall, 1974). On the other hand, the new Royal Society did attend to developments within medicine and encouraged medical men in their study of new science. It institutionalized the experimental method of scientific inquiry (Laslett, 1960). The organization's role was clearly agreed to be the service and improvement of the state and the citizens of the realm (Harrison, 2001). The newly established Royal Society became the leading scientific institution of the land and was regarded by its members as the embodiment of "Solomon's House" thereafter (Webster, 1967).

THE PHILOSOPHICAL TRANSACTIONS AND MEDICAL KNOWLEDGE

The Royal Society's serial publication *The Philosophical Transactions* was widely disseminated throughout Europe and the New World. It served as a vehicle for sharing the knowledge collected by observers in science and medicine, and also contained extensive reviews of new books on these topics as well. Medical correspondents communicated observations on diseases and cures. For many medical practitioners the publication offered the first opportunity to compare their own clinical experiences with those of physicians from all over the world (Porter, 1989). The medical historian Roy Porter has commented that not all the articles published by the Royal Society contributed much to any "progress of medical science." While the Royal College of Physicians at that time did little to encourage medical communication of ideas and shared experiences, the Royal Society fostered the careful but often random observation and reporting of clinical observations by medical practitioners (Porter, 1989). The mass of information published has been called a "budget of curiosities...justified by Bacon's notion that the philosopher might learn more from Nature's by-ways than from her plain and ordinary course" (Hall, 1974).

> The members sought empirical data, and thus the Society assiduously collected a hodgepodge of medical information about specific cures, the occurrence of monstrosities and reports of diseases, all in the hope of putting together a natural history...which would provide the foundation for generalizations and universal laws in the inductive manner of the Society's source of philosophical inspiration, Francis Bacon (Wear, 1995b).

This statement was certainly not meant as a criticism of the published data. In a new science, the practitioners did not have the theoretical knowledge to discern what was useful information; hence, they collected and recorded everything that seemed interesting. This represented the general plan for the Society offered by its first Secretary, Henry Oldenburg, in 1663. He told the members, "It is our business...to scrutinize the whole of nature and to investigate its activity and powers by means of observations and experiments; and then in the course of time to come out with a more solid philosophy and more ample amenities of civilization" (Hunter, M., 1981). And they were optimistic about the eventual success of this quest. "It is astonishing how quickly the discovery of natural laws bred a confidence that everything had a natural explanation" (Morgan, 1997b).

As a compendium of miscellaneous medical knowledge, the *Philosophical Transactions* served a very useful purpose by allowing physicians and other members to share observations and propose underlying causes of diseases seen in everyday life. At times, simple observations of unusual findings were presented. John Freke, a surgeon at St. Bartholomew's Hospital, reported the case of the boy who began to develop exostoses, bony growths along his back, starting at age three. He had no evidence of rickets, and the cause could not be discerned (Freke, 1739). Disease in a child was often assumed to result from injuries, illness or emotional stresses encountered by its mother during her pregnancy. Cyprianus reported a female child who was born after an easy labor and had a wound in her left breast, as deep as the intercostal muscles. At about seven months of the pregnancy, the mother remembered that she had heard the shocking story of a man who had murdered his wife by plunging a knife into her breast. It was therefore believed that the child received its wound "at the very moment that the mother was affrighted." The wound did not putrefy because air was excluded from the wound by the amniotic fluid (Cyprianus, 1695). William Gregory observed the case of a woman who visited a circus shortly after conceiving. She watched closely as a monkey wearing a hood performed with a bear. Shortly thereafter, she encountered a man with "a thin, pale and dismal aspect," and she thought that he looked like the face of a monkey. Eventually the women delivered a dead fetus looking just like "a hooded monkey" (Gregory, 1739). At other times the influence of the father appeared to be the factor resulting in disease in newborn children. Benjamin Cooke reported the case of a man who had lived in America for seven years, and returned to England "cachectic, anasarcous, and deep-tinged with jaundice." His wife then bore a child who developed jaundice and died at six months of age. She became pregnant again, developed jaundice herself at three months gestation but fortuitously delivered a healthy child, fair in color (Cooke, 1749).

The nature of infections during pregnancy was also investigated as a means of understanding transmission of disease from one generation to the next. Cromwell Mortimer (d 1752) studied medicine at Leyden and received the Cambridge M.D. in 1728. He practiced in London and was elected Fellow of the Royal Society in 1728. He served as its Secretary until his death and was actively involved in scientific activities throughout his life. He reported that a woman had viewed another woman with smallpox from a distance of 30-40 feet while pregnant. She never developed any signs of fright or disease. Two weeks later, she delivered a healthy male infant. But in one or two days, the child developed smallpox and died. Mortimer could not explain this chain of evidence:

> It is very surprising and wonderful to consider the different manner in which children while in their mothers' wombs, are affected by various accidents happening to their mothers. How the imagination only, affected by the disagreeableness of the sight, should convey the infection to this child...is, I own, what I am unable to account for, especially as there was no fright or surprise, and that the mother was under no apprehension of danger (Mortimer, 1749).

Another woman, who had previously had smallpox as a child, was exposed to the disease again when she was seven months pregnant. She delivered a female child with evidence of pox on the skin (Watson, 1749). A similar case resulted in a dead child also with evidence of active disease (Hunter, J., 1780). Yet another woman developed smallpox at seven months of her pregnancy. The child was born healthy, and eventually developed the disease himself five years later. It was therefore clear to these medical observers that:

> The child before its birth ought to be considered as a separate, as a distinct organization, and although wholly nourished by its mother's fluids, with regard to smallpox, it is liable to be affected in a very different manner; and at a very different time from its mother (Watson, 1749).

Such contemporary accounts indicated that exposure did not always produce clinical symptoms of disease in the offspring

Altered skin pigment was commonly seen in the darker races and could be an isolated finding, but sometimes was evident in several persons from the same family. William Byrd reported a boy born of Negro parents in Virginia, who had the expected dark skin until age three years. Then he began to develop dappled white spots on the chest. Each spot was about as large as a man's hand, and eventually spread to cover the entire body. The child was not sickly (Byrd, 1697). The cleric, John Bate, described another Negro from Virginia who had dark skin until age 25 years. The skin around the mouth and the fingernails then began to turn white, eventually spreading to involve about 80 percent of the entire body. The cause of this type of variation in skin tone observed in single individuals was quite unclear (Bate, 1759). On the other hand, familial cases of altered skin pigmentation did occur and were reported by James Parsons (b 1705), who had received the M.D. in Rheims in 1736. He was elected Fellow of the Royal Society in 1741 and practiced at the St. Giles' Infirmary in London. Parsons collected information on several Negro families with albino offspring who lacked all skin pigment. These reminded him of the "White Indians" describe by Wafer earlier in 1699. In one family, both parents were black, and one of three children was albino. In a second family, one parent was black, the other albino, and the child was as black as his father. Another similar family group produced one fair child with black areas on the thigh and buttock. In another case, an albino father and black mother produced a black son, who eventually married a black female. They had one albino son. Interestingly, the father then reported that "white" children had been born in other branches of his family (Parsons, 1765).

But what could explain the apparent transmission of a trait to offspring in some cases but not in others? Mark Akenside (b 1721) was a Leyden M.D. who was eventually appointed physician to Queen Charlotte in 1761. He examined a man who had numerous hard cutaneous tumors all over his body. When one was surgically removed, another one reappeared in the same place. Each seemed to originate from a subcutaneous gland. He thought that the recurrent tumors showed "the apparent consequence of an hereditary vice in the habit" (Akenside, 1768), and yet the family history revealed no other affected relatives.

While the members of the Royal Society shared many similar reports of medical curiosities, they could not shed much light on the underlying causes of the abnormalities being examined. In 1731, John Machin (d 1751), Professor of Anatomy at Gresham College and Secretary of the Royal Society, first reported the singular case of Edward Lambert, the "Porcupine Man, a different kind from any hitherto mentioned in histories of diseases." The child was a boy, aged 14 years, who had been born of normal parents. Numerous brothers and sisters appeared to be normal. The original report nicely summarized the physical findings:

> The skin seemed rather like a dusky coloured thick Case, exactly fitting every part of his body, made of rugged Bark, or Hide, with bristles in some places, which Case covering the whole of him excepting the Face, the Palms the Hands, and the Soles of the Feet, caused an appearance as if these parts alone were naked, and the rest cloathed...It is said he shed it once a year, about autumn at which time it usually grows to the thickness of three-Quarters of an inch, and then is thrust off by the new skin which is coming up underneath. The bristly parts, which were chiefly about the belly and the flanks, looked and rustled like the Bristles or Quills, of a Hedge-Hog, shorn off within an inch of the skin...his skin was clear at birth as in other children, and so it continued for about seven or eight weeks, after which without his being sick, it began to turn yellow, as if he had had the Jaundice; from which by degrees it changed black, and in a little Time afterwards thickened, and grew into the State it appeared in at present.

The boy was never sick. His mother did not experience any fright during the pregnancy; the cause of the remarkable skin condition was unknown (Machin, 1731).

By 1755, Edward had become the father of six sons, all affected exactly as he was. Lambert and one son were shown again at the Royal Society. Henry Baker (b 1678) was a prominent naturalist of the day, who reported now on the familial nature of the skin defect. He concluded:

> It appears, therefore, past all doubt, that a race of people may be propagated, by this man having such rough coats or coverings as himself, and if this should ever happen, and the accidental origin be forgotten, 'tis not improbable they might be deemed a different species of mankind: a consideration which would almost lead one to imagine that if mankind were all produced from one and the same stock, the black skins of the negroes, and many other differences of the kind, might possibly have been originating from the same accidental cause (Baker, 1755).

Baker thus proposed that a sudden change, a mutation, caused the altered skin covering that was then transmitted to the offspring. A new stock could then be generated. He also suggested that many other hereditary traits might have originated in the same "accidental" manner.

The father and sons Lambert toured the capitals of Europe and earned money in exhibitions. Peder Ascanius reported that the offspring had included both sons and daughters, and all had been afflicted with the same skin malady. E.A.W. Zimmerman recorded the same thing from Germany in 1778. Another German physician, W.G. Tylesius, interviewed men in the third generation of the family in 1792. Two brothers reported they had seven healthy sisters and claimed for the first time that nowhere in the history of the family had females ever been affected. While on tour in England, Dr. Girdlestone interviewed the family as well. They mentioned a third affected brother, and again claimed that all sisters were born normal (Girdlestone, 1802). Dr. Elliotson reported seeing the brothers' exhibition in Bond Street "at a shilling a piece." It was reported that all male offspring were affected (Elliotson, 1831). William Sedgwick (Sedgwick, 1861) and Charles Darwin (Darwin, 1868) later claimed that six generations of affected males existed, and that no females had ever been born affected. Since only males were affected, the horned skin, "ichthyosis," appeared to result from a gene on the Y chromosome, which was passed from father to all his sons during procreation, and to none of the daughters. This explanation has appeared in generations of textbooks on heredity since that time (Penrose and Stern, 1958).

In the twentieth century, the geneticists Lionel Penrose and Curt Stern collaborated with English clergymen to extract Lambert family history from church baptismal records in Suffolk. They found that, in fact, two females were affected in the second generation, and that the last affected male had occurred in the fourth generation. He died in childhood and had no offspring. The alleged fifth and six affected generations were pure fiction. Their conclusion was that the skin condition termed "ichthyosis hystrix" was a dominant trait and had appeared as a sudden mutation (Penrose and Stern, 1958). In fact, an analogous family was described by P.J. Martin in 1818. He observed a mother and daughter with ichthyosis like the Lambert family (Martin, 1818). His explanation for the sudden appearance of such an unusual deviation from the norm anticipated modern mutation theory and will be discussed in more detail later.

Color blindness was another familial trait examined by the Royal Society members. Joseph Huddart (b 1741) was a geographer who had surveyed the Indian Ocean for the East Indian Company. Huddart reported the case of a shoemaker who had known since early childhood that he could not distinguish a red stocking from a black one. Other children could differentiate cherries from leaves on a tree by color, while he could only discriminate them by differences in size and shape. The man had "two brothers in the same circumstances as to sight; and two other brothers and sisters who, as well as the parents, had nothing of this defect" (Huddart, 1777). Michael Lort (b 1725) was a clergyman who had been a Fellow of Royal Society since 1766. He noted the familial occurrence of color blindness in another example involving three generations. One affected man observed that "pink and pale blue appeared alike; full red and full green the same." Such a defect could be quite embarrassing in a social context. He had planned to give his daughter in marriage to a "genteel, worthy man." On the day before the wedding, the groom came to visit, wearing, as the bride's father supposed, a black coat. He said, "The groom must go back and change his colour." But the daughter protested that her father's eyes had deceived him, as the groom's coat was "a fine rich claret-coloured dress." The reason for this defect was clearly a "family failing." Three generations were affected: the "father has exactly the same impediment." The mother and one sister had normal color vision, while one sister and the male writer were imperfect. The affected sister had two affected sons and one normal daughter. The writer's own son and daughter had normal vision. His mother's brother had the same impediment, though his own mother had perfect color vision (Lort, 1778). Color blindness typically affected males much more commonly than females. This unusual family did have an affected woman who transmitted the defect to both of her sons. But in most instances, an unaffected female of a family known to have colorblind males would produce affected males and unaffected females. The defect was often said to "skip generations," being transmitted through unaffected females.

Over the course of the seventeenth century, the fortunes of the medical and scientific societies in England waxed and waned. The College of Physicians was an exclusive body, offering membership only to Oxford and Cambridge medical graduates. The Fellows did collaborate extensively with other nascent "scientists" on a wide range of medical and technological researches before the destruction of the College building in the Great Fire of 1666. In contrast, the Royal Society, from its inception, was inclusive, inviting membership from men of all interests for the betterment of mankind. The *Philosophical Transactions* disseminated ideas in the sciences not only in England, but also throughout the entire civilized world. The Fellows of the Royal Society certainly did report a virtual potpourri of medical curiosities. Birth defects, tumors, infections, abnormal skin and color blindness were noted in certain families to recur in successive generations. Some notion of hereditary disease thus evolved. By communicating a wide range of abnormalities of the human body, the members hoped to eventually discern natural laws on the causes of such human diseases.

Physicians in the next century would increasingly desire a more comprehensive scientific theory to explain the origin of diseases that would make them appear both knowledgeable and proficient as they treated their patients in daily medical practice.

Four

Medical Education and Practice, and a Theory of Heredity

English medicine of the eighteenth-century is often characterized as "static and stagnant" (Porter, 1995a). The leaders of organized medicine in the Royal College of Physicians continued to be conservative and exclusive. Fellowship was not available to religious dissenters or to physicians trained at medical schools other than Oxford or Cambridge.

On the other hand, the empirical approach to science fostered by Bacon in the seventeenth-century and applied during this era by the Royal Society encouraged the advancement of science in general. New theories to synthesize medical knowledge proliferated throughout the century and were designed to replace the ancient systems of Galen and Aristotle. In many repects, the new theories proved to be as speculative as the older ones regarding causes of disease. Clinical practice remained little changed over the decades. The therapies of diet and rest coupled with purging, cupping and bleeding remained the standard of care as physicians sought to help relieve their patients' symptoms (Franklin, 1974a; Risse, 1992; Porter, 1995b; Wear, 1992). John Floyer (b 1649) of Litchfield commented that the new theories of medicine had made but "little alteration in the practice of physic..." (Franklin, 1974b).

The expanding educated upper class in eighteenth-century England hoped that the application of the new science espoused by some would eventually improve medical practice. Having some form of comprehensive theory of disease also provided the physician with status as he practiced among more knowledgeable patients, who expected a rational explanation for their symptoms and for the proposed treatment plan (Risse, 1992). Physicians of the day considered these new ideas, while holding onto the tried-and-true remedies from the past (Franklin, 1974a). The historian, A.W. Franklin, has pointed out, however, that "real progress in clinical medicine had to await altered ways of thought, new concepts on the nature of disease, the idea that diseases were of different kinds, and new methods of judging the effectiveness of treatment" (Franklin, 1974c).

By the end of the eighteenth-century, preliminary changes had been initiated that eventually resulted in the flourishing of the scientific, rational medicine of the nineteenth-century. Nosology, the systematic classification of diseases, had been developed to group clinical syndromes with similar symptoms and thus suggest common underlying causes. Specific treatments like quinine and digitalis were being used to treat specific disease symptoms. Prevention of infectious disease such as smallpox by immunization was becoming a reality. Education of medical students, both at the traditional universities and at the newer London and Scottish schools, was changing dramatically. And, the communication of "new" medical knowledge via local medical societies and through the printed medical journals provided ongoing education for practitioners as they cared for their patients. The "static and stagnant" English medicine of 1700 was being transformed into a more dynamic and progressive practice after 1800 that actually made a difference in improving the quality of life for the growing population of the realm. The medical practitioner was coming to be viewed by patients as a scientist because he could actually do something to help alleviate, cure and sometimes even prevent human diseases (Corfield, 1995).

Health and Disease

Good health was viewed as the natural state of man. A balance between intrinsic factors, such as hereditary constitution, and external factors, such as diet, exercise, sleep and bowel habits were believed to be necessary to maintain wellness. Sickness was often perceived to result from neglect of the self, a personal deviation from the natural healthy status quo (Lawrence, C., 1994a). As such, sickness was often thought to be an avoidable evil. For example, a good constitution could be corrupted by excessive drink (Porter and Porter, 1988a). The role of the physician was to discern the nature of this imbalance, provide treatments to re-establish the patient's equilibrium, and then allow the natural healing powers of the individual to correct the defects (Risse, 1992; Lawrence, C., 1994a).

Although early in this era, the "new science" had done little to improve the practice of medicine, it did generate optimism for the future in the minds of both the physician and the lay-public. Because knowledge was viewed as power, the professional, learned physician appealed to the suffering populace. Daniel Cox of the Royal College of Physicians suggested as early as 1669 that: "...as for the cure of diseases, it seems highly probable that they who are best acquainted with the causes and symptoms of disease will apply medicines more properly than others that cannot so well distinguish, although possessed of the same remedies" (Wear, 1989). One hundred years later, an unsigned editorial from the College summarized the approach toward gaining that desired knowledge:

> The experience of many ages hath more than sufficiently shown that mere abstract reasonings have tended very little to the promoting of natural knowledge. By laying these aside, and attending carefully to what nature hath, either by chance work or upon experiment offered to our observation, a greater progress has been made in this part of Philosophy, since the beginning of the last century, than had been until that time from the days of Aristotle ("Editorial," 1768).

Such faith in the progress and eventual perfectibility of society was widespread during this era and demonstrated the power of "reason" (Risse, 1992).

The process of classifying different symptoms into consistent patterns among different patients defined nosology, a critical part of understanding underlying causes of disease. The irregular practitioner William Salmon (b 1644) had little medical education, but wrote learned treatises on medicine and enjoyed a long and successful career. He observed in his 1681 *Synopsis medicinae*, "...it is very necessary first to know what the disease is, before we proceed any further...before we offer to meddle or consider the cure" (Franklin, 1974d). One extensive attempt to understand specific types of disease was conducted by Thomas Sydenham (b 1624), who was educated at Oxford and

Leyden, and then developed a large clinical practice in London after the Restoration in 1660. He studied fevers in patients systematically for sixteen years and then attempted to classify disease by genus and species as a botanist classified plants. He concluded:

> In the first place it is necessary that all disease be reduced to definite and certain species, and that with the same care which one sees exhibited by botanists in their phytologies; since it happens, at present, that many diseases, although included in the same genus, mentioned with a common nomenclature, and resembling one another in several symptoms, are not withstanding, different in their natures and require a different medical treatment...Nature in the production of disease, is uniform and consistent...and the selfsame phenomena that you would observe in the sickness of a Socrates you would observe in the sickness of a simpleton. Just so the universal characters of a plant are extended to every individual of the species (Rather, 1974a).

Such careful classification of diseases was important, Sydenham believed, else "it would make the study of physic absolutely impossible, for if physicians cannot arrive at some distinction of diseases, we must act at random" (Risse, 1992b). Sydenham trusted only his own senses to study living patients and their symptoms. He apparently declined to use the microscope to study post-mortem tissues from his patients (Franklin, 1974e; Rather, 1974a). He then concluded:

> Now this great diversity [of fevers] appears both from the proper and peculiar symptoms incident to them and likewise from the very different cures which they respectively challenge. Both which do evince that they are of a quite different genus and nature one from another...(Meynell, 1991).

His findings that there were many different species of fevers thus had implications for treating the patient

Another contemporary physician, Thomas Willis, carried the analysis of disease one step further. He performed post-mortem examinations on as many of his patients as possible and attempted to correlate changes in anatomy with disease symptoms that he observed during life (Franklin, 1974a; Rather, 1974a). He commented in 1684, "...in delving the *Theory of Diseases*, leaving the old way, I have almost everywhere brought forth new hypotheses: but what being founded upon anatomical observations, and firmly established, better solve all Phenomena of the Sick" (Rather, 1974b). His method of inquiry reflected the inductive reasoning that characterized the new science of this era:

> ...for after I had not found in Books what might satisfie a mind desirous of Truth, I resolved with my self, research into living and breathing examples: and therefore sitting often times by the Sick, I was wont carefully to search out their cases, to weigh all the symptoms, and to put them, with exact diaries of the diseases, into writing; then diligently to meditate on these, and to compare some with others; and then began to adapt general Notions from particular events: and when by this means for a long time, observing the Accidents and Courses of Fevers I had busied myself, for the finding out forms of Reasons for their Cure, and at length a new Pathology of this Disease was conceived in my mind (Franklin, 1974a).

The importance of these preliminary attempts to define specific disease classes by Sydenham and Willis was to provide a thought construct for physicians of the eighteenth-century. By mid-century, William Cullen (b 1710), Professor of Medicine at Edinburgh, could state with certainty, "It is well-known to be necessary in order to successfully practice [medicine] that remedies be adopted not only to every genus but to every species, and even to every variety of disease" (Risse, 1992c). The role of the physician was thus to match his proposed therapy with each specific disease state. Cullen proposed that disease resulted from an imbalance in the nervous system. Too much excitement increased muscle tone, produced spasm of blood vessels and decreased circulation, resulting in altered chemical balance within the body. Conversely, a depressed nervous system resulted in decreased muscle tone, an impaired circulation and eventual collapse of the system. Treatments were therefore designed to re-establish the balanced state of the disordered nervous system. Calming agents for an overactive system included rest, a meat-less diet, bleeding, purging, sedatives and antispasmodic medications. Stimulants for an under-active state would include exercise, fresh air, meat and wine in the diet, warm baths and tonic medications (Risse, 1992a).

Medical Education

Variations in the traditional educational pathway leading to the profession of medicine evolved early in the eighteenth-century. The ancient universities at Oxford and Cambridge continued to provide ultraconservative, long and expensive courses for the few gentlemen with the time and money to complete the programs (King, 1958). Continental medical schools began to attract medical students away from England about this time. Herman Boerhaave (b 1668) had been appointed to the medical faculty at Leyden in 1701. He attempted to apply scientific findings to clinical medicine, and also encouraged the correlation of clinical signs with post-mortem findings (Booth, 1979; Risse, 1992a). He rapidly became the leading clinical professor of medicine in Europe during this era. His book *Institutiones Medicae* argued that the key to medical knowledge involved observation and experience: "...the art of Physic was anciently established by a faithful collection of facts observed, whose effects were afterwards explained, and their causes assigned by the assistance of reason..."(Cook, 2000a). He based his opinion on the prior work of Bacon and Harvey. Boerhaave thought that specific symptoms of a disease were the result of altered physiology. The same disease would be expected to produce the same symptoms in anyone. Treatments were then aimed at modifying such corporeal defects. This approach opposed the ancient assumption that each person was unique, and thus that the cause of the same sickness in different people would not be identical. Hence, it was traditionally assumed that a unique treatment would also be required for each individual (Cook, 2000b).

Boerhaave's style of teaching and the absence of a university religious test[3] encouraged many young English medical students to spend at least part of their time in training at Leyden or at one of the other leading European schools such as Paris, Bologna, Padua, Montpelier and Rome (King, 1958). A cadre of young Scottish students trained with Boerhaave and then carried continental ideas back home, establishing practices in Edinburgh and Glasgow. By 1726, the University of Edinburgh had established its own medical school with faculty trained on the Leyden model. The Royal Infirmary subsequently opened in 1729 to provide patient care and to foster clinical teaching of medical students (Walker, 1965; Lawrence, C., 1994a).

The three traditional professional corporations in London at this time did little to encourage medical education. Their leaders viewed their organizations as primarily licensing boards, rather than education institutions. The College of Physicians did sponsor several annual lectures on medical topics. The Apothecaries had discourses on medical botany. The Surgeons had occasional anatomical demonstrations performed on executed criminals (Lawrence, S.C., 1996a). But the lack of organized medical education in the capital fostered the development of teaching opportunities in private medical schools and within the confines of the large municipal hospitals that opened during the eighteenth century (Bynum, 1980; Cross, 1981a; Booth, 1979; Lawrence, S.C., 1995, 1996a).

Economic growth at this time expanded the number of individuals in the middle and upper classes who came to recognize that many infectious diseases appeared to originate among the poorer classes. Debilitated workers made poor employees for businesses. Enlightened self-interest therefore dictated that means be found to both isolate and, hopefully, cure the physical ills of the sick poor. Such charity would also teach the paupers gratitude for society's efforts to improve their physical and moral status (Porter, 1995a).

The two ancient hospitals, St. Bartholomew's and St. Thomas's, had survived since the twelfth century. As medical practice and education expanded, so too did the metropolitan hospitals. By 1750, Guy's, Westminster, St. George's, the London and Middlesex Hospitals all had been established with boards of governors composed of lay-people. Physicians and surgeons were appointed for life as voluntary medical staff to care for the poor patients (Lawrence, S.C., 1996a; Porter, 1995a). These medical men were viewed as the leaders of the profession at that time.

The hospitals became medical education centers because students could see many patients in a short period of time, observe the effects of different medications and surgical techniques, and correlate their clinical experience with post-mortem examinations. The metropolitan London population grew from 500,000 in 1700 to 1,500,000 in 1800. This concentration of people provided numerous opportunities for learning in medicine (Granshaw, 1992). Surgeons had walked the hospital wards with their apprentices at St. Thomas's as early as the sixteenth-century. As new hospitals opened in the 1800s, it became routine for paying groups of medical, surgical and apothecary students to work with practitioners in the hospitals and observe the many patients in the wards. Formal lectures to illustrate important clinical points were also begun in the hospitals. John Rutherford began such lectures at the Edinburgh Royal Infirmary in 1748. Over the next few decades, it became standard practice in the London hospitals as well (Lawrence, S.C., 1996a; Walker, 1965; Digby, 1994; Loudon, 1986). Operating theatres were built to demonstrate surgical procedures, and lecture halls were established to educate students in both medicine and surgery. In 1785, the London Hospital opened the first complete medical school with its own building (Lawrence, S.C., 1996a; Walker, 1965).

During this same period, while medical education became more "scientific," the London physicians began to act more like other educated men of the city. The Fellows of the Royal Society in particular were viewed by the public as scientists who met to exchange ideas, validate observations and thus advance science of the day. Science came to be accepted as an important instrument of progress in general. Educated people came to agree that the study of "the natural laws of the body" would surely result in improved health for society (Lawrence, C., 1994b).

Medical societies were begun by medical practitioners for analogous reasons to communicate new ideas, discuss difficult cases and build networks of professional colleagues. These organizations were quite different from the traditional Colleges in London. They were not exclusive, but rather sought to encourage physicians, surgeons and surgeon-apothecaries to come together to learn from each other. The first such local medical group was the Society for the Improvement of Medical Knowledge and was founded in Edinburgh in the 1730s (Booth, 1979; Bynum, 1980). By the end of the eighteenth century, at least sixteen new groups had formed in the London area alone. Some were comprised of staff members from specific hospitals, such as the Guy's Hospital Physical Society (from 1771) and the Middlesex Hospital Medical Society (from 1774), while others were open to any interested practitioner (Lawrence, S.C., 1996c; "Editorial," 1773).

Physicians of the day also sought to emulate their scientific colleagues by writing reports describing interesting medical cases. The *Philosophical Transactions* published by the Royal Society provided "an initial model" for the literary presentation of new ideas in both medicine and science in general during the century (Lawrence, S.C., 1996b; "Editorial," 1757). Physicians in the new medical societies began to publish their own journals, focusing exclusively on developments in their own specialty. The first volume of *Medical Observations and Inquiries* from the Society of Physicians in London explained the reason for a specifically medical journal. All agreed that the *Philosophical Transactions* had served as an important vehicle to communicate ideas in medicine: "...These are valuable treasures, that publick libraries cannot be without, and all learned men wish to profess; in the numerous volumes of which, many reports of medicine have been treated with utmost accuracy and ingenuity." But, many physicians did not have ready access to the *Transactions*, and "the greater share of all the tracts are not immediately relative to their proper business, but treat natural history, mechanicks, astronomy, abstract mathematics, etc." ("Editorial," 1757).

The first serial publications in the United Kingdom specifically devoted to medicine were *Medical Essays and Observations* (1733-1744) and the *Medical Observations* (1754-1765) published by the Edinburgh Society (Porter, 1995c; Bynum, 1980). The London societies followed suit after 1750. The journal *Medical Observations and Inquiries* (from 1757) has already been mentioned. The Royal College of Physicians initiated its *Medical Transactions* in 1754 (Porter, 1995c). The Medical Society of London published its own *Memoirs* from 1773. *Medical Communications* was the journal of the Society for the Improvement of Medical Knowledge (founded in 1782) ("Editorial," 1784). The editor from the Medical Society of London clearly identified the rationale for both the existence of such societies and the publication of the proceedings. Their aim was to enhance "the science which proposes the subtlest objects for its end, the preservation and restoration of health..." And that knowledge would be derived from comparing observations of professional colleagues. The members recognized that "deceased authors cannot solve our difficulties" ("Editorial," 1773). And London appeared to be the ideal location for such societies. The metropolis was growing rapidly. There were many hospitals and eminent physicians. The expansion of commerce enhanced communication of new and interesting medical ideas from the entire world ("Editorial," 1757).

On the Causes of Disease

Comparative study of animal species and extensive post-mortem examinations convinced John Hunter (b 1728) that human disease resulted from altered normal organ function, i.e., abnormal physiology. Previous concepts of disease argued that external entities "visited the body" and produced symptoms of fever, rash, diarrhea, etc. Hunter was trained as a surgeon and had been elected to the Royal Society as well. The more than 700 autopsies that he performed revealed the state or "disposition" of the internal organs affected in different disease states whose malfunction then resulted in the clinical signs and symptoms observed in the living patients. He noted, "the ultimate and visible effect of disease is action; but this is not the disease, for the action is only an effect, a sign, a symptom of disease" (Cross, 1981b). He labeled pathology as the "physiology of disease," the "perversion of the natural actions of the animal oeconomy" (Cross, 1981b).

The study of altered embryologic development was another means for learning about normal development of the different organ systems. Hunter observed:

> Besides having recourse to many of the inferior orders and animals for the elucidation of some of the phenomenon of the more complicated orders, we are also obliged to disease for many of our hints on the animal oeconomy, or for explaining the actions of parts, for the wrong action of a part often points out what the natural action was, and itself gives an idea of life. Disease often corrects our imaginations and opinions, and shows us that such and such parts cannot have the uses commonly attributed to them, and therefore brings us a step towards the knowledge of the true use. Monstrosities can contribute to rectify our opinions in the same if not a more intelligible manner. A monster is either from a deficiency of parts, which can be produced from art (and often is from necessity, as in operations), or else from a modification caused by the wrong arrangement or construction of parts, which will produce an unnatural action, by which means the natural action may be known (Cross, 1981c).

The disease classification (nosology) developed by William Cullen has already been mentioned. His scheme of disease as published in *First Lines in the Practice of Physic* in 1786 was not meant to define a fixed system. His nosology was a set of working ideas which he hoped would have heuristic value, by encouraging other physicians to observe their own patients carefully, in great detail, and then contribute to the progress of medical science (Risse, 1992a; King, 1958). Physicians of this era did attempt to define the causes of disease, utilizing a scheme of diseases as Cullen suggested, and viewing pathology, as Hunter proposed, as the result of abnormal functioning of the affected organs.

Contagion was generally agreed to be an important cause of much disease, transmitting symptoms from one person to another by contact. But sometimes the evidence argued against the contagiousness of certain disorders. John Pearson (b 1758) had been a student at St. George's and then studied with John Hunter. He was an example of the contemporary medical man who was also conversant with the best of science and was elected Fellow of the Royal Society in 1803. He observed that surgeons and their assistants were exposed to "the noxious effects of cancerous sores with perfect impunity." He therefore concluded that the risk of contagion from cancer was thus "so small as not to form an object of serious attention" (Pearson, 1793).

Other epidemic diseases did, however, appear to be transmitted easily from one person to another. William Heberden (b 1710) of London described the typical symptoms of measles and documented its passage from one affected person to another healthy person (Heberden, 1785). Smallpox was another common infection of both children and adults. It could even be passed from an infected mother to her unborn child in utero. John Hunter reported a woman in her sixth month of pregnancy who developed the disease. A dead child was delivered 23 days later with evidence of smallpox in the skin (Hunter, 1780). Another pregnant women also contracted the disease and eventually died. Her dead baby also showed evidence of the disease (Kite, 1795). William Turnbull (b 1729) documented the infectious nature of such neonatal cases by taking some pus from the wounds of the fetal skin and inoculating several older children. Typical symptoms of the disease subsequently developed in these children as well (Turnbull, 1795). But the contagion was not always so clear-cut. W. Watson described several instances where women had contracted smallpox in the past and hence were assumed to be in immune. But when exposed to persons with active disease during their pregnancies, they delivered babies with evidence of the disease. Another woman developed smallpox at seven months of the pregnancy. Her child was born healthy, and later developed smallpox at age five years. These variable results of exposure suggested that "the child before its birth ought to be considered as a separate, as a distinct organization; and although wholly surrounded by its mother fluids, with regard to the smallpox, it is liable to be affected in a very different manner, and at a different time from its mother" (Watson, 1749).

William Heberden received the Cambridge M.D. and practiced in London for many years. He was recognized as the most prominent physician of his day, and helped launch the *Medical Transactions* published by the College of Physicians. He was one of the growing number of physicians who were equally comfortable publishing results of their investigations in both the *Philosophical Transactions* and the more specialized medical journals that evolved during this time. He noted some similarity between chickenpox (varicella) and smallpox. Lay people assumed that the two were identical. Having had varicella, they might assume that they were likewise immune to smallpox, and avoid being vaccinated. To clarify the situation, Heberden described the clinical symptoms characteristic of chickenpox. He reported a family in which the mother had not had this disease. Two of her children became infected; she developed the same lesions nine days later, justifying the classification of chickenpox as infection. As with smallpox, those who had had chickenpox generally were immune. Heberden took some pus from a chicken pock and placed it within a small incision on the arm of a boy who had had chickenpox in the past; nothing happened, indicating that he was, indeed, immune (Heberden, 1768).

Notions on Constitution, Heredity and Disease

By the eighteenth century, some understanding of the interaction between individual constitution and one's health or disease had developed. Not all children exposed to smallpox or chickenpox developed symptoms of disease. Not all women exposed to frightful events during pregnancy produced children with defects noted at birth. Clearly sickness often produced different symptoms in different people, suggesting that the inherent properties of each individual, the constitution, might play an important role in producing symptoms of actual disease.

It was generally accepted at this time that one's "constitution" was inherited from parents. Hence, disease produced by corruption of the constitution could be analyzed by studying the family history of similar disease (Porter and Porter, 1988b). The modern usage of the notion of such constitution or "diathesis" evolved in France at the end of the eighteenth century. It came to mean "that state of the body which makes it acquire certain diseases" (Ackerknecht, 1982). The Societe Royal de Medicin in Paris sponsored an essay competition in 1788 to address the question of whether hereditary diseases actually existed. The participants shared their own observations from clinical practice rather than relying on quotations from ancient authorities (Lopez-Beltran, 2007a). The general impression was that predisposition or constitution was inherited, as well as certain specific and chronic hereditary diseases (Lopez-Beltran, 2007b).

In the early nineteenth century, an inherited predisposition would become widely accepted as an important cause of many different disorders. By 1800, British medical practitioners reported familial cases of cancer, gout, mental illness, rheumatism, syphilis, scrofula and rickets, suggesting that inherited constitution made these individuals susceptible to developing specific disease symptoms during their lives (Ackerknecht, 1982). James Jay observed in 1772, "Gout must be looked upon as a hereditary disease...A radical cure is not to be expected" (Waller, 2002a). The Edinburgh physician William Buchan recorded in his *Domestic Medicine* (1769) that children were "particularly prone to inherit the disease of the parent to whom they have the greatest similarity..." But sometimes reversions occurred, in which a child resembled a more distant relative: "So we shall find the constitution and disease of that child...in the nature of the progenitor whom it most resembles" (Wilson, 2003). Marmaduke Berdoe argued in 1772, "How absurd [are] all attempts to cure a confined gout" (Waller, 2002a). However, not all physicians so easily accepted the role of heredity in these diseases. William Cadogan questioned the role of inheritance and disease in *A Dissertation of the Gout* (1771). He observed:

> Those who insist that the gout is hereditary, because they see it sometimes, must argue very inconclusively; for if we compute the number of children who have it not, and women who have it not, together with those active and temperate men who are free from it, though born of gouty parents, the proportion will be found at least one hundred to one against that opinion (Waller, 2002b).

Scrofula, tuberculous swelling of the lymphatic glands in the neck, was also believed to be hereditary. However, the 1784 *Treatise on Struma or Scrofula* by Thomas White argued against the simple inheritance of such chronic disorders. "It frequently happens that children have the complaint whose parents do not appear to have been at any period of their lives afflicted..." In other families, both parents and children were affected. But, "even admitting one of the children of such [scrofulous] parents have struma, that is no proof that the disease originated in a hereditary taint or morbid predisposition, derived from the father or mother..." White thought, "If the disease were truly hereditary, none could expect to escape" (Waller, 2002c).

Nevertheless, both the general public and the medical profession agreed that children generally resembled their parents in many characteristics, and that features acquired by a parent often were transmitted to their own offspring. Oliver Goldsmith (b 1728) exemplified an educated layman of the day who observed the importance of heredity in producing diseases. Although known primarily as a poet and dramatist, he had entered the University of Edinburgh in 1752 to study medicine. He left after two years and practiced as an unlicensed physician until he achieved financial success as a writer. He noted in his 1774 work *Histories of the Earth* that artificial deformity such as flattening of the nose or binding of the feet

> ...in a course of ages shapes itself to the construct and assumes hereditary deformity. We find nothing more common in birth than for children to inherit the accidental deformities of their parents. We have many instances of squinting in the father, which he received from fright, communicated to the offspring; and I myself have seen a child distinctly marked by a scar, similar to the one the father received in battle...[These] can be continued or even increased through successive generations (Goldsmith, 1774).

Physicians had long noted the same disease symptoms in successive generations of certain families. John Hunter (d. 1809) was a prominent surgeon who developed a large London practice at St. George's Hospital. He prepared medical research reports for both the *Philosophical Transactions* and the *Medical Transactions.* He observed:

> The father begets a son like himself in every way in form of body, expression of countenance, colour of hair, and sound of voice...So also peculiar marks long continue to distinguish the same family of men. But this is particularly shown by the history of disorders; of which there are instances known to all in the cases of gout, scrofula, and madness. Again, diarrhea and unnatural dilatation of the arch of the aorta long infected the same family (Hunter, 1775).

The familial nature of certain diseases was obvious, but the mechanism for the transmission of such hereditary traits remained obscure. Hunter concluded, "...it is a fact that we cannot explain and yet there is no manner of doubt that peculiarities acquired by men do descend to their posterity" (Hunter, 1775). His Scottish colleague John Gregory agreed:

> How certain character or construction of mind can be transmitted from a parent to child is a question of more difficulty than importance. It is indeed equally difficult to account for the external resemblance of features, as for bodily diseases being transmitted from parent to child (Gregory, 1788).

English physicians of the day came to recognize the hereditary nature of these constitutional diseases. Subsequent family investigations would reveal the inheritance of specific physical defects and physiological disorders affecting virtually all the systems of the human body.

Numerous accounts appeared in the medical and scientific literature emphasizing the importance of heredity in causing unusual traits. In one example, the absence of skin pigment producing symptoms of albinism was noted in Negro families and was then reported to the Royal Society. But albinism also occurred in the Caucasian race. Charles Perceval reported an 11-year-old girl from King's County, Ireland, with fair hair, whiter than flax. The white of the eyes had a reddish cast, and the iris was devoid of pigment. It was not known whether other family members had a similar appearance, but the author intended to inquire (Perceval, 1790). In another example, hemophilia, the tendency to bleed easily, also appeared to run in families. George Fordyce (b 1736) was a prominent London physician at St. Thomas's Hospital and was elected Fellow of the Royal Society in 1776. He was an early leader in the Society for the Improvement of Medical and Chirurgical Knowledge after 1793. His 1784 work *Fragmenta Chirurgica et Medica* contained a brief mention of two individuals affected with a bleeding disorder. Hay, an army drummer, suffered repeated episodes of hemorrhage from trivial wounds. Lofton of Northampton experienced repeated episodes of epistaxis[4] as did his children (Fordyce, 1784).

George Armstrong, the author of an early pediatric textbook, described a family in which three baby boys had died of persistent projectile vomiting and dehydration at about three weeks of age. A post-mortem examination revealed spasm of the pyloric muscle with a distended stomach and empty intestines. This "pyloric stenosis" appeared to run in the family, curiously only affecting children in one generation (Armstrong, 1777). Like hemophilia, this disorder appeared to primarily affect male offspring.

J. Lucas, surgeon at the Leed's Infirmary, reported his experience with hereditary harelip (cleft lip). In one family, only one of thirteen children was affected, while in a second family four of five children were born with the same defect (Lucas, 1795). Lucas also observed cataracts present at birth in the eyes of several children from one family (Lucas, 1795). William Rowley, the London ophthalmologist, agreed that cataract was often of "an hereditary or congenital indisposition" (Rowley, 1790).

But in some cases, hereditary disease had a dynamic and not always hopeless outcome. Farar observed three children in the same family born with "opake cornea." When the first child was born and could not see, it was feared that permanent blindness would ensue. But by ten months of age, the corneas had become clear, and the child had good eyesight. The same thing happened with the second and third affected children (Farar, 1790). Lucas commented:

> The excellence of divine wisdom is not perhaps in any influence more forcibly displayed, than in demonstrating, that although various and even hereditary complaints may happen previous to birth, yet it is not within the search of human understanding to prognosticate events, the knowledge of which could only tend to increase the miseries of mankind, if not frequently be productive of more unhappy consequences (Lucas, 1795).

The medical literature of the time included other cases showing that disorders of the eye could be hereditary in some cases, and acquired in others. The oculist Benedict Duddell noted that the white Indian race reported by Wafer (Wafer, 1699) was almost blind in the light of day, but could see quite well by moonlight. The Countess of Remiremont suffered from the same disorder termed "day blindness." Duddell proposed that her problem resulted from the toxic effects of quicksilver in her system. The Countess had been prescribed a quicksilver[5] girdle for an inveterate itch. The doctor thought that the quicksilver passed via her blood into the aqueous humor of her eye, altering its function in daylight (Duddell, 1736).

The inability to distinguish individual colors had been recognized to run in families throughout the eighteenth-century. The most famous case of color blindness at this time was that of the chemist John Dalton. He did not recognize the deficit until, as an adult, he and his brother were examining colors of different plant leaves. The two of them thought that a laurel leaf was "a good match to a stick of red sealing wax" (Dalton, 1794). Another brother and sister in the family could distinguish many different colors, while the two affected brothers clearly could not. Dalton thought that the defect resulted from a blue tint of the vitreous humor of his eyes which resulted in selective absorption of red and green light (Dalton, 1794). After his death in 1844, his eyes were examined by Joseph Ransome, who found perfectly clear vitreous humor. The doctor then pierced the rear of the eye and viewed colors through the intact lens and vitreous without distortion. In his opinion the color defect occurred because of some malformation in the region of the brain that received nerve impulses from the eyes themselves (Neitz and Neitz, 1995).

Interestingly, the story of Dalton's color blindness has recently been updated using modern DNA technology. His eyes were air-dried after his death and then stored at the Manchester Literary and Philosophical Society. Samples from the dried retina were used recently to perform DNA analysis on the genes involved in color vision. There are normally three different photo pigments in three different retinal cone cells, with peak wavelength sensitivities of 420 nm (SW short wave), 530 nm (MW medium wave) and 560 nm (LW long wave). Normal color vision results from analysis by the optic cortex in the brain of the nerve impulses from the different cone cells of the retina. Typical color blindness results from defects in the genes coding for the MW or LW pigment proteins. The photo pigment genes are located on the X-chromosome in man. Normal individuals typically have 1-2 LW genes and 1-7 MW genes. The retinal samples from Dalton's eyes were found to contain one LW gene and lacked MW genes completely. This specific type of color blindness is termed deuteroanopia (Neitz and Neitz, 1995).

Even before the publication of Dalton's work, there was general awareness that color blindness could be a hereditary trait. King George III was interested in scientific and medical topics, and commented on this aspect of color blindness to Fanny Burney at court in 1785. He observed, "There are many people who have no eye for difference of colour. The Duke of Marlborough cannot tell scarlet from green...I do not find that this defect runs in his family, for Lady DiBeauclerk draws very finely" (Barrett, 1904). Elizabeth Beauclerk was the daughter of Diana Spencer, the sister of George Duke of Marlborough.

A Theory of Heredity

The latter half of the eighteenth century in England was a time of rapid economic growth in both agriculture and industry. Material wealth and general living standards improved because of political stability in the realm that encouraged the development of transportation systems of roads and canals at home, and oceanic shipping throughout the entire world. The intellectual climate was also fostered by society's "order, reasonableness and moderation" (Owen, 1974; Langford, 1992). The organized study of medicine, of the "natural laws of the body," was widely believed to have improved the general health of society (Lawrence, C., 1994a). Within the medical profession itself the trend was to favor reason over mere superstition, free-inquiry over dogmatism, and professional and personal experience over mere book learning. In 1793, Thomas Beddoes (b 1760), a prominent physician, wrote to his friend Erasmus Darwin his own opinion of these changes within the medical community, saying, "Many circumstances indeed seem to indicate that a great revolution in this part is at hand...You will agree with me in entertaining hope not only of a beneficial change in the practice of medicine, but in the constitution of the human race itself" (Porter, 1995d).

Erasmus Darwin (b 1731) was the grandfather of Charles Darwin and Francis Galton, both of whom would make significant contributions to knowledge of human heredity in the next century. Erasmus Darwin's father was a barrister who had a long-standing interest in nature and was elected Fellow of the Royal Society. He was a member of the Spalding Gentlemen's Society and enjoyed discussing literature and science with luminaries such as Alexander Pope and Isaac Newton.

The younger Darwin was sent to St. John's Cambridge in preparation for the study of medicine. He also attended lectures by John Hunter in London, and then enrolled at the University of Edinburgh in 1753. After two winter-terms there, he returned to Cambridge and received the M.B. degree in 1755. (It is unknown whether he ever received the M.D. degree during his lifetime.) He then established a medical practice in Litchfield near Birmingham. Although very busy with his medical practice, he became friends with local men who were interested in science and technology. The manufacturer Matthew Boulton , the chemist Joseph Priestley, the geologists John Michell and John Whitehurst, and inventors Benjamin Franklin and James Watt all became frequent guests at Darwin's house. He published his first scientific paper in the *Philosophical Transactions* in 1757 on the effect of electricity on vapor pressure, and pondered over the ancient bones of extinct creatures sent to him by his geologist colleagues. By the 1770s, he came to believe that a process of biological evolution must exist in which species change and become more complex over long periods of time. His biographer King-Hele argued that "Darwin could see the workings of nature more successfully than any of his contemporaries" (King-Hele, 1999a).

Erasmus Darwin was reluctant to publish his thoughts on evolution and heredity, fearing that such radical ideas would scandalize the general public and adversely affect his medical practice. Darwin's posthumous work, *The Temple of Nature* (1804), contained the most mature development of his conception about biologic change. He proposed that all living things were created by God, and "had been from the beginning in a perpetual state of improvement" (Darwin, 1804a). He thought that "all vegetables and animals now existing were originally derived from the smallest microscopic ones, formed by spontaneous vitality, and that they have, by innumerable reproductions, during innumerable centuries of time, gradually acquired the size, strength and excellence of form and faculties which they now possess..." (Darwin, 1804b). He also recognized that if such changes over time did occur, variation in plant and animal offspring had to exist. Darwin's study of plants had convinced him that asexual reproduction generally produced progeny identical to the parents (Darwin, 1804c); but "from the sexual or amatorial generation of plants new varieties or improvements are frequently obtained" (Darwin, 1800a).

Darwin then proposed a mechanism whereby characters of both parents could be transmitted from one generation to the next by sexual reproduction.

> First...redundant fibrils with formative appertencies[6] are produced by, or detached from various parts of the male animal, and circulating in his blood, are secreted by adapted glands, and constitute the seminal fluid; and that redundant molecules with formative aptitude are produced by, or detached from various parts, of the female, and circulating in the blood, are secreted by adapted glands, and form a reservoir in the ovary; and finally that when these formative fibrils become mixed together in the uterus, that they coalesce or enhance each other, and form different parts of the embryon...(Darwin, 1801a).

It was also clear that both parents contributed to the formation of the offspring.

> If the molecules secreted by the female organ...into the ovary of animals were supposed to consist of only unorganized or inanimate articles, and the fibrils secreted by the male organ only to possess formative appertencies to select and combine with them; the new embryon must probably have always resembled the father...But...the new offspring...must sometimes more resemble the male parent, and sometimes the female one, and sometimes be a combination of them both...(Darwin, 1801b).

The reason that the progeny resembled one parent more than the other depended therefore on the "qualities or activities of the fibrils or molecules at the time of their conjunction" (Darwin, 1800b).

Variation in the offspring resulted from the activity of these "formative fibrils" in the embryo. "These new fibrinous combinations acquire more appertencies, and produce molecules by their vital activity with new aptitudes or propensities; and thus gradually fabricate other secondary parts" (Darwin, 1801c). Darwin thought that variation could also result from characters acquired during the life of a parent that became hereditary and thus might be transmitted to the next generation.

> ...Add to these the various changes produced in the forms of mankind, by their early modes of exertion; or by the diseases occasioned by the habits of life; both of which became hereditary, and that through many generations...Many of these enormities of shape are propagated, and continued as a variety at least if not as a species of animal (Darwin, 1803).

Unlike Harvey, Darwin was willing to speculate about the existence and function of these "fibrils" which he could not see with his own eyes, but could imagine with his intellect.

Darwin thought that alcohol was not good for human health and observed that "hereditary disease" in England often resulted as a consequence of excessive spirit intake. In his opinion, gout, epilepsy, heart failure and insanity were due to over-indulgence. Excessive salt intake affected nervous and lymphatic absorption and could also result in scurvy, scrofula and consumption. Once acquired, he thought "the tendency to these diseases is certainly hereditary..." (Darwin, 1801d). Physicians could hopefully recognize these predispositions and counsel the patient to avoid exposure to such external triggers before symptoms of disease actually ensued (Wilson, 2003).

Darwin noted that organisms that reproduced asexually produced offspring identical with parents. They were not liable to "hereditary disease," if "these had been acquired by the parent from unfriendly climate or bad nourishment or accidental injury" (Darwin, 1804c). But, inbreeding among sexually reproducing lines increased the tendency to hereditary disease. "Where both parents are of families which are afflicted by the same hereditary disease, it is more likely to descend to their posterity" (Darwin, 1804d). It was common practice at that time for the upper classes in England to marry among themselves. Darwin offered a word of advice for young men in choosing a wife in such circumstances. "As many families become gradually extinct from hereditary diseases, as scrofula, consumption, epilepsy, mania, it is often hazardous to marry an heiress, and she is not infrequently the last of a diseased family" (Darwin, 1801e).

Darwin had never seen a cell through a microscope. He knew nothing of DNA or chromosomes as vehicles of inheritance. But his ability to imagine mechanisms for biologic information transfer from one generation to the next was far advanced for his age. Samuel Coleridge observed, "Dr. Darwin possesses, perhaps, a greater range of knowledge than any other man in Europe" (King-Hele, 1999b). Erasmus Darwin's theory of evolution from simple to more complex organisms based upon variety over time and generated by sexual reproduction was later expanded by his grandson Charles to form the basis for the modern theory of natural selection published in 1859. Likewise this early notion of pangenesis, in which physical molecules were secreted from different body parts, accumulated in the sexual organs, and then were transmitted via egg and sperm to form the embryo, became generally accepted fact in biology and medicine after Charles Darwin's "Provisional theory of Pangenesis" was published in 1868.

Erasmus Darwin thought about the natural world in a mechanical sense. He designed bridges, windmills and steering mechanisms for carriages. His model of physical "fibrils with formative appertencies" being carried by the blood from different body parts to the sexual organs, and physically being transmitted via egg and sperm to unite and form an "embryon" is remarkably prescient. Nobody saw a mammalian egg until the 1840s. Chromosomes, the "fibrils" carrying hereditary material, were unknown until the 1880s. And the chemical nature of the DNA in the chromosomes which actually carried the hereditary information was only elucidated after World War II. Darwin proposed that the fibrils in the embryo "coalesce or embraced each other," an analogy for the pairing of homologous chromosomes from male and female parents. Finally, in the developing embryo, the "fibrous combinations" produced new molecules with "new apptitudes" which "fabricate[d] other secondary parts." This model sounds strikingly like the generation of new protein molecules from genetic information coded by the DNA in the developing cells of the formative new organism.

Erasmus Darwin's understanding of the nature of heredity far surpassed that of anyone in his own or even the next century. In his day, he was also recognized as a highly competent medical practitioner. In the 1790s, he had treated the cousin of Lady Charlotte Finch, governess to the Royal household. King George III suffered from repeated bouts of a curious illness and had received little help from the London physicians. He requested help from the Midlands. "Why does not Dr. Darwin come to London? He shall be my physician if he comes..." (King-Hele, 1999a). But Darwin and his family did not like life in the metropolis and declined the Royal invitation (Browne, 1995). The King's recurrent illness seriously impaired his ability to govern the realm and more than once produced a constitutional crisis. The malady was known to run in the family. Would Dr. Darwin have managed his illness better than the learned London doctors? (Rushton, 2008).

Part II
Early Nineteenth Century Medicine and Heredity

Five

Science, Medicine and Society in England 1800-1860

With the defeat of Napoleon in 1815, Britain was once again able to trade more freely throughout Europe and the rest of the world. The British Empire possessed the largest military and merchant navy of the day, was the major commercial banker for the world, and produced more agricultural and manufactured goods than any other country. As the largest city in the world, London was the hub of the burgeoning English economy. Britain had emerged from the war pre-eminent because its economy had rapidly adapted to changes in transportation, technology and government regulation applied to production of goods and services. The country was becoming wealthier, urbanized and industrialized (Langford, 1969a).

The British government had a more liberal approach to regulating the economy compared to continental rulers. Britain had fewer tolls, guild restrictions and other legal boundaries that inhibited local and international trade. The Crown collected "reasonable" taxes and then allowed merchants to go about their business (Owen, 1974a). During the reign of George III, merchandise and agricultural output grew to such an extent that local needs were exceeded, permitting exports to the mass markets in Europe and the rest of the world (Owen, 1974b).

Industrial growth in Britain primarily involved expansion of three products—coal, iron and cotton. Coal production rose five-fold from 1782 to 1830, pig iron rose eight-fold, and cotton rose more than twenty-fold in the same period. The application of technology to develop mechanical spinning and looming machines permitted the evolution of the factory, the first phase of the Industrial Revolution (Beales, 1969a). The second phase of the revolution occurred during 1830-1850 with changes in the methods available for transporting goods and people from coach to barge to railroad. Britain was then able to produce and transport two-thirds of the world's cotton goods and one-half of its iron and steel (Beales, 1969b, c). The country thrived because, "Trade was the engine of growth." Britain was seen as "the workshop of the world," as well as its transporter and banker (Beales, 1969d).

The Crown also permitted significant religious freedom as well. Tolerance and moderation were prominent themes of the day (Langford, 1992b). Protestant dissenters had become politically successful as they supported the King rather than the Catholic Stuarts. Acts of Parliament gradually relaxed religious tests for trade certificates. Catholic citizens and other dissenters worshipped and prospered quietly, preferring material success to controversy in the realm of public religion (Owen, 1974c).

The relative political and religious freedom of the day allowed the lower classes to take on the trappings of the upper classes when they acquired the monetary means to do so. The rapid economic expansion of the Industrial Revolution provided the means for the English middle class to evolve after 1800 (Langford, 1992c). The working middle class became more comfortable and contented. Leisure time was spent on home life and hobbies rather than political ferment. The Revolution of 1848 strained continental societies, but simply did not occur in Britain (Matthew, 2000a).

By 1850, the majority of British people worked in towns rather than in isolated rural areas. Prince Albert sponsored the 1851 Exhibition at the Crystal Palace in London to show the entire world the wonders of modern English society. The 100,000 items on display fostered an increased national consciousness that science and technology were important factors in the economic and political success enjoyed by the country. Expansion of science, therefore, would logically improve the life of the people. Profits from the exhibition were, in fact, used to provide scholarships to endow students to further their education in the sciences (Matthew, 2000b; Tansey, 1994).

Enthusiasm for science swept through the country. Some degree of scientific knowledge seemed to be important for all those who wished to participate in the booming English economy. Attention to developments in science became a "fashionable posture which was socially acceptable" among the aristocracy. Public lectures and inexpensive mass publications allowed men of all classes to learn about developments in various aspects of science. During the first decades of the nineteenth century, English engineers, farmers and businessman applied new scientific ideas to the evolving technological society. The country was transformed from a traditional agricultural and class-defined society to one in which science and technology blossomed, and industrial opportunities abounded. Foreign observers were amazed at the expansion of manufacturing and transportation, and at the accumulation of personal wealth that improved the standard of living enjoyed by many (Foole, 1954; Youngson, 1979).

A general faith in science developed, assuming that the application of science would not only enhance progress in society but also virtually guarantee it. Science was not to be the theoretical pursuit of the wealthy or the privileged few. Rather, it was to be the means to further knowledge and hence to improve English society at large. The diffusion of scientific knowledge was viewed by many in almost a religious sense, in that it would help people to control "the passions," the irrational parts of life (Youngson, 1979; Foole, 1954).

The political diarist, Charles Greville (b 1794), reflected the opinion of many when he noted, "It has been a great privilege to have lived in the time which saw the production of steam, of electricity and now of ether—that is, of the development and application of them to human purposes, to the multiplication of enjoyments and the mitigation of pain" (Foole, 1954). The chemist, Humphrey Davy (b 1778), believed that applied science would assure the continued progress of civilization. He thought the "scientific glory of a country may be considered, in some measure, as an indication of its innate strength" (Foole, 1954). The physician and scientist, Robert Hunt (b 1807), agreed that the application of science would "advance the element of human happiness" throughout society (Foole, 1954). And, the astronomer, John Herschel (b 1792), believed that science would improve the lot of all citizens in the land, not just the wealthy. He thought science would allow improved utilization of natural resources, increase knowledge in general, and even improve art (Foole, 1954).

Despite this wide spread belief that progress in science would benefit all aspects of life in English society, public health at this time continued to present major problems. The endemic diseases of urban life—smallpox, typhoid, typhus, malaria and cholera—killed thousands of all classes each year. In 1834, Edwin Chadwick (b 1800) was appointed Secretary of the Poor Law Commission and employed physicians to survey the health and living conditions in cities throughout the United Kingdom. His 1842 report titled *General Report on the Sanitary Conditions of the Labouring Classes* concluded that such epidemic diseases resulted from contagion—the filth of crowded urban living conditions. The solution to the problem would require the application of modern technology to provide clean drinking water and effective sewers for waste, the removal of refuse from public thoroughfares, and the reduction of industrial waste as well. The 1858 Public Health Act created a General Board of Health in the Privy Council that could function as an adviser to the government for "comprehensive and scientific legislation" designed to improve public health (Fee and Porter, 1992).

Science and Institutions

The new social class of educated, upwardly mobile men in British society was quite distinct from the traditional gentleman-class comprised of Oxford and Cambridge graduates. The democratization of society at large was also reflected by change and conflict within the scientific and medical institutions that had existed little changed for centuries in London society. Trained scientists, for example, were recommended as members of the Board of Directors for the British Museum, rather than the nobles or churchman who traditionally had operated that organization (Desmond, 1989). Learned societies were formed throughout the land, such as the Lunar Society of Birmingham, in which men of science, medicine and industry could meet to discuss and collaborate on the application of new scientific developments to better human life. Class lines were crossed, allowing for individual achievement (or failure) by action rather than by birth (Langford, 1992d).

After decades of intellectual slumber, the Royal Society was revitalized to some extent under the presidency of Joseph Banks (b 1743). He assumed the post in 1778 and fostered collaboration between scientists and engineers on applying theory to solve the practical problems of the day (Langford, 1992d). But, Banks kept a tight rein on the chair, and only he decided what problems would be discussed and who would be invited to join the elite membership of the society. The Fellows at this time were mostly upper class men interested in science, mostly amateurs to one degree or another, who rarely produced any new science. Of the 300 members at that time, 79 were physicians, and only 24 had published at least one scientific paper in the *Transactions*. There were 21 surgeon members, and a mere 10 had published. The great majority of members, however, published nothing (Williams, 1961). Membership in the Royal Society nevertheless did enhance the social and professional status of medical men. One critic noted that the initials "F.R.S." after the doctor's name actually meant "Fees Raised Since." Members became widely known throughout the broader community, as one commentator called the Royal Society a "medical advertising office" (MacLeod, 1983a).

By 1820, the status of the Royal Society had become even worse. Augustus Granville (b 1783) was a physician with a large London practice who surveyed the 651 Fellows at the time. He was dismayed to find that only about 20 percent were active scientists. The 58 physician and surgeon members also contributed little to the role of the Society to advance science in England (MacLeod, 1983b). When Banks died in 1820, the Ruling Board offered the presidential chair to Prince Augustus Duke of Sussex (b 1773) who had obvious social connections but knew little about science. He also suffered from porphyria and often exhibited odd behaviors. His own royal brothers often wondered whether his intellect "might be deranged" (Rohl, Warren and Hunt, 1999).

The appointment of such an unsuitable candidate to lead the pre-eminent scientific society of the land dismayed those members who feared for the continuation of scientific advancement in England. The mathematician, Charles Babbage (b 1792), had been elected F.R.S. as a very young man in 1816. He attended other scientific meetings in Italy and Germany over the next decade and was impressed with the respect paid to scientific societies in those countries. Their work was often supported by grants from the respective governments. In England, science was primarily an amateur profession. Babbage feared that continental science would soon outpace English work because it was publicly supported. The ranks of professional scientists might continue to grow somewhat in England, but unless their economic base expanded, their impact on society would be minimal (Williams, 1961).

In 1830, Babbage published his ideas in *Reflections on the Decline of Science in England and Some of its Causes.* He argued that there was little teaching of science at the great English universities. The Royal Society had become a social organization and was moribund (Williams, 1961; Orange, 1972a). The Scottish scientist, David Brewster (b 1781), had found that on the English campuses, "There is not one man in all eight universities of Great Britain who is at present known to be employed in any train of original research." Brewster thought, "It is a disgrace to men of science and to the Royal Society, the natural guardian of the new science, that they have not combined in a vigorous attempt to raise public feeling on the subject" [of science] (Williams, 1961; Orange, 1972a).

Pleas from within the organization to limit the membership of non-professional scientists in the Royal Society were not accepted by the ruling council (Williams, 1961). Brewster then wrote to Babbage in February 1831, "The Royal Society seems to be gone—so is that of Edinburgh, and the Royal Irish Academy has been long ago at an end. This is therefore the time for a general effort. I hope you will not be backward in giving your aid to such an occasion" (Orange, 1972b). That occasion was to be the founding meeting at York later the same year of the British Association for the Advancement of Science (B.A.A.S.). The 325 men who attended that first session represented a broad range of scientific interests. They agreed that the new association would "give a stronger impulse and more systematic direction to scientific inquiry, to obtain a greater degree of rational attention to the object of science, and of a removal of those [factors] which impede its progress, and to promote the intercourse of the cultivators of science with one another, and with foreign philosophers" (Orange, 1972c).

The B.A.A.S. did succeed in its purpose, extending an influence even to its parent organization, the Royal Society. One of the early leaders of the new society was Spencer Compton, Second Marquis of Northampton, a widely respected mineralogist and archeologist. When he later succeeded to the Presidency of the Royal Society in 1838, Compton was able to begin a program of bridging the gap between the conservative and progressive members of the organization. He observed to Granville a few years later, "You see, dear Doctor, that we are accepting little by little your suggestions; all the rest will come by and by" (MacLeod, 1983c).

By 1850, the Royal Society had become more representative of the English community at large. It was a group that combined the traditional—"the dignity of monarchy"—and the modern—"the representative power of a broader republic" (MacLeod, 1983d). The President governed through a cabinet rather than as an autocrat.

The Times of London observed in 1848, "The Royal Society, like all other institutions, must take account of the fact that democratic principles now govern the world in all civilized communities. The chief scientific society must in all matters itself be scientific" (MacLeod, 1983e). In this transformation, the Society was strengthened and became more able to effect the translation of basic science into useful industry for the state (MacLeod, 1983f).

The medical community of the day was also undergoing a process of democratization and professionalization as well. Changes in the Royal Colleges and Parliamentary Acts combined to create a "respectable professional image" of the medical practitioner, recognizing his status by ability rather than strictly by birth (MacLeod, 1983g; Waddington, 1984a). Physicians also eagerly joined the local literary, philosophical and scientific societies which developed in towns throughout the land, because belonging helped legitimize their social and intellectual positions in the community (Durey, 1983). If science was really advancing, the medical practitioners wanted to be identified as part of that general movement in society.

Nonetheless, family ties still counted. The middle-class medical practitioner did not belong to "society." A professional of any type was identified with a certain class by right of birth or family connection. Middle-class professionals—the vast majority of practicing physicians—knew their place in society and were viewed in general as examples of "sobriety, thrift, hard work, piety and respectability" (Hibbert, 1987a). Concern for one's social standing was "an almost universal preoccupation in middle-class society" (Hibbert, 1987b). The status of physicians was, in fact, enhanced by government actions such as the Medical Act of 1858 that required practitioners to pass prescribed examinations before being licensed to serve in the community (Hibbert, 1987c).

By the early nineteenth-century, three distinct branches of medicine had evolved in Britain. The three chartered Colleges—the Royal College of Physicians, the Royal Colleges of Surgeons and the Worshipful Society of Apothecaries—each granted licenses to practice medicine. The R.C.P. was the most prestigious, and almost all of its members were graduates of Oxford or Cambridge. These physicians were expected first to be educated gentleman. They may have encountered little in the way of medical training at the universities, but were fluent in Latin and Greek. These Fellows comprised about 3 percent of all practitioners in the United Kingdom at the time (Waddington, 1984b).

Surgeons were the practical medical men who were trained by apprenticeship and a few lectures on medical topics. They drained the abscesses and set the fractures. And apothecaries were shopkeepers who prepared medications on orders from physicians or surgeons. However, the reality of medical practice in most parts of the country blurred the distinction between the three types of practitioners. Physicians were supposed to diagnose internal conditions and then prescribe medications to be prepared by apothecaries. Except in upper class London society, the physicians often practiced minor surgery and may have dispensed some medications directly to their patients if an apothecary was not nearby. Likewise, the surgeons not only drained the abscesses and set fractures, but also diagnosed and prescribed for minor medical conditions as well. Sir Anthony Carlisle (b 1768) was a practicing surgeon and member of the Council at the Royal College of Surgeons from 1815 until his death. He noted in 1834, "the distinction between what ought to belong to a physician and what belongs to the surgeon are quite indefinable." In that same year it was estimated that only 200 of the 6000 members of the R.C.S. limited their practice strictly to surgery (Waddington, 1984c).

As the middle-class economy evolved in Britain, its members' demands for medical care also grew. Typically, most citizens could not afford the high fees charged by prominent physicians and surgeons. A third class of general medical practitioners then evolved to meet these needs. By the 1830s, at least 90 percent of medical care was being provided by these "general practitioners" who were licensed first as apothecaries and often secondarily as surgeons. The Apothecaries Act of 1815 had defined the educational and practical experiences required to receive a license from that organization to practice medicine. Most Licentiates of the Society of Apothecaries also took a second examination required to become members (but not Fellows) of the Royal College of Surgeons (Loudon, 1984). These men became the "ordinary attendants in everyday life" healing medical illness, delivering babies and performing minor surgery for the majority of the people (Loudon, 1992; Waddington, 1977; Hill, 1985).

By 1850, more than 90 percent of the medical practitioners in United Kingdom were not recognized as Fellows by either the Royal College of Physicians or the Royal College of Surgeons. The existing colleges had little reason to consider any changes in their membership requirements. The status of physicians and surgeons rested on their university education and positions in prominent hospitals, not on any scientific training in medicine. Reform clearly would mean loss of power for these lofty practitioners (Loudon, 1992). Leaders in the Colleges were generally appointed by social rank rather than by familiarity with science. The general practitioners argued that such approaches smothered incentives to "scientific improvements" in medical practice. The old corporations were called "obsolete-effete-moribund." As members of the new emerging middle-class, the general practitioners viewed science and its enhancement to be an "intrinsically desirable commodity" which would enhance the lot of society at large, and, at the same time, confer prestige to the science-interested practitioners as well. In this manner, the general practitioner expected to become more credible in the eyes of the public (Warner, 1991a; Youngson, 1979; Shortt, 1983).

During the same time, many within the medical profession—surgeons, physicians and general practitioners—had come to an agreement on what constituted a recognized member of each profession. A basic scientific education in anatomy, physiology, pharmacology, medicine, surgery and midwifery plus hospital-based clinical training was imperative. The 1858 Medical Act provided the mechanism to review and license these qualified practitioners for public service. Possession of the license to practice assured the public that the medical man was both qualified and "safe" (Poynter, 1966; Lawrence, C., 1994; Poynter, 1961; Walker, 1965; Loudon, 1992).

The claim that "scientific medicine" would benefit society at large had been assumed, but not universally accepted. The medical historian A.J. Youngson noted that medical progress did not occur at the same rapid rate as other sciences and technologies. English medical practice of 1840 did not differ very much from that of 1740 (Youngson, 1979). Most people agreed that professional recognition and enhanced social status in the eyes of the public clearly resulted from scientific education and the licensing of medical practitioners. As medical practice became more "scientific," many assumed that human suffering would be alleviated (Shortt, 1983). Analysis of the results of British scientific medicine may now be examined to determine if that hope was at all justified.

TRADITION AND CHANGE IN BRITISH MEDICINE BEFORE 1860

The scientific physician in Britain in this era was more influenced by knowledge gained by direct clinical observation or experimentation than by dogma promulgated by authoritative physician leaders in the Colleges. The application of rational treatment experiments and arithmetical presentation of the results actually evolved during the late eighteenth-century in England, a generation before it became more widely known in the Parisian medical schools after 1820 (Trohler, 2000a; Weisz, 2001).

Young British physicians, often trained at the Scottish medical schools and traveled to Paris in the early 1800s because the style of clinical education there appealed to their nascent interests in "scientific medicine." Developing clinical experience convinced them that physical signs and symptoms reflected changes in the structure and function of the internal organs, and thus constituted a rational and empirically based understanding of human "disease." One such physician was James Hope (b 1801), who had studied at Edinburgh, Paris and London. He was an early advocate in England of auscultation to understand altered physiology in the human heart. He correlated heart murmurs with changes in the heart valves and vessels that he later observed at post-mortem examination. Hope concluded in 1839, "I am satisfied that the process of thought which passes through the mind at the bedside and in the postmortem theater is from symptom to lesion" (Hope, 1839). In the eyes of the medical practitioners, and eventually the general public, the modern physician thus was able to at least diagnose disease in a more "scientific" fashion (Woodward, 1961).

However, becoming a scientific practitioner did not appeal to all medical men. Those in positions of power within the medical community—at the Colleges or major hospitals—tended to doubt the importance of such clinical-pathological correlations in the work of medicine, which to them meant taking care of the patients' ill symptoms. Such new ideas were viewed as threatening to the status quo because they questioned the abilities of the current leading practitioners to manage specific medical conditions in a competent fashion (Trohler, 2000b). For example, William Sanders (b 1743) had been educated at Edinburgh and then developed a large London practice. He lectured at Guy's Hospital and was physician to the Prince Regent (later George IV) after 1807. He doubted the usefulness of such human experimentation, because each human was unique. He thought that each person would respond "differently when placed under similar situations and exposed to the action of the same occasional causes." As each individual would respond differently, comparison of large numbers of people treated in the same fashion would be fruitless (Lawrence, S.C., 1996). If the leaders of medicine, who wrote books and articles read by general practitioners, did not espouse the scientific and rational aspects of medical practice, then the work-a-day general practitioners would understandably be reluctant to immediately apply new ideas to their own practice of medicine (Shortt, 1983). Science might appeal to them as a good thing in general, but whether it could really change medical practice for the better remained an open question.

Other voices in the British medical community began to argue that this rational empiricism should, in fact, alter clinical practice and would eventually improve the outcome for individual patients. William Black (b 1749) had been educated at Leyden and established an extensive London practice. He presented the results of his study of human disease using "medical arithmetick" to the Medical Society of London and later published the material in a 1789 book titled *Arithmetical and Medical Analysis of Diseases and*

Mortality of the Human Species. He argued that quantitative methods could be applied to large numbers of humans to understand how diseases flourished. He observed:

> Physicians had been too long running astray in speculative or frivolous employments of philosophical drudgery...Medical arithmetick establishes on a solid foundation a multitude of the fundamental principles...of medical architecture; and erects platforms for completing the entire superstructure...In its most extensive application...[it] may be termed what trigonometry, geometry and the telescope are to the arithmetician and astronomer, or the compass and quadrant to the navigator.

Black thought this approach would "prove our superiority" over the dogmatists in medicine throughout the world (Trohler, 2000c).

The development of large hospitals and outpatient dispensaries in England at this time permitted physicians interested in such "medical arithmetick" to try different therapies on large numbers of patients within a reasonable time frame and then to analyze their successes and failures. The treatment of ague [intermittent fever] traditionally involved bleeding, blistering and purging, and sometimes the use of Peruvian bark [quinine]. Several physicians in the late eighteenth-century attempted to apply a more rational approach to treatment, hoping to improve the outcome, which often was rather dismal. James Lind (b 1716) had been apprenticed as a surgeon and eventually obtained the M.D. degree from Edinburgh in 1748. He was appointed naval surgeon at the Haslar Hospital and collected treatment outcomes from ague sufferers who had received tartar, opium, blistering, and then bark. In 1765, he reported only two deaths among 500 patients so treated. Another surgeon of the same era, John Lettsom (b 1774) had received the Leyden M.D. and worked at the general dispensary in Aldersgate Street in London. He used bark alone in his patients with agues and recorded mortality of only one in 38 for the season 1773-1774. John Millar (b 1733) was another Edinburgh graduate who worked at the Westminster General Dispensary in London. He treated ague with Peruvian bark alone and recorded death of only 1 in 110 patients. Millar later collected statistics on ague and its treatment among British soldiers stationed in North America during 1788-1791. The traditional purging, bleeding and blistering typically did not save many of the patients. Peruvian bark, on the other hand, allowed the vast majority of soldiers to recover and then return to duty. Millar argued that the comparison of treated and untreated cases of the same disease could provide a truer assessment of whether any treatment actually helped patients to survive. He noted:

> Detached cases, however numerous and attested, are insufficient to support general conclusions; but, by recording every case in a public and extensive practice, and comparing the success of various methods of cure with the unassisted efforts of nature more useful information may be obtained; and the dignity of the profession may be vindicated from vague declarations and groundless aspersions (Trohler, 2000d).

The use of a control group of untreated patients allowed for the calculation of the effect of any particular treatment. Millar believed, "It will be proper to ascertain the ordinary termination of disease when left to the unassisted efforts of the constitution" (Trohler, 2000e). This rational and empiric approach to medical therapy could then be applied to assess the efficacy of other proposed treatments for disease which were evolving at the same time.

Attempts to prevent the scourge of smallpox flourished in England after the Prince of Wales (later George II) allowed two of his children to be vaccinated in 1720. The technique used was potentially fatal, as patients occasionally became seriously ill from live virus vaccination and developed the disease itself. The country doctor and apothecary Robert Sutton (b 1708) almost lost one of his own sons to smallpox vaccination and then sought a safer means of preventing the disease without harming the patients. He perfected an improved technique after a trial with a small number of patients and rapidly became well known for his accomplishments. The upper classes accepted Sutton's prophylaxis and experienced a significant decline in smallpox mortality after 1750. Wider application of vaccination protected more than 300,000 people by 1776. Statistics from Maidstone in Kent revealed the success of such treatment with a reduction of mortality from 252 persons in the period 1752-1763 to a mere two persons from 1792-1801 (Bynum, 1980).

Diseases of the heart also appeared to respond to more rational treatments. William Withering (b 1741) was another Edinburgh physician who practiced in the Birmingham area and was a member with Erasmus Darwin in the Lunar Society. He was an accomplished botanist and had heard of the use of the plant foxglove to treat "dropsy" from an old countrywoman. He found it useful in treating angina pectoris and heart failure, but did not report his findings to the medical community until he had studied its effects for fifteen years. He eventually collected 163 cases from his own clinical experience and noted:

> It would have been an easy task to have given selective cases, whose successful treatment would have spoken strongly in favour of the medicine, and perhaps been flattering to my own reputation. But Truth and Science would condemn the procedure. I have therefore mentioned every case...proper and improper, successful or otherwise (Trohler, 2000f).

But, widespread application of such developments did not always follow easily in the broader medical community.

Therapeutic change came very slowly because men in official positions failed to perceive that the application of scientific medicine really made much difference in the lives of the patients. The British Navy was aware of the work by James Lind on the prevention of scurvy using a diet rich in fruit by 1750. During three voyages around the world spanning the years 1768 to 1779, Captain James Cook's naval surgeons gave their charges a diet enhanced by sauerkraut, mustard, oranges and lemon juice. When his fleets returned to England, not one seaman had succumbed to the ravages of scurvy. In 1776, Cook presented a public report on his experiences to date with such antiscorbutics in preserving the health of seaman. The Royal Society awarded him the Copley Medal for the outstanding presentation of the year (Davis, 1998; Keynes, 1997). Official recognition of this advance, however, did not come until the end of the century with the influence of Gilbert Blane. Trained at Edinburgh and Glasgow, he entered naval service as physician to Admiral Rodney on his West Indies cruises during the 1780s. Blane had advised the medical staff of an East Indian Company fleet to provide fruit juice daily to the seamen. When the fleet arrived in Madras after a nineteen-week voyage without a single case of scurvy, the Admiralty finally agreed with Blane's contention that the disease could be prevented and the health of the seamen preserved during long voyages. Because of Blane's official position within the Admiralty, the use of fresh fruit and fruit juices on a regular basis within the British Navy was finally mandated in 1795 (Trohler, 2000g).

A more respectful opinion had begun to evolve regarding science and its usefulness within the medical community with the advent of the nineteenth-century. John Bostock (b 1773) was another Edinburgh physician who eventually practiced in London. He was a lecturer at Guy's Hospital and Fellow of the Royal Society. In 1833 he expressed the opinion of the state of science in English medicine as producing a

> ...most beneficial influence in the general state of medical practice. If it has, on some occasions, produced fluctuation of opinion, and in others indecision or inertness, it has tended to sweep away much error, and to purify the science from many of the antiquated doctrines and practices that still maintain their ground (Trohler, 2000h).

The Professor of Medicine at King's College London, Francis Hawkinson (b 1794), who was also physician to King William IV, agreed that the application of arithmetic had benefited medicine and had changed the way people thought, both within the profession and in the general public.

> Statistics had become the key to several sciences...And there is reason to believe that careful cultivation of it, in reference to the natural history of man in health and disease, would materially assist the completion of the philosophy of medicine...Medical statistics affords the most convincing proofs of the efficacy of medicine...If we form a statistical comparison of fever treated by art, with the results of fever consigned to the care of nature, we shall derive an indisputable conclusion in favour of our profession (Trohler, 2000h).

The scientific approach in medicine, then, identified a view of the world deemed desirable for a modern physician. In the eyes of the public, this scientific outlook characterized the physician as a man of learning and improved his social status (Haigh, 1991). Medical men in England at this time did not view science merely as an intellectual pursuit, as an end in itself. While British physicians might be attracted to the clinical sciences as performed in the hospitals of Paris, their professional interests were fundamentally different. The French physicians were more interested in studying the processes of disease rather than attempting to find and apply treatments that actually helped the patients suffering from various diseases. One observer noted, "It is remarkable, that with all the light to be derived from morbid anatomy, the treatment of disease should be so deplorably bad in that country." The French were primarily interested in clinical science, while the English were more interested in applying that science to treating the patient. One English observer wrote, "We are indisputably the best practitioners in the world." British medical education was designed to produce physicians "who wish to become not mere philosophers, but skillful and useful practitioners" (Warner, 1991b). British physicians of the era were confident in their use of treatments that had been systematically tested on large numbers of patients. This form of scientific knowledge was then to be applied to the general good of the populace (Corfield, 1995).

Six

Heredity and Medicine 1800-1860

In 1813 the *Philosophical Transactions* reported a new variety of sheep from America. The unusual animal appeared suddenly among a flock near Boston, Massachusetts in 1791. It had a long body and short legs. Local people thought it looked like an otter, a common mammal on the banks of the Charles River at the time. Some thought that this "caprice of nature" was caused by a pregnant female sheep being frightened by an otter during gestation. Such maternal impressions were frequently cited as causes of many different types of defects present at birth in both animals and humans.

David Humphreys, the Royal Society correspondent from America, also reported that the "singularity of form seems to be confirmed in the blood," because he had observed the character in successive generations after it first appeared. The variant propagated its "deformity and decrepitude until these characteristics had become constitutional and hereditary." The new breed of sheep was called Ancon. If both parents were affected, all offspring were also affected. When one parent was Ancon and the other a normal-appearing sheep, the offspring never had blended characteristics of both parents. Instead the offspring were fully like only one parent, Ancon or normal (Humphreys, 1813).

Botanists from England reported similar findings after breeding different varieties of plants during the same period. The President of the Horticultural Society of London, Thomas Knight, was actively involved in the production of disease resistant stock in fruit trees and vines. His work on the garden pea was notable because he also found no evidence of blending inheritance. When he crossed gray and white seed varieties, the first generation was all white. Crossing these with white, the offspring had both white and gray varieties (Knight, 1823). John Goss reported similar findings to the Horticultural Society in his crosses of pea varieties with blue and white seeds. The first generation had only white seeds. Crossing of these produced a second generation with some pods containing blue peas, some containing white, and others with both white and blue seeds. In subsequent generations, blue seed varieties only produced peas with blue seeds. The white seed varieties produced some offspring with only white, and some with white and blue seeds. No intermediate colors were observed (Goss, 1822). Alexander Seton examined crosses of green and white peas. The first generation produced only green seeds. Crossing these produced offspring with green or white seeds. Seton noted, "They were all completely either of one colour or of the other, none of them being an intermediate tint" (Seton, 1824). These results from both animal and plant breeding suggested segregation of characters in the offspring, rather than a mere blending of characters.

If there were regular patterns for the inheritance of specific traits in plants and animals, perhaps similar laws could be discerned in the human population as well. If such rules existed, they would have enormous implications for medical practice, because it was generally believed, by both the medical profession and the public at large, that heredity played an important role in causing many different human diseases (Waller, 2001).

Anthony Carlisle (b 1768) was a prominent London surgeon. He was also a Fellow of the Royal Society and surgeon to the Prince Regent, who later became King George IV. Carlisle observed the transmission of digital anomalies from one generation to the next in a family and urged his medical colleagues to report such findings.

> Accumulation of facts must always be desirable, that more reasonable deductions may be established concerning the laws which direct this interesting part of creation...Though the causes which govern the production of organic monstrosities or which direct the hereditary continuance of them, may forever remain unknown, it still seems desirable to ascertain the variety of these deviations.

He reasoned that rules for human inheritance must exist. "There is doubtless a general system in the areas of nature, as is abundantly evinced by the regular series of monstrosities exhibited in both animals and vegetables" (Carlisle, 1814).

Observations made by other physicians clearly showed that variations did appear occasionally among humans, and that these could then be transmitted to subsequent generations. William Lawrence (b 1783) was a surgeon at St. Bart's Hospital and another Fellow of the Royal Society. In 1822 he published *Lectures on the Natural History of Man* and noted the same point made by Carlisle. He believed all physicians would agree that there was:

> ...the occasional production of an offspring with different characters from those of the parent, as a native or congenital variety, and the propagation of such varieties by generation. It is impossible in the present state of physiological knowledge to show how this is affected (Zirkle, 1946).

Most offspring generally resembled their parents in many characteristics. John Elliotson was Professor of the Practice of Medicine at the University of London and physician at Guy's and St. Thomas's Hospitals. His observations argued that animals "have a general tendency to produce offspring resembling themselves and progenitors, in form, structure, composition and all qualities...The varieties, and the minutest peculiarities of the individual in both structure and composition are transmitted" (Elliotson, 1840a). While physicians accepted the fact that inheritance of both normal and abnormal traits did occur, they had no ability to predict outcomes of specific marriages (Waller, 2001).

From a medical point of view such varieties were important because they were often not benign, but, in fact, predisposed certain individuals to the ravages of disease. John Robertson in his *Institutes of Health*, published in 1817, expressed the opinion:

> There are particular individuals, whose constitution is, from the commencement of their existence, much more subject to one kind of morbid affection than another, at least to one particular class of disease, whose distinguishing features bear some resemblance to each other (Hurst, 1927).

The Irish physician, J. Osborne, observed that the structural differences handed down in families provided the "strongest predisposition for certain diseases, and thus hereditary diseases will appear to rise from hereditary similarity of structure..." (Osborne, 1835). In a lecture delivered at King's College London during the academic year 1836-1837, T. Watson also argued that an inherited predisposition to certain diseases did exist. The most frequent diseases of this type were scrofula, gout, asthma and mania (Watson, 1844).

One model discussed by physicians at this time proposed that factors in the blood were the hereditary elements. Horatio Prater thought that disease could become hereditary when some deep-seated change occurred in the globules of the blood. These then circulated to all the tissues and deposited diseased material throughout the body. Such diseased globules could then be transmitted to offspring, making them liable to develop such hereditary diseases as cancer, scrofula, epilepsy or insanity. There was no cure for hereditary disease, as the globules were always in the blood. But recurrence, perhaps, could be prevented. If the trait came from the father's side, each infant should be nursed by its mother, as her milk might contain the same globules as the blood. The healthy milk from the mother might counteract the diseased elements from the father. But if the trait was on the mother's side, then the child should be given to a wet nurse. This might prevent further transmission of disease elements in breast milk to the baby, and hopefully ameliorate the maternal hereditary defect (Prater, 1842).

Some individuals in the general educated public were, however, skeptical about such claims relating heredity to disease. The historian, Henry Buckle, noted:

> We often hear of hereditary talents, hereditary vices, and hereditary virtues, but whoever will actually examine the evidence will find that we have no proof of their existence. The way in which they are commonly proved is in the highest degree illogical, the usual course being for writers to collect instances of some mental peculiarity found in a parent and in his child, and then to infer the peculiarity was bequeathed. By this reasoning we might demonstrate any proposition, since in all large fields of inquiry there are sufficient number of empirical coincidences to make a plausible case in favor of whatever view a man chooses to advocate. But this is not the way in which truth is discerned; and we ought to inquire not only how many instances there are of hereditary talents, etc., but how many instances there are of such qualities not being hereditary (Buckle, 1857).

The medical writer George Lewes responded to Buckle's concern by noting that bodily organization was certainly inherited, as parents and children resembled each other in many respects. He argued:

> It must be admitted that many of the cases collected to prove hereditary transmission have been allowed to pass unchallenged by criticism, and many of them are worthless as evidence...there can be no doubt that organisations are inherited...unless parents transmitted to offspring their organisations, their peculiarities and excellencies, there would be no such thing as a breed or a race... (Lewes, 1859a).

He thought that the physical arrangement carried with it "tendencies and aptitudes" for health or sickness. Children were compounded with features from both parents—the male's eye color, the female's chin. The influence of one parent could enhance or mask manifestation of the trait inherited from the other parent, and sometimes one parent could predominate in many body parts. The problem in understanding this process resulted from the fact that no known formula could explain the outcome for specific cases (Lewes, 1859b).

The diseases that doctors often characterized as "hereditary" were also typically chronic and incurable, such as gout or scrofula. Could it be that labeling a disorder as "hereditary" removed all hope that the physician could effect a cure for the patient's ill? George Henning utterly criticized such fatalistic medical care:

> It is a fact, on every account worthy of observation, that gout or mania, scrofula and phthisis, together with epilepsy are the only diseases...which are acknowledged to be

> incurable by the means of medicine, and are the only ones that have acquired the character of being inheritable. A fact that begets some suspicion that the medical world has taken sanctuary under this term hereditary, to shelter themselves from the opprobrium of not having devised remedies for these obstinate maladies. For surely, if it can be rendered plausible, that these infirmities are so intimately blended, by nature, so interwoven, as it were, with our fabric, as to be inextricable from it by any art, we vindicate our profession from censure, although we add nothing to the reputation of it (Waller, 2002a).

If one's constitution, or fabric, was hereditary, then specific predispositions to these "inherited" disease tendencies were transmitted in certain families. Labeling these disorders as "hereditary" was thus a face-saving explanation for the fact that the medical professionals of the day could not alter the underlying defective constitution and really effect cures of such inherited diseases. Therapy was therefore felt to be frustrating and often useless (Waller, 2002b).

Monographs in Human Heredity

Four physicians in this era attempted to provide a more detailed scheme to understand the transmission of normal and abnormal traits from parent to child. Their collective efforts constituted the first monographs in the English language to consider human heredity.

One of these men was Joseph Adams (b 1756) who began his medical career as an apothecary. He attended medical lectures at both St. Bart's and St. George's Hospitals in London, and became friends with John Hunter. He learned the importance of evidence rather than mere opinion in medicine. In 1796, Adams was awarded the M.D. degree from the University of Aberdeen. He subsequently established a flourishing London practice and was admitted to the Royal College of Physicians on order of its President, Lucas Popys, in 1809. Adams later served as President of both the Medical Society of London and the London Philosophical Society (Motulsky, 1959; Emery, 1989).

Adam's work titled *A Treatise on the Supposed Hereditary Properties of Diseases based on Clinical Observations* was issued in 1814 and summarized a lifetime of observations. His purpose was to educate not only the medical community, but also the general public at large, because many citizens had developed great apprehension about contracting marriage, fearing that the transmission of hereditary disorders would cause "misery to posterity" (Adams, J., 1814a). Adams differentiated two broad classes of peculiarity: those of a family nature were confined to the children of one generation, i.e., brothers and sisters; while those of a hereditary nature were passed from one generation to another (Adams, J., 1814b). There also appeared to be two different types of susceptibility to such disease in families. If disease symptoms appeared without any triggering event, a disposition to disease was present. When external causes appeared to induce symptoms of disease, then a predisposition to disease was said to be evident (Adams, J., 1814c).

Diseases present at birth were labeled "congenital;" they were often familial but not hereditary. Hydrocephalus, cataract and deafness were given as examples of dispositions that were familial and congenital (Adams, J., 1814d). Hereditary disease such as gout might be a disposition in some families without any known triggers, while in other families, it was clearly a predisposition and only appeared with a rich diet and sedentary lifestyle (Adams, J., 1814e).

Adam's observations suggested that congenital diseases were rarely hereditary. Deafness and cataract often appeared among siblings of particular families. But when they married, their children were consistently unaffected (Adams, J., 1814f). In contrast, dispositions often were hereditary. Blindness and angina pectoris were observed in many family members, and symptoms often appeared at a certain stage of life. If children in such families passed the typical age of disease and were unaffected, they could expect to remain free of the disease for the rest of their lifetime (Adams, J., 1814g).

As predispositions required external factors to bring on disease symptoms, Adams suggested, "We may hope to avoid it by avoiding such causes." If children in such families with predispositions consistently and carefully eschewed the trigger factors, they could expect to remain healthy. Adams thought in this way nature tended to correct itself of hereditary defects over time (Adams, J., 1814h).

Adams also noted that inbreeding tended to increase the likelihood of certain features. He observed that "many endemic peculiarities found in certain sequestered districts, which heretofore had been imparted to the water...actually resulted from inbreeding" (Adams, J., 1814i). He presented a model in which hereditary disease could become established in an isolated area and then proliferate due to close breeding. He thought that idiocy was an example of such a hereditary disorder.

> May we not impute its general precedence in the secluded spot to the accidental settlement of a family, in which it was hereditary to produce ideots [*sic*], and the frequent intermarriage of their descendants, which is very likely to happen, where poverty and wildness of the country would prevent migration from or colonization among them? (Adams, J., 1814j).

Because of this fact, Adams was concerned about the possibility of such individuals becoming more common in succeeding generations. He suggested a means for dealing with "family peculiarities" that he thought would benefit both individuals and society at large. He suggested the establishment of registers in which such traits would be "accurately traced and faithfully recorded." Such information had to be handled with a "delicacy sensitive to the subject" (Adams, J., 1814k), but could be used to guide prospective marriage partners and remove some of the dread associated with the specter of hereditary diseases.

In 1838, another book was published in London with the wordy, but informative title *Intermarriage; on the Mode in which, and the causes why, Beauty, Health and Intellect, result from certain unions, and Deformity, Disease and Insanity, from Others* (Walker, 1839a). The author was Alexander Walker (b 1779) who attended medical school in Edinburgh, but apparently never received his degree. He also studied anatomy at St. Bart's Hospital in London and then supported himself by teaching medical students and writing books on anatomy and physiology (King, 1970). Walker had compiled a mass of information on heredity from plant and animal breeders, and was convinced that the laws of nature operated in man as well. He dedicated the book to T.A. Knight, President of the Horticultural Society of London.

On the first page, Walker clearly stated his purpose in writing. His aim was to establish a new science, one,

> which, for the first time, points out and explains all the natural laws that, according to each particular choice in intermarriage, determine the precise form and qualities of the progeny—which unfolds the mode in which, and the causes why beauty, health and intellect result from certain unions, and deformity, disease and insanity from others—and which enables us, under all given conditions, and with absolute

> certainty, to predict the degree and kind of these which must result from each intermarriage (Walker, 1839b)

Clearly, children typically resembled their parents. Walker observed, "There never was a child that did not strikingly resemble both its real parents" (Walker, 1839c). Tall parents had tall children. Polydactyly was present in four successive generations of a family he recorded. Idiocy was passed through a five-generation family. The "porcupine" skin condition was evident in at least three generations of the Lambert family (Walker, 1839d). Walker observed, "Like produces like, not in general, but in details" (Walker, 1839e). The variety of diseases that he believed were hereditary in nature is outlined in Table 6.1.

Table 6.1
Walker and Hereditary Disposition to Disease

Scrofula	Consumption
Gout	Insanity
Rheumatism	Bladder stone
Hare lip	Squint
Hernia	Club foot
Cataract	Aneurism

Reference: Walker, 1839f

Walker was convinced he had discerned biological laws that could predict "the organization of parents [and how it] affects that of children as it regulates the organs which each parent respectively bestows—the mode in which like begets like" (Walker, 1839g). In his system, one parent typically contributed the anterior portion of the head, the organs of sense and the internal nutritive systems. The other parent usually contributed the posterior part of the head, the lower part of the face, and the locomotor system (Walker, 1839h).

The mechanism of transmission was not always perfect, however. Occasionally a feature reappeared in a child that was not present in a parent, but had been evident in a more distant ancestor. These "atavisms" were difficult to understand. Walker thought that the ability to explain such differences precisely would require an understanding of "the theory of generation" which might never occur, even in the future (Walker, 1839i). But, the laws he described were accurate enough to predict the likely outcome of specific marriage crossings. Two individuals who were sane themselves could produce insane progeny according to the theory. For example, if in one parent, the "forehead and the observing, imitating and other faculties were very affected" and in the other parent, the "backhead and the exciting faculties, the passions and the will" were equally defective, the offspring might receive the defective forehead from one parent and the defective backhead from the other parent, producing idiocy. Chances of inheriting insanity and sanity would be equal. If one parent had one portion of the head well developed, and the other had neither portion intact, Walker thought the offspring had "one chance of sanity against three of insanity or defect." Conversely if one parent had both portions of the head well developed and the other had only one portion defective, there would be "three chances of sanity against one of defect" (Walker, 1839j). Walker here suggested segregation of such traits with numerical probabilities of disease, given different classes of parentage. The British medical community was made aware of Walker's work by a report that appeared in the *British and Foreign Medical Review* in 1839. The reviewer commended the author's attempt to apply lessons learned from plant and animal breeding to the broader understanding of human heredity ("Intermarriage," 1839).

A third monograph titled *A Pathological and Philosophical Essay on Hereditary Disease* appeared in 1843. The author, Julius Steinau, had emigrated from Germany and wished to present his ideas to the English-speaking world. He restricted the term "hereditary" to the transmission of a character from parent to child over several generations. Many diseases had been labeled "hereditary" which, in fact, were due to noxious influences during pregnancy. Steinau gave an example of a pregnant woman who was frightened by a beggar with a club foot, felt pity for him, and then delivered a child also affected with club foot (Steinau, 1843a). He thought that family diseases—those present in siblings but not in parents—were often due to such "bad regimens" during pregnancy. He believed that family diseases could become hereditary, but rarely so (Steinau, 1843b). On the other hand, his observations suggested that deformities acquired by one parent during life often could be transmitted to offspring (Steinau, 1843c).

Whether disposition to disease or the disease itself was inherited clearly was controversial. Steinau observed that external features such as abnormalities of the eye or fingers were inherited directly, while internal diseases often developed later in life and could be triggered by factors after birth. When such disease did develop, it was often at the corresponding age in the parent and affected children (Steinau, 1843d). The human disorders Steinau thought fit the definition of hereditary diseases are summarized in Table 6.2.

Table 6.2
Steinau and Hereditary Diseases

Early balding	Scrofula
Early graying	Phthisis
Leprosy	Rachitis
Herpes	Epilepsy
Ichthyosis	Hemophilia
Hernia	Dropsy
Cataract	Gout
Blindness	Bladder stone
Night blindness	Apoplexy
Aneurysm	Syphilis
Helminthiasis	

Reference: Steinau, 1843a

Steinau believed that one could learn little from observing a few cases of different hereditary disease. He argued for the use of statistics to form a "perfectly satisfactory answer in studying heredity" (Steinau, 1843e). He also followed Walker in postulating a mathematical model to predict the frequency of hereditary disease in specific marriages. He proposed that if inbreeding was a cause of hereditary disease, "...a fair application of mathematics to physiology" would show its effect "in the ratio of the squares of the number of marriages" (Steinau, 1843f).

James Whitehead (b 1812) wrote the last English monograph on human heredity in this period. *On the Transmission from Parent to Offspring of Some Forms of Disease and of Morbid Taints and Tendencies* was first published in 1851, and a second edition appeared in 1857. Whitehead qualified first as a surgeon and then received the M.D. from the University of St. Andrews in 1850. He developed a large practice at the Manchester Clinical Hospital for Women and Children. Whitehead cited cases of disease present at birth because of maternal impressions during pregnancy. One pregnant woman was apprehensive about eye disease because her sister's child was blind in the left eye. She subsequently had five children, and all had defective development of the left eye. Another woman had delivered three healthy children, but during the sixth month of her last pregnancy, she fainted after seeing a child with double harelip and cleft palate. Three months later, her own child was born with the same defect (Whitehead, 1857a). Whitehead thought that such defects, once evident in the family, could become hereditary and recur in subsequent generations. Characters acquired by parents during the course of their life were also liable to become hereditary. He observed a man who had three healthy children and then injured his leg in an accident. His fourth child was born with a defective and shortened corresponding leg (Whitehead, 1857b).

However, the primary focus of Whitehead's work was diathases, a susceptibility to disease of a particular nature; it was disease in a "latent form" (Whitehead, 1857c). Symptoms of such diseases were rarely seen at birth. The predisposition to disease was inherited, and often required some environmental factor to begin the process toward actual disease later in life (Whitehead, 1857d).

Several diseases mentioned by Whitehead in which heredity played an important causative role are recorded in Table 6.3. The various forms of tuberculosis were of particular importance, in his opinion. He noted, "The transmission of these two forms of disease (scrofula and phthisis) constitute a fact as well-established as any in the history of medicine." He cited cases where scrofulous material was purposely placed in wounds of healthy people, and no new disease developed. Clearly heredity, rather than contagion, was all-important in the large number of familial cases of these diseases. Whitehead was also not very optimistic about treatment for the hereditary diseases. He felt symptoms could be ameliorated by careful diet and a "genial climate" (Whitehead, 1857e), but the best course would be prevention. If disease diathesis was present in the offspring of an affected parent, the tendency to disease should be recognized before symptoms occurred, and all inciting factors then carefully avoided (Whitehead, 1857f).

Table 6.3
Whitehead and Common Hereditary Diseases

Scrofula	Gout
Rachitis	Quinsy
Phthisis	Erysipelas
Cancer	Rheumatism
Mania	Bladder stone
Epilepsy	Cataract
Apoplexy	Deafness
Paralysis	Syphilis
Dental diseases	Cutaneous syphilis
Asthma	Dropsy

Reference: Whitehead, 1857a

The medical arithmetic used by the English physicians in the latter eighteenth century (described in Chapter 5) focused on treatment outcomes. In 1814, Pierre-Simon Laplace published a work in Paris in which he suggested that mathematical regularities in nature actually implied physical causality. French physicians, especially in mental health, then sought to apply such "statistics" to the study of the causes of human disease. As such, practicing physicians appeared to act like "scientists" and enhanced their social status in the eyes of modern citizens (Cartron, 2003). Etienne Esquinol practiced as a moral physician, "medicins des alienistes," among the thousands of mentally ill in the state hospitals around Paris in the 1820s. The French government kept careful records of patient family history that allowed him to collect large amounts of data. Esquinol believed:

> ...the tabular forms of statistics established with daily notes taken down during several years, on a great number of aliens in the same conditions, will give comparative terms with other tabular forms obtained from observations of sick living in opposed climates and subjected to different morals, laws, and treatments.

He was confident that such analyses would point toward the underlying causes of mental illness (Cartron, 2007). The rationale for this approach to causality was a summary of each physician's own clinical experiences. He observed:

> What is experience if not observation of facts, often repeated and stored in memory? But sometimes memory is unreliable. Statistics record and don't forget. Before a physician puts forward a prognosis, he has done a mental calculus of probability and solved a statistical problem. Notice that he has observed the same symptoms, ten, thirty, a hundred times in the same circumstances and from this, he draws his conclusion. If medicine had paid attention to this tool of progress, it would have acquired a great number of positive truths. It would not be taxed with being a conjectural science lacking strong principles (Lopez-Beltran, 2006).

By 1838, Esquinol reported that when the family history of mental illness was known, he had been able to accurately predict the onset of madness in the children born of affected parents years before symptoms of disease actually appeared. Such information had enormous implications for potential preventive treatment of such mental disorders (Cartron, 2007).

After 1800, most French physicians, like their English colleagues, agreed that individuals inherited a fixed constitution, including weaknesses or predispositions, that could develop into actual disease, if triggered by external factors (Cartron, 2003). But exactly how heredity transmitted these predispositions remained a mystery. As early as 1817, Antoine Petit urged physicians to carefully tabulate their experience with the so-called "hereditary" diseases. He hoped that such collective statistics over time could aid in the formulation of theories of human hereditary mechanism. Over the next twenty years, Antoine Portal and Emmanuel Fodere also wrote monographs on human heredity and disease. As in England, a French "hereditarian" wave was evident, emphasizing the importance of heredity as a causative factor in much of human disease, both mental and physical (Lopez-Beltran, 2003a).

The historian Lopez-Beltran has observed how the term "heredite" came to be used as a noun in French medical literature after 1830, rather than its traditional convention as an adjective (Lopez-Beltran, 2003b). In 1834, D.A. Lereboullet noted in his *De l'Heredite dans le Maladies* that heredity had been accepted as the "transmission of particular dispositions that tend to reproduce in children the same character their parents had at the same age..." (Lopez-Beltran, 2003c). The work of Prosper Lucas summarized the opinion of French physicians in the 1840s that heredity encompassed both conservation of body type and change of individual peculiarities (Lopez-Beltran, 2004). The application of statistics to human disease then convinced many physicians that heredity was an important cause of specific human ills. Lucas's 1847 *Traite de l'Heredite Naturalle* became well known in both France and England (Lucas, 1847a). The work reflected the collective opinion in the medical world in both countries that hereditary diseases, both mental and physical, did exist, but that the intricacies of hereditary transmission of such characters, both normal and pathological, remained largely unknown (Lopez-Beltran, 2006).

SPECIFIC "HEREDITARY" DISEASES

The proliferation of medical journals in the United Kingdom after 1800 fostered rapid and widespread communication of clinical observations throughout the profession. Physicians increasingly shared reports of families affected with characteristic patterns of disease. The fact that several members of these families shared the same abnormalities suggested that heredity was an important underlying cause of such traits. As the monographs on human heredity also became more widely known, physicians began to more frequently consider the possibility that many human ills were hereditary and could be transmitted from one generation to the next.

EYE DISEASES

Physicians in the early nineteenth century noted numerous examples of eye disease that appeared to run in families. J. Saunders had studied surgery at Guy's and St. Thomas's Hospitals in London. In 1805, he established the London Dispensary for Curing

Diseases of the Eye and Ear. He soon discovered several families with cataract. There were different types of cataract, and the specific appearance of each was consistent among members of affected families. In one report, all parents appeared to be healthy, but in four different families, several children developed cataracts at a young age. There were respectively: two brothers, two twin brothers, two sisters and one brother, and one sister and three brothers affected (Saunders, 1811). Four other families noted by William Adams in the following year had a different pattern of illness: both parents and offspring were affected. In one of these families, father and son had cataracts; in another, the father and two children were affected; and in a third family, the paternal grandfather, the father and five of seven children were affected. But, in an additional family, normal parents produced two affected sisters and one affected brother (Adams, W., 1812). There were different types of cataracts in the different families, and clearly different patterns of inheritance were involved.

Adams achieved prominence in his profession and was appointed oculist to the Prince Regent (later George IV). Subsequent studies again showed that the same type of cataract recurred in the same family. In some examples, the parents had normal eyes while children were affected: in one family three of four siblings; in another three of five sisters; and in a third two brothers and one sister. Other families had several successive generations that were affected (Adams, W., 1817).

Clinical observations suggested that not all cataracts were hereditary; they could develop after eye injuries. However, in many other cases, physicians commonly noted that this lens abnormality "runs through families and appears to be hereditary" (Green, 1824; Lawrence, 1827). Dyer reported a family with an affected grandfather, three of his sons, and two affected grandsons (Dyer, 1846). Streatfield from the Royal London Ophthalmic Hospital noted a family with an affected mother, three of her brothers and one son. His observations also revealed that all the affected individuals had grey irises and light brown hair, suggesting that the three traits might have a common hereditary mechanism (Streatfield, 1857a).

A later royal oculist to Queen Victoria, W.W. Cooper, who practiced at the North London Eye Hospital, recorded a family with a more severe eye anomaly. A son and two younger sisters had microphthalmia [miniature eyes] and aniridia [absent iris]. A fourth child and both parents were, however, quite healthy. The mother explained her understanding of the defect as a fright she had endured while pregnant with the first child. She had met a man with very small and peculiar eyes and then carried that face in her mind daily until her confinement. Cooper thought it was an open question as to the actual cause of the defect in the three subsequent children (Cooper, 1857). Another family with the unusual structural eye disease anophthalmia [the absence of the eyeball] was noted by James Briggs. He studied successive family members as children were born from 1813 to 1826. Once again, the parents were healthy, but two girls and two boys of seven total children were affected with the anomaly (Sorsby, 1934).

The color of the iris also appeared to have a hereditary basis. A peculiar spotted iris—brown irregular pigment spots on a yellow iris background like a tortoiseshell cat eye—was particularly common in County Wexford. At least three generations were affected, involving both males and females. One affected woman reportedly had nineteen affected children. A titled person in the area had the same peculiarity, having had an ancestor who married a daughter from the same family (Osborne, 1835).

Streatfield reported several generations of families with segmental defects in the iris [coloboma irides]. Two distinct patterns of inheritance were observed. There could be direct transmission of the character from grandparent to parent to child. Conversely, within the same family the character could skip a generation. An affected grandparent could have an unaffected child, who then married and had both affected and unaffected offspring (Streatfield, 1857b).

Squint or esotropia [turning in of the eye due to muscle imbalance] was also observed to run in families. Henry Holland, physician to Queen Victoria, noted one family in which both parents were affected, and all five of their children had the same eye disease (Holland, 1857). Streatfield noted a different pattern of inheritance for esotropia in another family in which two unaffected sisters had two of five, and six of nine affected children, respectively. Prior generations had had no evidence of eye disease (Streatfield, 1857c). Holland also recorded a family with unusually long eyelids. Direct inheritance was evident as the father and seven of ten children were affected (Holland, 1857).

The functional characteristics of the eye also appeared to be impacted by heredity. Blindness [amaurosis] was known to run in families, but not directly from parent to child in many cases. Holland reported one family with normal parents, though the mother's ancestors had been blind. Indirect heredity was evident as the couple produced four of five blind children (Holland, 1857).

The phenomenon of color blindness in John Dalton and his brother has been noted in the previous chapter. More afflicted families were reported after 1800 as well. Nicholl investigated the color vision in four generations of a family. One young boy could only perceive red, yellow and purple colors. He had a brother and four sisters with normal color sense, as did his parents. But, the maternal grandfather and maternal great-uncle demonstrated the same inability to perceive those specific colors (Nicholl, 1816). A second family, again, had unaffected parents. One unaffected son had a daughter with defective color vision, followed by seven normal-seeing children. Two affected brothers were born next. One had five children, three sons and two daughters, all having normal color vision (Nicholl, 1818). The phrenologist, George Combe, became interested in color perception when he met a man who told him an unusual story. The man had wanted to purchase a beautiful green gown for his wife. One day, while walking in town, he observed a lady on the street with what he perceived as just the shade of green dress he wanted for his own wife. But she was astonished at his choice of colors and assured him that, in fact, the gown was a drab brown and not the magnificent green he had wanted (Usher, 1911). The man in question had two children, a son and a daughter, both with normal color vision. The daughter subsequently produced three sons with color blindness and four unaffected daughters. Combe concluded that this defect affected only the power to perceive color, as the vision itself was quite acute. As a phrenologist, he believed that the lack of color sense was due to a defect in that portion of the brain that recognized colors (Combe, 1825).

Subsequent reports documented the overwhelming male predominance in this disorder of color vision. Typically, an affected male had an unaffected daughter, who married and produced affected sons herself. Browne observed two unaffected sisters borne of an affected father, who both then produced affected males (Bronner, 1856). However, color blind females did occasionally appear. Wilson noted that a countess inherited the trait from her father and produced both affected and unaffected sons. More characteristically, several males in one generation were affected. In one example, six brothers were all color blind. Wilson surveyed the general English population for color blindness and found 5.6% of males affected. Female cases were much rarer. The familial nature of the disorder clearly demonstrated that it was hereditary (Wilson, 1855). The unusual pattern of affected males and unaffected carrier females was characteristic of what later came to be called sex-limited heredity.

Skin Diseases

Unusual features of the skin and hair characteristic of certain families were also recorded in the medical literature of this era. Relatives of the well-known Lambert family with ichthyosis hystrix resurfaced in London, both in carnivals and in more sober medical meetings. John Elliotson reported that he had seen the grandson of Edward Lambert, the porcupine man, at a carnival in Bond Street. The public was charged "a shilling apiece" (Elliotson, 1831). Two years later, family members were presented at the Westminster Medical Society. Four generations of males were said to be affected, while all the females had normal skin. The direct male-to-male transmission of this form of ichthyosis appeared to be quite unique (Pettigrew, 1833). Another family with a similar skin condition, but a different pattern of heredity was observed by P.J. Martin. He thought such "heredity defects in man, sometimes, good or bad, in animals and vegetables, arise accidentally, and are gradually worn out and lost again, or suddenly lost, like a particular kind of apple, or the supernumerary claw of a fowl's foot, by the extermination of the race." Since these defects were not widely distributed throughout the population, such mechanisms of extinction then tended to maintain the "common course of nature" (Martin, 1818). These "mutations" rarely survived long within a large population.

One particularly striking accident of nature was noted by Hamilton in 1827 as the "hairy men of Ava." The Governor General of India had visited Ava, a province in Burma, the previous year and had been presented a young man who lived in the Royal court. Since childhood, this individual had been covered from head to toe with long shaggy hair. Only his hands were free of hair. He also lacked many teeth. His parents had had normal skin, hair and teeth. The young man subsequently married a woman chosen by the King, and produced several children. One daughter inherited the condition from her father (Hamilton, 1827). A subsequent visit to the Court revealed a third affected generation, as the affected daughter had married and produced two affected sons. One of the sons later had an affected daughter. A revolution in 1885 drove the family away from the Royal Palace. An Italian officer, Captain Paperno, who served as military adviser to the Court, rescued the family and subsequently took them on tour in London and Paris. They may also have visited the United States. Four generations, involving both males and females, were affected with this disorder labeled hypertrichosis lanuginosa (Bondeson, 1996). Direct heredity was evident.

Physicians in this generation agreed with William Harvey that much could be learned from such alterations of the normal human condition. "...Practical medicine... may hope to receive additions from the study of these exceptional cases of original structure and function," wrote John Thurnan, surgeon at Westminster Hospital. He observed another family in which individuals had absent teeth, hair and sweat glands—a form of ectodermal dysplasia. Two maternal male cousins showed the same clinical picture of almost complete absence of body hair, absence of tears and perspiration, soft delicate skin, and only four teeth. Microscopic examination of the skin confirmed deficient fat and sweat glands (Thurnan, 1831).

The lack of skin pigment [albinism] also appeared to run in families, particularly of Negro origin. Indirect heredity was the mode in most cases. Thomson noted one family with normally pigmented parents who produced four males and one female of similar coloration, while three male and one female children were albino (Thomson, 1858). Another family with a similar pattern of inheritance was notable because the parents were cousins (Hamilton, 1827).

Abnormal growths on the skin were also noted to run in families. A "fungoid tumour" was observed in a grandfather, his two brothers, a son and several grand children. The tumor had a bluish character and appeared scattered throughout the skin fields. Because three generations were affected, Norris expressed the opinion, "This disease is hereditary" (Norris, 1820). Direct transmission of this type of melanoma was evident in the given example.

Bone and Muscle Diseases

Many defects of bones and joints also appeared to run in families. Carlisle was one of the first physicians to present results of a family with polydactyly [extra fingers and toes], using a pedigree table to show relationships among the individuals, as he said, according to "the methods of the genealogists." The family demonstrated transmission of extra digits from great grandmother to all eleven of her children. One affected daughter then had three affected sons and one affected daughter. One of the affected sons subsequently had two affected daughters, while another affected son produced one affected and one unaffected twin (Carlisle, 1814). Another three-generation family demonstrated polydactyly in a grandfather, his son and daughter, and nine of ten children born of the son ("A many toed and fingered family," 1834). Direct heredity was the rule in such families.

In 1840, the New Zealand Company purchased the Chatham Islands in the South Pacific. Natives there were noted to have "an excess of toes, so as to have six or more on each foot." Dieffenbach thought this was a trait "common among other savage nations" (Dieffenbach, 1841). However, Watson recorded an English family with four generations of individuals having six toes and six fingers. He did note instances where the trait sometimes skipped a generation. "Peculiarities not possessed by a parent may nonetheless be transmitted by him." Watson urged other physicians to study similar cases because he believed that an understanding of heredity and disease was important for everyone. "I need surely say a word respecting the importance to medical man, and indeed to all man, of a knowledge of the hereditary tendencies." He thought that society should regulate marriage choices in cases where such "hereditary tendencies" were present in the families (Watson, 1848a).

Abnormal structures of the digits were also present in successive generations of other families. Elliotson recorded two examples of contractures involving specific digits. Direct inheritance was usually evident. One family had a father and four sons with contractures of the fifth digits. In another family, a mother and two sons were affected with contractures involving the second digit (Elliotson, 1840b). Syndactyly [webbing of digits] was noted in five successive generations of one family. In two more families, the anomaly skipped a generation, and then reappeared in two subsequent generations (Thomson, 1858). In all cases, both males and females were affected, and direct inheritance was the rule.

Members of the families with digital anomalies sometimes suggested specific causes for such unusual malformations. In one case, brachydactyly [shortened digits] suddenly appeared in a daughter born of normal parents. The same anomaly was subsequently evident in the next six generations of her offspring. Family members explained that the original case had occurred because of the action of the mother during pregnancy. The wife had stolen an apple from her husband's orchard. The husband was angered and cursed the thief, whomever he or she might be, wishing that the perpetrator's fingers be chopped off. His own daughter was then born with defective, shortened digits (MacKinder, 1857).

Such maternal impressions were widely assumed to cause many defects present at birth. An even more striking example was noted in a family from Oxbridge. The local surgeon observed a woman and her two daughters with very unusual hands. The thumbs were normal, the ring finger had two phalanges, while the other fingers had only one phalanx each. For nine successive generations, almost all the females in the family reportedly had been born with the same condition. Tradition in the family gave a familiar explanation for the origin of the defect many years ago. A parson had an orchard and eagerly anticipated enjoying the fruit from the trees. He ordered his gardener to forbid anyone from touching the developing fruit. Suddenly one day, all the apples from one particular tree disappeared. The gardener denied any wrongdoing. The parson confronted his pregnant wife who also denied taking the fruit. The husband did not believe her and angrily stated that if she had done the evil deed, he hoped that her baby would be born without fingers. Hence "the fingerless race began ten generations before!" (Kellie, 1808; "Letter," 1808).

Abnormalities of bone formation also were found to run in families. Two sisters had unusually brittle bones. One had suffered 31 fractures in the first 14 years of her life. Both girls also were noted to have blue-grey color of the iris (Arnott, 1833). Excess bony growths [exostoses] also appeared to be hereditary. One family had four affected children (Curling, 1851). James Paget, who became Queen Victoria's physician, reported another family with two normal sisters. One produced an affected son and grandson; the second bore an affected daughter and three affected sons (Paget, 1853a). Another interesting family with exostoses was noted by E. Stanley. A woman had married normal men twice and had an affected son by each husband. In this case, he thought, "The hereditary predisposition, whatever it be, is delivered from the maternal side..." of the family in a direct pattern (Stanley, 1853).

Another abnormality inherited from the maternal side the family, but with a different pattern for heredity was investigated by Edward Meryon. He studied medicine at University College London, and subsequently lectured on anatomy at St. Thomas's Hospital Medical School while also developing an extensive practice in London (Emery and Emery, 1995a). His 1836 book, titled *The Physical and Intellectual Constitution of Man Considered,* revealed his opinion on causality of certain diseases. He did not accept the commonly held opinion that acquired characters often become hereditary. He argued that centuries of foot binding in China, for example, had not altered the size of the feet of babies born in that country (Emery and Emery, 1995a). Hereditary disease did exist in specific families, and sometimes an entire family would possess the same physical "peculiarities" (Meryon, 1836a). Hereditary transmission of such peculiarities could pass from either side of the family, "the offspring [could] assume the characteristics of either one of the parents" (Meryon, 1836b), rather than a mere blending of features.

Meryon presented a family with a rare type of muscle degeneration to the Royal Medical and Chirurgical Society late in 1851. The normal parents produced six healthy daughters, one normal son, and three sons with the same unusual muscle disorder. The affected boys were healthy at birth and walked at the normal age. Tripping and weakness in the leg muscles with enlargement of the calf muscles became evident by the early teen years. The boys subsequently died of respiratory muscle failure. Benjamin Brodie also knew of the family and mentioned that the brother of the mother had died with a similar clinical condition. Meryon performed an autopsy on one of the boys. The brain, spinal cord and peripheral nerves were intact. Fatty degeneration of the skeletal muscles, especially in the lower legs, was evident by microscopic examination. The same clinical picture was also noted in two other unrelated families. In both of these cases, the parents were healthy. One family produced one healthy daughter and three affected sons. The other produced two healthy daughters and three affected sons. In discussions at the medical meeting, Dr. Hawkins mentioned another family in which the mother's brother had been affected, as were her two sons in the next generation (Meryon, 1851, 1852).

Meryon collected more family histories of muscle disorders and summarized his findings in a later book titled *Practical and Pathological Researches in the Various Forms of Paralysis* (Meryon, 1864). One family, in particular, demonstrated the fact that unaffected females appeared to transmit the anomaly. Three sisters had several unaffected daughters, but four of their sons were affected with the degenerative muscle disorder. Microscopic analysis of the muscles again revealed fatty granular degeneration. As in previous cases, nervous structures appear to be intact (Emery and Emery, 1995b). Heredity of the character was clearly of the sex-limited type.

The detailed clinical, microscopic and hereditary analysis of this degenerative muscle disorder has surely documented that Meryon was the definer of this so-called "hypertrophic muscular paralysis." Subsequent medical authors have generally attributed Guillaume Benjamin Duchenne in Paris with the delineation of the syndrome. The malady is now routinely called Duchenne muscular dystrophy, although he did not see a case of this disorder until 1858. He coined the term "paralysie pseudohypertrophique" later in 1868. Meryon's seminal contribution to understanding the nature of this hereditary disease has been almost forgotten (Bach, 2000).

Neurological Diseases

Neurological diseases also were being recognized as having a hereditary component to their causality. Edward Sieveking, a prominent London physician and early advocate of the use of bromides as medications to control epilepsy, surveyed his own patient population and found a positive family history for seizures in approximately 11% of all cases (Sieveking, 1858). Henry Holland observed a family with tremor in three successive generations (Holland, 1857).

Heart and Lung Diseases

The cardiac and pulmonary systems also were involved in diseases that appeared to run in certain families. Angina pectoris caused severe chest pain in a young man who died within one hour. His father had had a similar demise. Post-mortem examinations of both men revealed a single coronary artery and thin myocardium in the ventricle (Latham, 1846). Henry Holland was familiar with another family with a similar history, having angina and cardiac death in three successive generations (Holland, 1857). Other abnormalities of the vascular system included a family in which several successive generations had individuals in which the radial artery twisted aberrantly to the backside of the radius in the forearm (Burns, 1809).

Many medical authors at this time observed that the predisposition to develop asthma was hereditary (Watson, 1848b). Holland reported the disease in three successive generations of one family (Holland, 1857). Direct heredity was evident in such cases.

Systemic Diseases

Scrofula was a common form of tuberculosis in England at this time and involved enlarged lymph nodes in the neck that often formed abscesses. Similar lesions could appear in the bones and joints. Contagion did not appear to be involved in causing this condition. Repeated attempts to produce disease by implanting pus from scrofulous lymph nodes into healthy human tissues failed (Lomax, 1977). The general consensus at the time was that children could be born with "an hereditary disposition to the complaint." External exciting causes were believed to allow development of actual disease in susceptible persons. These external stimuli might involve abnormal diet, climate or other illnesses that increased debility, allowing scrofula to develop. By avoiding such exciting causes, one could potentially prevent symptoms of the disease altogether (Lomax, 1977). The risk of developing disease depended on individual heredity. Children were felt to inherit "the constitution of their parents. If a parent is scrofulous, the child will often show similar symptoms. If two affected persons marry, a great proportion of the children will be born with a scrofulous disposition" ("Surgical Lecture," 1824).

The notion of inherited predisposition to the tuberculous disorders was, however, controversial. James Clark noted in his 1834 *Treatise on Tubercular Phthisis*, "that pulmonary consumption is a hereditary disease—in other words that the tuberculous constitution is transmitted from parent to child, is in fact not controverted" (Waller, 2002a). Alexander Tweedie prepared an article on "Hereditary Predisposition" for the 1847 edition of the *Cyclopedia of Practical Medicine*, edited by John Forbes. He concluded that "the hereditary predisposition to scrofula, consumption, gout and insanity is a part of the medical creed" (Waller, 2002b). On the other hand, Benjamin Phillips reviewed the family histories of 2023 children afflicted with scrofula. His 1846 treatise on *Scrofula: Its Nature, Its Causes, Its Prevalence and the Principles of Treatment* found that when one parent was also affected, the offspring had only 4% greater likelihood of disease than those children born of healthy parents (Waller, 2002d). But scrofula and phthisis were very common diseases in mid-century England. Henry Holland concluded in 1846 "...in individual cases, and in masses of cases, it is very frequently difficult, and sometimes impossible, to determine when the disease is transmitted hereditarily and when it has been acquired" (Waller, 2002e).

A similar hereditary predisposition to developing leprosy was also widely believed to exist. Numerous cases of parent to child transmission were noted by many medical authors. J. Simpson, Professor at Midwifery at the University of Edinburgh, observed, "Few facts in the history of tubercular leprosy seem to be more universally admitted by all writers on the disease, both ancient and modern, than the transmission of the predisposition to it from parent to offspring." The trait could lie dormant for one or two generations and then reappear. Simpson cited families with two brothers who had an uncle also affected. But in another example, direct transmission was evident. A mother, brother and sister in one family were all affected (Simpson, 1842).

Hereditary predisposition also appeared to underlie the uncomfortable, painful swelling of the joints called gout. A man with the "gouty habit" tended to have children who would be "more likely to be attacked with this complaint" than those who never had such heredity. Once again, avoiding exciting causes could decrease the likelihood of actually developing disease symptoms. In one family, a man with gout had three sons. Two were affected, but one escaped due to "extreme care and attention" to his daily habits ("Surgical Lecture," 1824). Charles Scudamore was a surgeon who practiced at Guy's and St. Thomas's Hospitals in London. He completed a study of 522 of his own patients with gout and concluded that heredity was an important factor in causing the disease. In this population, 64% of the patients had other family members affected. In 141 cases the disease was transmitted from the father, in 59 cases the mother transmitted it, and in 24 cases, both parents were affected; either one could then transmit the predisposition to their children (Scudamore, 1823). Alfred Garrod, Professor at University College Hospital, and later physician to Queen Victoria, subsequently discovered the mechanism of gouty pain in the joints. Elevated levels of uric acid in the blood caused crystals to precipitate in the joints and caused intense pain and inflammation. His own patient population also had at least 50% with one or both parents affected. In one family, he found the eldest son in four successive generations affected by the gout (Garrod, 1859), suggesting direct heredity. William Gairdner surveyed the family histories of his gouty patients and noted that the disorder "does not always descend from father to son in uninterrupted succession, but often passes over a generation or two...It rarely however fails to revive its dominion even in a 3rd or 4th generation" (Waller, 2002f).

While cancer frequently appeared in several members of a certain family, whether the disease was actually hereditary was poorly understood. As early as 1806, one author raised the question of whether a cancerous predisposition was inherited by children born of an affected parent. If it were shown to be true, perhaps the outcome could be modified by judicious diet, medicine or education in lifestyle. If, in fact, there were no hereditary predisposition to cancer, such a fact would certainly relieve the minds of many family members in such situations from their "perpetual apprehension" about developing cancer themselves ("Institution for investigating the nature of cancer," 1806). James Paget reviewed his own cancer cases in the 1850s and concluded that in general about one in six had a positive family history for the disease (Paget, 1853b). He thought that typically what was inherited was a predisposition, "a tendency to the production of those conditions which finally manifest themselves as a cancerous growth" (Paget, 1853c). Paget later divided his cases among cancerous and non-cancerous tumors. Of 254 with cancer, 24% had affected relatives; and of 147 with non-cancerous tumors, 18% had affected relatives. Certain types of cancer appeared to have a more pronounced hereditary predisposition, especially breast and epithelial [skin-related] forms (Paget, 1857).

Other Disorders

Cleft lip ["hare lip"] often occurred with cleft palate among several members of certain families. The Irish surgeon, John Houston, observed two affected siblings in a family with normal parents (Houston, 1842). Several years later, Bellingham noted a four-generation family with one great-grandfather having a cleft lip. One unaffected son in this example produced a son with cleft lip, and several unaffected sons had two affected grandchildren—one with cleft lip, and one with cleft lip and cleft palate. Another branch of the family had two grandsons affected with cleft lip alone (Bellingham, 1855).

Bladder stone was particularly common in the Norwich region in England at this time. Alexander Marcet, physician at Guy's Hospital in London, reviewed reports from 506 operations done at the Norfolk and Norwich Hospital from 1772-1812 (Marcet, 1817). Marcet and his colleague, John Yelloly, who actually practiced in Norwich, observed the frequent familial occurrence of the stone. Yelloly mentioned one family in his practice in which the grandfather was operated upon twice, as was the father and two of his sons, all living in the Norwich area. Such an "instance of a calculous tendency in three continuous generations" certainly suggested a hereditary predisposition to bladder stone (Yelloly, 1829). Direct heredity appeared to be the rule in these cases.

Hemophilia, the tendency to easy bruising, spontaneous and severe hemorrhage, and bleeding into joints and other internal structures, commonly affected several children in one generation of certain families. In 1835, J. Osborne, the President of the College of Physicians of Ireland, presented a family with normal parents, and three affected sons and one unaffected daughter. Why males were primarily affected was unclear. Osborne noted, "The descent of peculiar features in families, has never been examined, so as to afford the pathologist proper data for ascertaining the laws of hereditary diseases..." (Osborne, 1835). Earlier reports had emphasized the repeated occurrence of affected males in many generations. Davis reported one family with two affected boys. The mother stated that on her side of the family, no males had reached adulthood, although the females were quite healthy. But, if the females married, their sons "inherited from them this family curse, while their daughters were equally free from it" (Davis, T., 1826). Another family had four affected sons, as well as two healthy sons and four healthy daughters. The brother of the unaffected mother was also a bleeder (Burnes, 1840). The life of hemophiliac boys was quite gruesome at this time. In one family, a brother bit his tongue and bled to death. Another brother died of hemorrhage after losing a tooth, and two others died after lacerations on the scalp. A fifth brother survived, but had had similar episodes of severe hemorrhage after minor accidents (Lane, 1840).

The hereditary nature of hemophilia was illustrated by another large family history compiled by Lane in 1840. Five brothers had died of uncontrollable bleeding. One unaffected sister had two affected sons. Another unaffected sister had two affected and one normal son, and a third unaffected sister bore two affected sons and two healthy daughters (Lane, 1840). Treatment was attempted with occasional success in such cases of massive bleeding. One boy had had episodes of recurrent hemorrhage. At age 11 years, he underwent strabismus surgery and bled for six days. As a last resort, he received a blood transfusion from an unrelated young woman and survived (Lane, 1840). In another family, two unaffected sisters each produced affected males and unaffected females. It was obvious that the sisters had transmitted the bleeding tendency to their sons: "The history of the sisters and the death of the boys together with the improbability of each sister meeting with a husband affected with this rather rare complaint, fix its origin without doubt" (Wilmot, 1841). Sex-limited heredity was evident in such families.

British physicians were well aware of the existence of other bleeder families in the United States and Germany. Such families in these countries exhibited the same pattern of heredity: the females were generally healthy, but passed the trait to their sons. ("Hereditary tendency to hemorrhage," 1826; Cochrane, 1841). All observers agreed: "The most remarkable characteristic of the disease is its hereditary tendency." The law of heredity in such cases was called "very singular" (Pickells, 1852). The rules for heredity in hemophilia were:

1. Only males were subject to disease;
2. The father of a bleeder was always free from the disease;
3. The son of a bleeder was never affected by it;
4. The bleeder normally inherited the "diathesis" from his maternal grandfather (Lane, 1840).

Both the medical community and the lay-public were beginning to recognize the likelihood of transmitting such serious and potentially fatal diseases. James Clark advised careful choice of marriage partners and lifestyle in cases where such hereditary diseases were evident, hoping "the predisposition which is so often entailed on...offspring might be checked, and even extinguished" (Waller, 2002g). In some of these cases, Benjamin Phillips advised abstinence. However, when marriage was contemplated, " a young lady will have her chance of marrying very much lessened if an impression exists that she is scrofulous herself or comes from a scrofulous family" (Waller, 2001). Because many believed such diseases to be hereditary, "...one of the most important points in choosing a wife, is to ascertain that she is exempt from scrofula" (Waller, 2001).

THE ORIGIN OF VARIATIONS

It was widely believed in both medical and lay communities that acquired characters could become hereditary. Although physicians such as Meryon had pointed out the absence of any data in favor of such a proposition, the numerous tales of lesions acquired by injury and then reappearing in offspring, or of maternal impressions during pregnancy, generally convinced most people of the day that such mechanisms did indeed operate. Everard Home trained with John Hunter and practiced surgery at St. George's Hospital. In 1818, he was appointed surgeon to King George III. Ten years later, he reported finding nerves in the human umbilical cord which he believed communicated with uterine nerves via the placenta during pregnancy. Hence, there was a potential communication between the maternal and fetal brains that could transmit impressions from mother to child. For example, in one case a woman at the seventh month of pregnancy developed tertian fever [every third day]. The fetus suffered paroxysms on a "distinct schedule" as well (Home, 1828a).

Many were also of the opinion that "frights" of the mother during pregnancy often resulted in abnormal offspring. In one case, a woman experiencing her tenth pregnancy was robbed by a man with a harelip. Her baby was born with a similar defect. Another woman allowed her dog to place its paws on her abdomen during pregnancy. Her child was subsequently born with marks like paw prints on its skin. A woman was frightened during early pregnancy by a man having only one arm; her child was born lacking one arm. Another woman had a similar fright. Her child in that pregnancy appeared to be normal, but a subsequent child was born with only one arm (Home, 1828b). Yet another child was born with eyes like a ferret after his mother was scared by such an animal during pregnancy. All subsequent children in the family were born similarly affected and then became blind at puberty (Wright, 1830).

The hearing sense was also believed to be sensitive to such frights during pregnancy. One expectant mother encountered a terrified, screaming child. Her baby was then born deaf and screamed when excited. A deaf beggar frightened another woman during three successive pregnancies. She delivered three deaf children. She never saw the beggar again and bore healthy children thereafter. Finally, another woman's house overlooked the playground of a deaf and dumb institution. She listened to the odd noises made by the affected children during her pregnancy and delivered a deaf child. The fact of living in one particular house in a rural county appeared to be the common cause of deafness in three different families. In one instance, a married couple occupied the house and produced a deaf child. A second and third family subsequently resided in the same house and also had deaf children (Buxton, 1859).

There were also concerns that the general health of the public could be affected in a similar manner. While walking down the street in London, one woman in her sixth week of pregnancy saw a boy running around without a shirt. He had been born without arms; her child was subsequently born lacking both arms. The author of this note thought it "both cruel and disgraceful to allow this child to run at large without its being properly clothed, so as to hide its deformity; because in so much as it has been sufficient to affect one pregnant woman, there is no reason why it should not similarly effect hundreds of other women who pass by a busy street" (Davis, R., 1850).

Injuries acquired by the father during his life were also reported to pass to the next generation. For example, one father who was a sailor in the Royal Navy had eight healthy children. He was then wounded in battle, losing his right arm and right eye. When he recovered and returned home, the next child born in the family also lacked the right arm and right eye (Langworthy, 1850).

The importance of heredity as a cause for much human disease was widely recognized by the medical profession by mid-century. The 1851 medical student guide for obtaining the clinical history from patients at Guy's Hospital in London specifically recommended that attention should be paid to both hereditary and acquired tendencies "...as well as predisposing or exciting causes of disease..." (Newman, 1957). But the mechanism of heredity was poorly understood. James Paget observed, "We cannot understand the transmission of a tendency or disposition...independently of all material conditions" (Paget, 1853c). Many were of the opinion that there had to be such a material connection between the generations that carried hereditary information from both the male and female sides of the family. Those factors united to form the child who could share features of one or both of his parents (Lopez-Beltran, 2006; Muller-Wille and Rheinberger, 2005).

The development of the microscope allowed physicians interested in reproduction to perceive how such hereditary transmission might actually occur. Martin Barry completed his medical studies at the University of Edinburgh and then worked on embryology with Tiedemann at the University of Heidelberg. In 1843, he recovered eggs from the fallopian tubes of female rabbits after cohabitation with males. Microscopic study showed spermatozoa within the eggs themselves (Barry, 1843). Several years later, the London surgeon George Newport actually observed the penetration of frog egg membranes by spermatozoa, and then described subsequent cell division as the fertilized zygote formed the early embryonic frog (Newport, 1852, 1854). These observations were important because they modeled potential mechanisms for human heredity. Prosper Lucas proposed in 1847 that the laws of inheritance were identical in both humans and animals (Lucas, 1847b).

Jonathan Hutchinson was a young surgeon in London at this time studying eye disease at the Royal London Ophthalmic Hospital. He was developing a life-long interest in heredity and disease, and wrote a brief summary of the knowledge on this topic in 1857. He noted that, generally, children resembled their parents, but variation certainly did occur. He thought that acquired characters could be inherited, and that this was the source of variation that might improve the human race in the future. But, he was forced to admit that while everyone, it seemed, had a theory on heredity, there actually was but little knowledge of how factors were transferred from one generation to the next (Hutchinson, J., 1857; Hutchinson, H., 1946). Henry Holland was of the same opinion when he noted with dismay that there was "no single reference in the medical literature on heredity and disease" (Holland, 1857).

Physicians in this era certainly were interested in mechanisms for heredity. Their collection of pedigrees and observations on the patterns of inheritance described in this chapter provided a more systematic basis for future understanding in this area. Preliminary attempts to define mathematical ratios of affected and unaffected offspring born of specific parents would also be applied to a more detailed understanding of how heredity worked in the future. The wish of many physicians for such a theory of heredity was, in fact, being addressed by one of Holland's distant cousins, the naturalist Charles Darwin.

Seven
Charles Darwin and a Provisional Theory of Heredity

The publication of *The Origin of Species* in 1859 made Charles Darwin the most prominent naturalist in England. The book was the culmination of decades of work on material he had begun to collect as a young man on the HMS *Beagle* expedition around the world. He spent the five years of the voyage studying fossils of extinct animals and plants, as well as observing behaviors of living birds and lizards on tropical isles. He became convinced that species were not fixed, but that variation in nature did occur on a regular basis. The hereditary transmission of such variation from one generation to the next provided the vehicle whereby the species could change over time. Darwin recognized early in his study of organic evolution that heredity played an important and necessary role in transmitting variation to future generations.

Charles Darwin was born in 1809. His father, Robert, was a prominent physician in Shrewsbury, and his mother was Susanna Wedgwood Darwin, the daughter of Joshua Wedgwood, founder of the china company in Staffordshire. Both parents came from well-connected families in the Midlands and were solidly upper class in local society (Browne, E.J., 1995a). Charles grew up in a family with a long tradition of medical service. His grandfather was Erasmus Darwin, probably the most knowledgeable naturalist and physician of the prior century. His father was very large, over six feet tall and weighed more than 24 stone. Despite his looming physical appearance, Robert was a sensitive person. Charles noted later in life, "The most remarkable power which my father possessed was that of reading the characters and even the thoughts of those whom he saw for even a short time. We had many instances of this power, some of which seemed supernatural" (Katz-Sidlow, 1998). Charles thought that his father was "incomparably the best observer whom I ever knew" (King-Hele, 2003). Robert used these skills of sensitivity and careful inspection of patients to develop a very profitable medical practice, although behind that success, he was a man of contradictions. Robert told his son:

> At first he hated his profession so much that if he had even been sure of the smallest pittance, or if his father had given him any choice, nothing should have induced him to follow it [medicine]. To the end of his life, the thought of a surgical operation almost sickened him, and he could scarcely endure to see a person bled—a horror which he transmitted to me (Barlow, 1959a).

During his youthful observation of his father's medical practice, Charles did not appear inclined to follow in the family tradition. Robert was, in fact, quite disappointed with his son, thinking that he wasted his time. He commented, "You care for nothing but shooting, dogs and rat-catching; and you will be a disgrace to yourself and your family" (Katz-Sidlow, 1998). Charles did attempt to please his father and accompanied the doctor as he attended the poor in the area around Shrewsbury the summer after he finished school (Bowlby, 1990a). The young Darwin discussed the cases with his father and learned how to compound medicines for them. He noted, "At one time I had at least a dozen patients, and I felt keen interest in the work" (Barlow, 1959b).

The following October in 1825, Charles agreed to accompany his older brother, Erasmus, to the medical school at Edinburgh, where Erasmus had already begun his studies. Charles only remained there for two academic years, November 1825 until June 1827. During the first year, he took lecture courses on different aspects of medicine and made ward rounds in the hospital. He wrote to his sister Caroline that the lectures were "long and stupid." He was disgusted by human anatomy class. But the "clinical lectures, which means lectures on sick people in the hospitals—these I like very much" (Darwin, 1826). He read extensively during that first year, not only on clinical medicine, but on broader aspects of zoology and botany as well (Bowlby, 1990b).

After completing the first year of medical studies, Darwin's interests had begun to shift away from the practice of medicine. As his experience with sick patients increased, he found his own sensitive nature did not react well to dealing with serious illnesses in other people. He noted that some of the hospital cases "distressed me a great deal" (Barlow, 1959b). He observed two "very bad operations" in the hospital in that era before anesthesia. One involved a small child. Darwin was so horrified by what he saw that he rushed from the operating theater and never attended hospital rounds again. Such cases "fairly haunted me for many a long year," he later wrote (Barlow, 1959c). About the same time, he became convinced that his father planned to leave him "property enough to subsist on with some comfort." This belief was "sufficient to check any strenuous effort to learn medicine" (Barlow, 1959d; Bowlby, 1990b; Platt, 1959). For the rest of his life, Darwin continued to be interested in medicine as a science, but not as a profession.

When the second year of medical school began, Charles attended only two lecture classes—one on the practice of medicine and a second on natural history that examined geology, zoology and botany. This was where his interests really resided. He joined the student natural history society and began to study local marine invertebrates. He reported his observations to the student society, demonstrating keen skills of observation in the natural world, very much like those of his father in the medical world (Bowlby, 1990c). When he left Edinburgh in the spring of 1827, Darwin had learned rudiments of human anatomy and physiology, as well as some techniques for field biology. He definitely had lost interest in becoming a physician but he was also not inclined to become a mere country gentleman, "an idle, sporting man" (Bowlby, 1990c).

Darwin did not seem suited for life in the military or the law because of his sensitive nature. He had already decided against a medical career. The next logical path for a young man with reasonably independent means was the clergy. Darwin agreed that the role of the country parson sounded agreeable to him. He worked with a tutor and successfully passed the examinations for admission to Cambridge University for the term beginning January 1828. While meeting the minimal course requirements there, he spent most of his time reading extensively in natural history, and studying rocks and beetles in the countryside around the university. In fact, he only attended one lecture course on botany in 1828. This comprised his entire formal education in the sciences while at Cambridge (Bowlby, 1990d; Browne, E.J., 1995b). During the summer of 1831, Darwin accompanied Adam Sedgwick, Professor of Geology at Cambridge, on an extensive field trip through Wales to study and map geological formations (Bowlby, 1990e). The life of a country parson with an extensive interest in natural history studies seemed to be the ideal position for young Darwin.

Shortly after his return from Wales, Darwin was offered a position as naturalist on HMS *Beagle* that planned to make a voyage to investigate the natural history of South America. Darwin accepted immediately, and the ship sailed in December 1831. The trip was expected to last two years, but it actually was five years before Darwin returned home to England (Browne, E.J., 1995c). Eventually he would study not only South America, but also the Galapagos Islands and Australia as the ship sailed across the Pacific.

During the months away from home, collecting fossil plants and animals, hunting and preserving birds and other animals, collecting rocks from seashores and mountains, Darwin found that his plans were changing. He wrote to a friend early in the voyage, "I often conjecture what will become of me; my wishes would certainly make me a country clergymen" (Bowlby, 1990f). As time went on, he began to realize that he was now drawn more to natural history rather than to natural theology. He wrote to his mother Caroline:

> I think it would be a pity having gone so far, not to go on and do all in my power in this my favorite pursuit...I trust and believe that the time spent on this voyage...will produce its full worth in natural history. And it appears to me, the doing of what little one can do to increase the general stock of knowledge is as respectable an object of life, as one can in any likelihood pursue (Bowlby, 1990f).

By February 1836, his sister, Susan, expressed the opinion of the family, "There are but small hopes of you still going into the Church. I think you must turn Professor at Cambridge" (Bowlby, 1990g).

Robert Darwin was finally pleased with his son's career plans. The idea of ordination was removed from consideration when the younger Darwin returned to England. Dr. Darwin gave his son a stipend of 400 pounds per year in early 1837 which allowed Charles to settle in Cambridge and begin writing up his observations on natural history which had been collected during the *Beagle* expedition (Bowlby, 1990h; Browne, E.J., 1995d). As he began to organize his own thoughts on the history of species, one of the first things Charles did was to review the writings on evolution produced by his grandfather, Erasmus. Charles wrote that he found there a "vivid imagination." Erasmus had "great originality of thought...a prophetic spirit in both medicine and in the mechanical arts." He valued "experiments and the use of hypotheses," showing he had "the true spirit of a philosopher." But the younger Darwin believed that Erasmus also had the "overpowering tendency to theorize and generalize" (Colp, 1986). Charles felt that his grandfather often speculated beyond the available facts in natural history. As his own career developed, he hoped that the "prophetic spirit in science" was something he could achieve as well (Colp, 1986).

Darwin next opened a series of notebooks outlining questions on evolution and heredity which he hoped to answer in his studies of the natural world. He had become convinced that natural species were not fixed and that variation over time did indeed occur. His 1837 *Red Notebook* indicated that sexual reproduction was clearly important as "the physiological vehicle of organic change" (Kohn, 1980a). He argued that sexual reproduction spread variability throughout the species. As such, variability could be adaptive, and certain individuals would more likely survive to reproduce again. Such heritable variability was then the engine of evolutionary change (Kohn, 1980b). Certainly not all variation was adaptive. Some characters had been maintained in the species for many generations because they had been useful in the distant past and now were neutral. Darwin thought that a too large or too small change would disrupt the stability of an organism. Heredity provided a mechanism for accumulating small changes over time in the species: "By a succession of generations, these small changes become multiplied, and great change can be effected" (Kohn, 1980c). Hence, over time, heredity allowed one species to change enough to be recognized eventually as a distinct new species.

Darwin, like most of his contemporaries, believed that acquired characters could become hereditary. He thought that the changing world altered the adult organism in some way that eventually modified the egg or the embryo, and resulted in changed offspring. Such change could be adaptive and permit the offspring to then respond to changes in the environment. In *Notebook B*, Darwin postulated that over time such changes might allow one "...generation to adapt and alter the race to [the] changing world" (Ospovat, 1981).

A brief 1842 essay summarized his thoughts at that time on heredity and evolution. Several factors were outlined that he planned to address in subsequent work. The major problem Darwin encountered was blending inheritance—the tendency of offspring to demonstrate characters intermediate between those of their parents. This was generally the rule for inheritance accepted by authorities of the period. Exceptions did occur, such as reversions, which were the reappearance of characters seen in prior generations and not in the immediate parents. If blending inheritance was the general rule in nature, any slight variation in an individual would tend to be lost in crossing with the general population stock in the next generation. Darwin worried, "If varieties be allowed freely to cross, such varieties will be constantly demolished. Any small tendencies in them to vary will be constantly counteracted." This aspect of heredity would then doom any variation from surviving in subsequent generations and hence lose any potential adaptability. If the environment induced biologic variations that would only rarely be successfully transmitted to the offspring, Darwin knew that this would not create "the beautiful and complex adaptations" he envisioned as one species changed into another over time (Vorzimmer, 1963).

Two years later in a larger essay, Darwin postulated that social isolation was one mechanism to protect loss of variation from a population. In a small group, he felt it was more likely that variants could be transmitted. He also proposed three other factors that would tend to decrease the blending aspect of heredity. His observations suggested that "at whatever period of life a peculiarity appears...it tends to reappear in the offspring at the corresponding period of life" (Vorzimmer, 1963). And he also believed that the longer a variant existed within a population, the more likely it was to become a regular feature of subsequent generations. In this manner, the power of inheritance would be enhanced (Vorzimmer, 1963). Lastly, Darwin introduced the idea that the environment could make an individual unusually liable to vary. He felt some individuals in a population would be "plastic," i.e., more liable to vary in greater degree than the regular slight variations occurring in other members of the species (Bowler, 1974). The more variation induced within a population, within the limits of stability required of all organisms to survive and reproduce, the better the chance of such variation being transmitted to offspring in the future.

While hypotheses were all well and good, Darwin could not stop there as his grandfather had done. He moved on to collect as much data from the natural world as he could to show that the variations which occurred in animals and plants could indeed become hereditary and appear in subsequent generations as required for his notion of evolution—that one species could be transmuted into another. He asked those who knew about the breeding of plants and animals for their opinions in this regard. His coachman gave him material on the breeding of hounds. Country friends provided information on their experiences with breeding pigs, horses and hares, as well as grapes, flowers and trees (Browne, E.J., 1995e; Secord, 1985). Darwin met Mary Anne Whitby who cultivated silkworms in Hampshire. She had observed a black eye-browed variant of the silkworm caterpillar. Darwin asked her to cross the variants and was pleased to hear that the unusual character could be inherited (Darwin, 1847). He later asked Mrs. Whitby to report to him "anything remarkable on the hereditary principle..." that she saw in her silkworm population (Darwin, 1849).

Darwin also installed gardens and greenhouses on his own country estate and began plant-breeding experiments (Secord, 1985). He later became interested in the breeding of pigeons as a means to study effects of inheritance and variation. He became friends with William Tegetmeier, who had graduated from University College London in medicine, but had become bored with country medical practice (Merrington, 1976; Richardson, 1916). Tegetmeier then developed a reputation as a well-respected pigeon breeder in London and supplied Darwin with different races of birds for his own breeding studies. Darwin also asked Tegetmeier to perform crosses of specific races over many years. The men wrote over 160 letters back and forth detailing the results of their breeding studies. Darwin's results challenged several well-accepted notions about variation and heredity in these animals.

As early as 1838, William Yarrell had suggested to Darwin the notion of "hereditary inertia." Breeders often felt that once two races were crossed, the older, more established one would contribute the most characters to the offspring. When Darwin tested this notion with his own pigeons, he found no evidence that Yarrell's hypothesis was correct. Breeders also generally believed that the male parent tended to transmit external features while the female parent influenced development of internal features. Darwin dissected offspring from dozens of pigeon crosses and found no evidence that this notion was correct either (Bartley, 1992). The results of his years of work on plant and animal breeding further convinced Darwin that heredity and evolution were intertwined. Without a well-organized mechanism of heredity to ensure continuity from one generation to the next, there was no way for small variations to accumulate over time and eventually result in changes as one older species changed into a new species.

Darwin's natural history studies had also convinced him that blending inheritance was not the general result of sexual reproduction in plants and animals. In 1858, he noted to the naturalist Thomas Huxley:

> Approaching the subject [of evolution] from the side which attracts me most, viz. inheritance, I have lately been inclined to speculate...that fertilization will turn out to be a sort of mixture and not true fusion, of two distinct individuals, as each parent has its parent and ancestors. I can understand on no other view the way in which crossed forms go back to so large an extent to ancestral forms (Clark, 1984a).

Darwin subsequently focused more intensely on heredity as he pondered the species question. He noted to the botanist J.D. Hooker in 1859, "Though of course inheritance is of fundamental importance to us, for if a variation be not inherited, it is of no significance to us" (Darwin, 1859a). Although Darwin recognized the importance of heredity in his scheme of organic evolution, when he published his ideas in *The Origin of Species* in 1859, he was not at all sure how such transmission, in fact, took place. In the very first section, he admitted to his readers:

> The laws governing inheritance are for the most part unknown. No one can say why the same peculiarity in different individuals of the same species, is sometimes inherited and sometimes not so; why the child often reverts in certain characters to his grandfather or grandmother or more remote ancestors; why a peculiarity is often transmitted from one sex to both sexes, or to one sex alone, more commonly but not exclusively to the like sex (Darwin, 1963a).

Darwin also observed the frequent recurrence of a character in several generations of human families as well. He thought this "...cannot be due to a coincidence, but must be consequential on the members of the same family inheriting <u>something</u> in common in their constitution" [emphasis added] (Darwin, 1859b). This statement implies the hereditary transmission of some physical element from one generation to the next. In *Origin*, he admitted, "Our ignorance of the laws of variation is profound" (Darwin, 1963b). A year later, Darwin noted to Maxwell Masters, surgeon and botanist, "The laws of inheritance seem to be determined to puzzle everyone" (Darwin 1860).

Darwin had come to recognize that most variation in nature was minor, such as differences between individuals in a population. Extensive variations, "sports," "saltations," or "monsters" were usually sterile and hence did not reproduce. From an evolutionary point of view, these were of no consequence for subsequent generations.

The process of natural selection, Darwin believed, worked on small minor variations in populations over extended periods of time (Vorzimmer, 1963; Bowler, 1974). Toward the end of *Origin*, Darwin summarized this concept as:

> Inheritance, that cause which alone...produces organisms quite like each other or as we see in cases of varieties, nearly alike. The dissimilarity of the inhabitants of different regions may be attributed to modification through variation and natural selection, or probably to a subordinate degree to the definite influence of different physical conditions (Darwin, 1963c).

Heredity always involved the tension between faithfully maintaining the species type from one generation to another, as well as occasionally transmitting variations that occurred in the population, usually due to altered environmental factors which somehow influenced the reproductive cells, and hence the offspring (Webster, 1992).

During the 1860s, Darwin focused his attention on developing a comprehensive mechanism to explain how hereditary transmission worked. He wanted a theory that would explain the myriad examples of hereditary variation that he had collected over the years from plants, animals and humans. The manuscript which eventually explained his theory of heredity was completed between January and April 1863 ("Variation," 1999). Darwin then sent a copy to T.H. Huxley, biologist and physician, for his comments the following month. Darwin reworked and expanded the material into a final chapter called "Pangenesis" that was presented to the public in 1868 as part of a two-volume work titled *The Variation of Animals and Plants under Domestication.* By the end of this extensive project, Darwin was both exhausted and pleased with the outcome. He had been thinking about heredity for years, as already noted. He commented to Charles Lyell, the geologist:

> I do not know whether you ever had the feeling of having thought so much over a subject that you had lost all power of guiding it. This is my case with Pangenesis (which is 26 or 27 years old), but I am inclined to think that if it be admitted as a probable hypothesis it will be a somewhat important step in Biology (Robinson, 1979).

Darwin had reason to be pleased with his theory because it did appear to explain in great detail the different forms of heredity he had observed in nature. Modern historians of science regard "Pangenesis" as "the very first attempt at a really comprehensive elucidation of the transmission process" based upon not only theory, but experimental results and field observations collected over many years of work (Lefevre, 2005). Darwin wrote to Hooker, "This hypothesis serves as a useful connecting link for various grand classes of physiological facts, which at present stand absolutely isolated" (Clark, 1984a). To Asa Gray, Professor of Biology at Harvard, he noted, "I think it contains a great truth" (Browne, J., 2002a).

Darwin had assembled diverse examples of not only plants and animal heredity, but also human material. His sources of human data ranged from observations made by his own father in the course of medical practice, from reports of other prominent medical men who he came to know, from the burgeoning medical literature, and from reports by missionaries and anthropologists exploring the secrets of societies in the four corners of the globe. Darwin compiled so much human hereditary material that he considered preparing a separate work on human variation; but he never found the time to complete this project (Browne, J., 2002b).

Through family medical connections, Darwin became friends and correspondent with many of the leading physicians of the day. Henry Holland and J. S. Burton-Sanderson were old friends. Henry Bence-Jones and Andrew Clark served as his personal physicians. The pharmacologist, J. S. Brunton, and the surgeons, William Bowman and James Paget, also were interested in Darwin's work on human variation. Darwin noted to Paget after a dinner meeting, "It was very kind of you to bear in mind my strong wish to learn any facts on inheritance at corresponding ages, and a correlation of growth" (Darwin, 1859b).

Darwin's library collection and annotations of books he read clearly indicated that he closely followed developments in the medical sciences and gleaned as much material as possible from them for use in his own work. He was well versed in the human heredity studies of the French physicians prior to 1860, and annotated his own copy of Prosper Lucas's text (Lopez-Beltran, 2003). One source which proved "particularly valuable and interesting," according to Darwin, was a series of seven articles published in the *British and Foreign Medico-Chirurgical Review* from 1861 to 1867. The author, William Sedgwick, had studied at University College Hospital and then practiced medicine in London. Sedgwick devoted serious time and effort to the study of hereditary human disease, and published his work during this decade. Darwin used several examples of human variation from this material and carefully considered Sedgwick's opinions on the mechanism of human heredity (Sedgwick, 1896; "Obituary of William Sedgwick," 1905).

Darwin presented numerous examples on human heredity and variation in Chapter XII of *Variation*. The various characters and their sources in both the first 1868 and subsequent 1878 editions of this work are summarized in Table 7.1. His first example was the well-known Lambert family recorded in the prior century as the "porcupine" men with scaly skin. The family had now been followed for at least three generations. Only males reportedly exhibited the unusual skin quality. There were other examples of more mundane features which also could be transmitted. Dr. Hodgkin recorded an English family in which individuals over many generations were born with a forelock of another color than the rest of the hair on the head. Darwin himself was familiar with a three-generation family affected by a characteristic white forelock.

Habits and gestures also appeared to be hereditary. The German naturalist, Hofacker, noted that several generations of specific families had almost identical handwriting. Characteristic gait, facial gestures and hand motions also were observed in successive generations of particular families.

Darwin also accumulated information on many other medical conditions which illustrated the power of heredity through his numerous physician contacts. Garrod noted heredity in about half of his series of patients with gout. Insanity affected five males in one generation and two males in a subsequent generation of one unfortunate family. Disorders of the eye often ran in families. Darwin was aware of one family in which parents and many of their children suffered from ptosis, drooping of the eyelids. An elongated eyelid was noted in a father and seven of his children. Errors of visual refraction also were noted in parents and their offspring. Amaurosis [blindness] and aniredemia [absence of the iris] were observed in three generations of different families. Coloboma irides [cleft iris] was seen in four generations, but only males were affected. Conversely, color blindness was noted in five generations of one family, but only females were affected in this unusual instance. Night blindness affected individuals of both sexes in a six-generation family recorded from France. Heterochromia irides [different colored iris in each eye] was noted in a mother and 21 of her children.

Abnormalities of the hands and feet commonly recurred in successive generations. Polydactyly often appeared in parents and children. Deficient phalanges of the hands and feet were observed in a three-generation family. Of 16 affected individuals, only one was female. But in another family, supposedly extending over 10 generations, only females were affected with a similar anomaly. Clinodactyly [incurving of the fifth finger] was observed only in males of a family recorded by the German-English physician, Steinau. Abnormalities of the internal organ structure and function also could be

Table 7.1
Human Hereditary Variation

Trait	Reference	First ed. p.	Second ed. p.
Porcupine man	Baker	12-13	448
Different colored hair lock	Hodgkin	14	449
White forelock	C. Darwin	14	449
Handwriting	Hofacker	15	450
Gait, gesture, voice	Hunter	15	450
Gait, gesture, voice	Carlisle	15	450
Habits	R. Darwin	15	450
Crossing leg habit	De Buzareignues	15	450
Finger motion	C. Darwin	15	450-451
Gout	Garrod	16	451
Insanity	Sedgwick	16	451
Suicide	Sedgwick	16	451
Ptosis	C. Darwin	17	452
Ptosis	Wade		452
Eyelid fold	Carlisle	17	452
Elongated eyelid	Holland	17	452
Eyebrow hair length	Paget	17	452
Hypermetropia	Bowman	17	452
Myopia	Bowman	18	453
Squinting	Bowman	18	453
Cataract	Bowman	18	453
Amaurosis	Sedgwick	18	453
Aniridia	Sedgwick	18	453-454
Coloboma irides	Sedgwick	18	454
Corneal opacity	Sedgwick	18	454
Microphthalmia	Sedgwick	18	454
Ectopia lentis	Portal	19	454
Dayblindness	Sedgwick	19	454
Night blindness	Sedgwick	19	454
Color blindness	Sedgwick	19	454

Table 7.1, *Continued*
Human Hereditary Variation

Trait	Reference	First ed. p.	Second ed. p.
Albinism	Sedgwick	19	454
Heterochromia irides	Sedgwick	19	454
Polydactyly	Struthers	22-23	457
Polydactyly	Wilder, Huxley		457
Absent digits	Ogle		458
Clinodactyly	Struthers		459
Diabetes	Holland	27	460
Death with peculiar coma	R. Darwin	28	460
Albinism	Devay	28	460
Deafness	Sedgwick	34	466
Cleft lip and palate	Sproule	36	466
Hydrocoele	Holland	72	27
Colorblindness	Sedgwick	93	48-49
Colorblindness	Earle	93	48-49
Hemophilia	Sedgwick	94	49
Deficient phalanges	Sedgwick	95	49
Hairy family	Crawfurd	98	53
St. Vitus dance	Lucas	99	54
Amaurosis	Sedgwick	100	54
Amaurosis	Lucas	100	54
Deafness	Sedgwick	100	55
Insanity	Sedgwick	100	55
Insanity	Lucas, Piorry	100	55
Apoplexy	Lucas	100	55
Asthma	Lucas	101	55
Clinodactyly	Lucas	101	55
Clinodactyly	Lucas, Sedgwick, Steinau	101	55
Pityriasis versicolor	Sedgwick	101	55
Migraine headache	Sedgwick	101	55
Cancer	Paget	102	56
Cataract	Bowman	102	56

Reference: Darwin, 1868c, 1893a

hereditary. Diabetes was seen repeatedly in certain families. Holland noted three brothers affected. Robert Darwin gave the report of four brothers in one family who each lapsed into coma, between 60 and 70 years of age, and then died. The French physician F.M. DeVay studied albinism. Two brothers married two sisters who were their first cousins. They produced seven children between them, all albinos.

Darwin was particularly intrigued by Sedgwick's reports of hereditary characters that primarily affected only one sex. Although the physician had reported one five-generation family with 13 females affected by color blindness, at least 90% of other affected families he investigated had only males exhibiting this trait. The same pattern was generally found regarding hemophilia. Through five generations, only males had the bleeding disorder, although it appeared to be transmitted through unaffected females. In another example, deafness occurred only in males of three consecutive generations. Insanity and suicide plagued three generations of males in another family noted by the French physician Prosper Lucas. A skin condition, pityriasis versicolor, resembled hemophilia in its inheritance with only males being affected and unaffected females appearing to transmit the trait. Finally, migraine headaches plagued ten males in three generations of one family in which all the females escaped this agonizing malady.

Darwin summarized his theory of inheritance in Chapter XXVII of *Variation.* He realized that, despite his best efforts to be inclusive, his "view is merely a provisional hypothesis, a speculation, but until a better one is advanced, it may be serviceable by bringing together a multitude of facts which are at present left disconnected by any efficient cause" (Darwin, 1868d). The basic tenet of the "hypothesis of Pangenesis" was:

> The whole organisation, in the sense of every separate atom or unit reproduces itself. Hence ovules and pollen grains—the fertilized seed or egg, as well as buds—include and consist of a multitude of germs thrown off from each separate atom of the organism (Darwin, 1868d).

He envisioned cells releasing "minute granules or atoms, which circulate freely throughout the system, and when supplied with proper nutrients, multiplying by self-division, subsequently being developed into cells like those from which they were derived." These "gemmules" were concentrated in the female ovary or the male testis and represented the physical vehicles whereby "every single character possessed by the parent" could be transmitted to the subsequent generation (Darwin, 1868e). Darwin thought:

> So it must be with the separate constituent elements of the germ cells, that is the many gemmules or atoms of protoplasm thrown off from each tissue and cell during its development. By the multiplication and presentation in an undeveloped state of these gemmules, I account for all latent characters (Olby, 1963).

Gemmules therefore had a real physical existence if they could be passed through many generations and then become active and produce traits in subsequent offspring. Even earlier, Darwin had become aware of the idea of the French naturalist Charles Naudin who proposed that a hybrid was really a "living mosaic." Darwin noted to Huxley:

> Propagation by true fertilization will turn out to be a sort of mixture, and not true fusion, of two distinct individuals, or rather of innumerable individuals, as each parent has its parents and ancestors. I can understand on no other view the way in which crossed forms go back to so large an extent to ancestral forms...
> (Geison, 1969).

Darwin then reiterated the same point he had made in 1859:

> If the occurrence of the same unusual character in the child and parent cannot be attributed to both having been exposed to the same unusual conditions, then...the result cannot be due to mere coincidence, but must be consequent on the members of the same family inheriting <u>something</u> in common in their constitution [emphasis added] (Darwin, 1868e).

In making such a comment, Darwin essentially accepted heredity as the result of physical particles that were transmitted through reproduction and then maintained their properties for subsequent action (De Beer, 1964).

Darwin thought that variation tended to be more common in organisms that reproduced sexually compared to those using asexual or budding techniques (Darwin, 1868f). He also observed, "hybrids...are generally intermediate in character between the two parent-forms, yet occasionally they closely resemble one parent in one part and the other parent in another part, or even in the whole structure" (Darwin, 1868g). Darwin's own observations on plant hybrids had helped him see that offspring were, in fact, not always intermediate between the two parents. For example, he had crossed the painted lady and purple varieties of sweet peas. When he examined the offspring he found both parental types, and no intermediates (Darwin, 1866). As he had noted in human examples of disease, one sex sometimes "has a stronger power of transmission than the other" (Darwin, 1868f). Gemmules derived from one parent could be "superabundant in number" or have some other advantage in affinity or vigor compared to those of the other parent (Darwin, 1868g). Clearly, every character from each parent was present in either an active or latent form in each generation. When hybrids were inbred, traits of one of the grandparents often reappeared, demonstrating the existence of the gemmules in the parents without expression, but still being capable of transmission to the offspring (Darwin, 1868f).

Transmission and development of a character were certainly two distinct processes. In one example, a grandfather might transmit a character through his unaffected daughter to his grandson who then developed the character in question. Why certain traits commonly appeared in only one sex was quite unknown, although it was a well-known occurrence (Darwin, 1868h). Latent characters could thus be transmitted for several generations and then reappear as a "reversion," either because of the variation engendered by sexual reproduction or because of a change in the environment faced by the offspring (Darwin, 1868i). Darwin commented to Hooker in 1863, "When one thinks of a latent character being handed down, hidden for a thousand or ten thousand generations, and then suddenly appearing, one is quite bewildered at the host of characters written in invisible ink in the germ" (Geison, 1969).

Darwin next argued that external forces affected the cells of each organism and altered the type or quantity of gemmules produced by each tissue.

> If from changed conditions...any part of the body should become permanently modified, the gemmules, which were merely minute portions of the contents of the cells forming the part, would naturally reproduce the same modification. Subsequently some normal and altered gemmules would circulate in the organism and be transmitted to the offspring (Darwin, 1868j).

The same reasoning was used to explain the inheritance of acquired characters, such as an injury or a structure altered by use or disuse. Such factors were expected to alter the gemmules produced by the particular organ involved. Darwin thought that inheritance of acquired characters was more the rule than the exception (Darwin, 1868k). There might be no apparent alteration in structure for several generations until the altered gemmules "became sufficiently numerous to overpower and supplant the old gemmules" (Darwin, 1868l).

In Darwin's theory, variability was due to one of two factors. A character could result from deficiency or superabundance or redevelopment of a dormant trait. In such cases, there were no changes in the gemmules themselves. Secondly, the organism itself may have been modified by altered environment, use or disuse, and thus could produce altered gemmules. When multiplied, these could then result in altered structures in subsequent generations.

When *Variation* was completed, Darwin thought that his Pangenesis theory of inheritance was both true and important for the general world of biology, because it explained a wide range of observations on heredity from diverse aspects of the natural world (Browne, J., 2002c). If nothing else, he hoped the theory would encourage other naturalists to think and experiment along the same lines.

> But if anyone should hereafter be led to make observations by which some such hypothesis could be established, I shall have done good service, as an astonishing number of isolated facts can thus be connected together and rendered intelligible (Clark, 1984b).

Despite his high expectations, *Variation,* and Pangenesis in particular, did not produce the praise for all his efforts that Darwin had hoped to receive. The physical scientist Fleming Jenkin noted, "Darwin's theory is an ingenious and plausible speculation...with some faint half-truths, marking at once the ignorance of the age and the ability of the philosopher" (Clark, 1984c). In February 1868, Darwin noted to Hooker, "I fear Pangenesis is still born. Bates says he has read it twice, and is not sure that he understands it...Old Sir H. Holland says he read it twice, and thinks it very tough, but believes that sooner or later something akin to it will be accepted" (Darwin, 1868b). But later that same year Darwin advised Hooker not to "touch on Pangenesis." The botanist, George Bentham, was "hostile;" and the biologist Victor Carus was "dead against it" (Darwin, 1868a). The surgeon, James Paget, also read it and commented to Darwin:

> I expect to be made even more than I am now ashamed of my ignorance (and I fear I may add that of my profession, too) on the influence of variations and mixtures of diseases. But I hope that my deeper shame may be the beginning of deeper knowledge (Paget, S., 1903; Towers, 1968).

Darwin was disappointed at this initial reception, but not utterly dismayed. He commented, "...I feel sure if Pangenesis is now still born, it will, thank God, at some future time reappear, begotten by some other father, and christened by some other name" (Darwin, 1868b).

After the publication of *Variation* in 1868, Darwin next focused his attention on human evolution. A second edition of the work did appear in 1878, but only minor changes were made. He used essentially the same human examples of hereditary traits and diseases, only adding several more recent accounts of anomalies of the hands (Table 7.1). The Pangenesis chapter was also essentially unchanged although Darwin was now more impressed than ever with the number of complex molecules each gemmule must carry. An egg or sperm had to contain a vast number of gemmules that could be transmitted to the next generation (Darwin, 1893b). He again observed that hybrids often were intermediate between the characters of their parents, though occasionally they did resemble one parent more than the other. The gemmules derived from one parent could have had an advantage in number, vigor or affinity; one form could then become prepotent (Darwin, 1893c).

Darwin lived until 1882. Although he did not publish any further detailed study of human heredity, he continued to collect material from physicians and other naturalists in England and abroad. George Rolleston, physician and Professor of Anatomy at Oxford, sent Darwin information about a man who lost one eye due to infection. Fifteen years later, he married and produced two sons, both having one eye smaller than the other (Rolleston, 1861). This fact appeared to support Darwin's notion that acquired characters could become hereditary. W. S. Wade provided Darwin with the family history of a coal miner who acquired narrowed eyelids "after having fits as a child." No prior family members demonstrated that trait, and yet two of his three children were similarly affected (Wade, 1873). W. W. Keen, a physician from the Jefferson Medical College in Philadelphia, presented contradicting information on the heredity of acquired characters to Darwin. He noted that Jews had practiced circumcision for more than 3000 years, and yet newborn Jewish boys still were born with normal sized foreskins. Keen felt this was an historical argument against Darwin's notion that acquired characters often became hereditary over time (Keen, 1874). Other evidence against the heredity of acquirements came from Lawson Tait, a surgeon in Birmingham. He told Darwin about the supposed spinal cord lesions in mice produced by the French physician, Edouard Brown-Sequard. Some of the offspring of such surgically traumatized animals developed epilepsy that was then transmitted to some of their pups. Tait thought such reports "quite worthless." His own observations indicated that many different factors, even something as simple as altered diet, could induce seizures in experimental animals (Tait, 1881).

James Paget also sent Darwin articles on inherited malformations. He pointed out that, within a family, not all offspring necessarily inherited the same disease. They tended to develop related diseases of the same body system—nerves, skin, and intestinal tract (Paget, J., 1863). Horace Dobell was a physician at the Royal Hospital for Diseases of the Chest in London. He was particularly interested in heredity and respiratory disorders. Dobell sent Darwin a family history form he had devised, asking for comments on its completeness in elucidating a detailed family history from each patient (Dobell, 1863a). Darwin replied that the "the importance of hereditary transmission [of disease] can hardly be exaggerated under every point of view..." He thoroughly endorsed the use of the genealogy form to show any distant relationship between family members. And he asked Dobell to send him "any remarkable cases of inheritance..." (Darwin, 1863). Dobell subsequently provided Darwin with information on several families with inherited anomalies of the hands (Dobell, 1863b). Darwin also corresponded with William Ogle, physician and naturalist. They were working on the family history of twins born with clinodactyly and misplaced teeth (Ogle, 1869). The potential ill effects of inbreeding were considered in letters between Darwin and the Oxford physician, Gilbert Child. They agreed that the available data was conflicting. Child thought in general close breeding did not result in degeneracy (Child, 1869). Darwin's mind continued to ask pointed questions on heredity throughout the latter portion of his life. Even in the last year of his life, Darwin corresponded with W. T. Van Dyck, Lecturer in Zoology at the Protestant College in Beirut, Lebanon. Darwin was requesting information "on peculiarities of any kind affecting the milk teeth of children" (Van Dyck, 1882). He commented to the Swiss botanist Alphonse de Candalle, "...How mysterious a subject is that of generation" (Darwin, 1873).

Darwin had many close friends in the medical profession. He read the medical literature and collected numerous examples of human heredity that he then used to illustrate his pangenesis theory of inheritance. Although many within the profession did not understand the details of Darwin's work, they did appreciate the man's reputation within English science. He was elected to honorary membership in several medical societies and was awarded three honorary medical degrees during his lifetime. William

Gairdner, Professor of Medicine at the University of Glasgow and Physician to Queen Victoria, summarized the medical profession's opinion of Charles Darwin when he delivered a eulogy upon the naturalist's death in 1882. Gairdner summarized Darwin's importance to natural science of that era by calling him "the man of the century" (Towers, 1968).

Part III
Later Nineteenth Century Medicine and Heredity

Eight

Francis Galton and the Beginning of the Science of Human Heredity

By the middle of the nineteenth century, English medical education was stagnant, but innovations in both clinical and laboratory medicine were developing in France and Germany. English medical students flocked to these foreign hospitals and clinics where freedom of thought was encouraged. By the 1840s, Paris was considered by many to be the "best teaching centre in the world" (Booth, 1979). There was a general trend on the Continent for new discoveries to take place in the laboratory, not on the hospital ward. The correlation of physical signs and symptoms with pathologic lesions noted in subsequent post-mortem examinations had become a powerful tool toward understanding human disease, even before 1850. Led by Claude Bernard in Paris, the study of disease processes next became a laboratory science. He argued that medicine began in the hospital, but the physicians who wanted to become true scientists then carried their questions about disease to the laboratory. Bernard said:

> I consider hospitals only as the entrance to scientific medicine, they are the first field of observation which a physician enters; but the true sanctuary of medical science is a laboratory; only thus can he seek explanations of life in the normal and pathological state by means of experimental analysis (Bernard, 1865).

The physician there would "seek to account for what he has observed in his patients by study with experimental animals to assess the origin of morbid lesions or the actions of medications" (Cunningham, 1992).

About the same time in Germany, physicians began to quantify human physiological functions with the clinical thermometer to measure temperature, spirometer to measure lung function and sphygnomanometer to measure blood pressure. Clinical tests on body fluids such as urine and blood were developed to assess normal and abnormal function. The ophthalmoscope allowed examination of the interior of the living eye, and the laryngoscope was developed to examine the throat as well. The microscope was increasingly utilized to detect changes in microanatomy associated with disease states (Keele, 1968a).

British physicians took advantage of these Continental opportunities to learn new approaches to scientific medicine and later returned to England. Lionel Beale was one such young physician who then organized a course on clinical microscopy at King's College in London after 1854 (Keele, 1968a). George Harley had studied with Bernard in Paris and then established himself at the University College London. His classes in histology and physiology attempted to demonstrate in the laboratory each fact presented to students in lecture. Similar programs developed during the 1860s at the medical schools in Edinburgh, Manchester, King's College in London, Glasgow and Liverpool (Bonner, 1995a).

The 1858 Medical Act established the General Medical Council (G.M.C.) to establish minimal educational requirements for competent physicians and surgeons throughout the United Kingdom. The G.M.C. was supposed to recommend training in the sciences which could be both safely and usefully applied to the daily practice of medicine (Ellis, 1966). During the 1860s, the G.M.C. responded to increased interest in the sciences by advising that medical students expand their understanding of the natural world by specifically encouraging laboratory courses in chemistry and microscopy (Bonner, 1995a). By 1885, five years of medical training were required including courses in physics, chemistry and biology. Medical students were not expected to become scientists. Instead, they were exposed to knowledge that was deemed useful for the practice of medicine. The curriculum was supposed to be a summation: to state scientific conclusions, rather than "the connection of facts and reasoning...that is science itself" (Ellis, 1966).

The application of scientific ideas to medicine in Britain at this time was quite controversial. It argued against the traditional physician of good social breeding who understood his patient's personal life and learned from clinical experience over the years in practice. The physician of the day was expected to be first a gentleman of good social standing. Application of scientific principles could be done by any practitioner, even those of middle-class origin (Romano, 1997). The historian A.J. Youngson observed, "A struggle [existed] between the new attitudes of scientific observation, experiment, reasoning and innovation, and old attitudes of classical culture and conservatism" (Youngson, 1979). Some even went so far as to argue that applying science to all of medicine would foster an "intellectual revolution" (Bonner, 1995b). Perhaps, but would such a revolution be desirable for the practice of English medicine?

John Brown of Edinburgh was a practicing physician as well as an essayist. He recognized the tension between the old and the new in medicine during the 1860s and recommended keeping an open mind:

> Let us avail ourselves of the unmatched advantages of modern science... let us convey into our heads as much as we safely can of new knowledge of chemistry, statistics, the microscope, the stethoscope, and all new helps and methods; but let us go on with the old serious diligence, the experientia as well as the experimenta...Young men have now almost the whole field to themselves. Chemistry and physiology have become to all men above forty, impossible sciences. The young man teaches and talks, the old learns and is mute. In this intensely scientific age, we need some wise heads to tell us what not to learn, or to unlearn, fully as much as what we learn (Keele, 1968b).

Brown always emphasized the tension of medical practice as both an art and as a science.

The leading scientific organization of this era, the B.A.A.S., was also becoming interested in medicine as a science. One commentator noted that the organization had traditionally avoided medical topics. But as medicine was increasingly both an important and yet an "inexact science," it was hoped that "experiment and induction [would become] as indispensable here as elsewhere" in the natural sciences. Development of medicine along scientific lines would allow it to become more systematic rather than relying on "authority or antiquity" as the source of its knowledge ("Editorial," 1863).

In 1880, John Bradbury, Professor of Medicine at Cambridge, spoke before the British Medical Association on the relationship between science and medicine. He was convinced that discoveries in biology had greatly influenced medicine over the prior decade. He urged the teaching of medical students in laboratory science, and "exact methods of investigation," because he was convinced this would foster further advances in medicine itself (Bradbury, 1880). One observer at the International Medical Congress expressed the same opinion in 1881:

> [The Congress] has demonstrated to the world the progress that medicine has recently made, that it is advancing because it has become more scientific, and that the only great advances in store for it must result from the successful application of the same methods ("Medical Congress," 1881).

Thomas L. Brunton, who had studied pharmacology in Vienna, Berlin and Leipzig, and then established a pharmacology research laboratory at St. Bart's Hospital, voiced a similar opinion. He attended the 1897 International Medical Congress and noted, "Practical medicine depends on physiology, pharmacology and pathology, but all three are becoming more like divisions of the modern science of chemistry" (Brunton, 1897).

However, many other practitioners within the English medical profession were concerned that medicine would be consumed and then subsumed by the broader natural sciences. Medicine was viewed by many in the profession to be a unique art, albeit aided by science. William Gull, prominent physician at Guy's Hospital, who also attended the Royal family, expressed this concern nicely in 1868. He thought that a scientific understanding of disease processes was important. But he was concerned that the medical school curriculum should be protected "against assaults on the side of science...lest we betray it by accepting a too chemical-physical limit to our thought" (Bonner, 1995c). By the 1880s, the scientific emphasis in medicine was frustrating some of the more senior practitioners. Samuel Gee, a well-respected consultant at St. Bart's Hospital, had completed the M.D. in 1865. When he returned to the same institution in 1888, he told the medical students there to "forget all your physiology. Physiology is an experimental science—and a very good thing no doubt in its proper place. Medicine is not a science, but an empirical art" (Bonner, 1995d). The Professor of Surgery at Cambridge, George Humphrey, commented in 1892 that medical education should pay more attention to principles and less to the details of any subject. In the "accessory subjects" such as chemistry, biology and physics, a grounding in principles was the key, and the details then should be used to illustrate those principles. He was afraid that the medical student was being "overladen and worried and his spirit broken..." by attempting to learn all the details of all the sciences applied to medical training (Humphrey, 1892). In summary, there was concern that medical education would involve the "wholesale conversion of bedside practice into a science" (Bonner, 1995e).

While the application of science to medicine had aided the understanding of disease processes, it had actually done little to effect change within the art of medicine, which meant taking care of and treating the patient's ills. T.L. Brunton from St. Bart's noted that progress in actually treating disease was slow:

> As we review the rapid progress made in recent years by physiology, pathology and other departments of medical science, and compare it with the slow advance of therapeutics, we experience a growing dissatisfaction with our present empirical methods of treatment, which consisting of the mere tentative administration of drugs without a definite knowledge of their action, must necessarily retard progress (Keele, 1968).

William Jenner, Professor at University College London and physician to the Royal family, also commented to the British Medical Association:

> The spirits of many have been dampened by the modern advances in the science of medicine which have led to skepticism in regard to the medical powers of medicine as an art; and especially to the medical powers of drugs (Keele, 1968).

Twenty years later the same opinion was expressed by John Bristowe of St. Thomas's Hospital who was a well-known teacher and microscopist. He commented, "The great aim of medical art is the cure of disease. Unfortunately, however, a direct cure (at all events a direct cure by means of drugs) in the great majority of cases is totally impossible" (Bynum, 1995; Bristowe, 1887).

Despite these negative attitudes of some leaders in medicine, general practitioners, physicians and surgeons alike educated themselves about the application of science to the practice of medicine. An increasing number of medical journals circulated throughout the Empire. Local medical societies met for professional comradeship and the sharing of clinical observations and opinions. Travel to France, Germany or Austria became considerably easier with the advent of steamships and railroads. An increasing number of English physicians regularly traveled abroad to visit clinics and hear lectures delivered by Continental leaders in medicine (Newman, 1961).

Medical professionals came to be recognized by the community as members of an educated social class, distinct from the traditional Oxford or Cambridge medical graduate who was first a gentleman, and then a physician. Long before medical science made much difference in medical treatment, physicians in the city and the country espoused science because it defined them as a class of individuals with "specialized expertise." That slowly came to count more in the society of the day than one's birth status, and allowed a "vehicle for social mobility" within the greater community. Medicine and its practitioners gained prestige, not because of enhanced ability to treat disease, but because the general public believed in the "science" embraced by the physicians and the surgeons (Loudon, 1984; Shortt, 1983). In fact, after 1888 developments in bacteriology finally allowed accurate diagnosis of many important human diseases. The successful treatment of some of them further convinced medical practitioners and the general public that laboratory science coupled with medical art were both essential for the health of the nation (Bonner, 1995f).

Physicians in this era of growing scientific knowledge also attempted to apply theories of heredity to better understand the nature of diseases that appeared to be transmitted from one generation to the next. As discussed in Chapter 7, the leading theory on heredity was the "Provisional Theory of Pangenesis," published by Charles Darwin in 1868 (Darwin, 1868). Physicians became familiar with the work as it used many examples from the medical literature to illustrate Darwin's points, but it was "difficult, to put it mildly, for an ordinary mind to grasp," so commented W.C. Johnston, pathologist from McGill University, as he spoke before the Medico-Chirurgical Society of Montreal (Johnston, 1886).

A young English scientist who had almost completed training to become a physician would now attempt to use experimental techniques to validate the tenets of Darwin's theory. In so doing, Francis Galton, Darwin's cousin, began a life-long career that would eventually establish human heredity as a science in its own right. Galton was born in 1822, thirteen years after his illustrious cousin, Charles. He was the last of nine children. His mother, Violette, was a daughter of Erasmus Darwin, and his father, Samuel, was a prominent manufacturer and banker in Birmingham. The senior Galton was an avid amateur scientist and a friend of local professionals such as Joseph Priestley and James Watt (Forrest, 1974a). The educational experience of the youngest Galton paralleled that of his cousin. He, too, experienced little success in several boarding schools, and eventually was sent to the Birmingham General Hospital as a medical student at age sixteen. He learned how to formulate medications and made hospital rounds. He worked very hard, even staying there during school holidays (Forrest, 1974b; Pearson, 1914a). Galton assisted at several surgical operations in those days before anesthesia. He survived these experiences better than Darwin did, and wrote to his father stating that he was learning not to be squeamish and to focus on the procedures themselves (Galton, 1838a). By the middle of the first term, he was identifying himself as "Dr." in letters to his family. He also mentioned that street children near the hospital often called after him, "There goes the Doctor!" (Galton, 1838b).

After a year at Birmingham, Galton transferred to King's College in London. He took lecture classes in chemistry and physiology, and spent a great deal of time in the anatomy room (Forrest, 1974c). He also became proficient in using the microscope (Pearson, 1914b). The following year, he decided to enroll at Cambridge to study mathematics, believing this would improve his powers of observation and skills as a physician. He told his father that he definitely planned to return to King's College after Cambridge to complete his medical studies (Galton, 1839).

Galton enrolled in the mathematical tripos at Trinity College Cambridge in October 1840. He worked diligently there and enjoyed his tutorials immensely (Forrest, 1974d). He also read anatomy, chemistry and forensic medicine. By the beginning of his third year at Trinity, however, Galton's health broke down. He suffered severe headaches, dizziness and could not concentrate on the work. He had to forego the rigors of the tripos and qualified for a poll degree in mathematics (Keynes, 1993).

Although he continued to state that he planned to complete medical training, Galton, in fact, was becoming more and more disillusioned about medical practice. He felt it would be necessary to become a "humbug" if he were to succeed as a physician in practice (Forrest, 1974e; Keynes, 1993). His father died in 1844, and Francis decided to halt medical studies, "being much upset and wanting for a healthier life" (Galton, 1908). He inherited sufficient wealth to be independent of any profession and noted, "I was therefore free, and I eagerly desired a complete change" (Pearson, 1914c).

At this point in his young life, Galton had had a rather varied educational experience. He knew more mathematics than most biologists, more biology than most mathematicians, and more pathology, anatomy and physiology than either one (Keynes, 1993). What he lacked was a specific aim in life to which he could apply these talents. During the 1850s, he embarked on several excursions to Africa and subsequently presented careful measurements of longitude, latitude and altitude to the Royal Geographical Society in London. He was elected Fellow of the Royal Society in 1856 based on these studies (Gillham, 2001a).

Galton read Darwin's *The Origin of Species* when it was published in 1859. He wrote to his cousin in the emotion of that moment, "I have laid it down in the full enjoyment of the feeling that one rarely experiences after boyish days, having been initiated into an entirely new province of knowledge..." (Galton, 1859). He became intrigued by the notion that change could be transmitted from one generation to the next, and then sought to apply such an investigation to human talent. Galton collected life histories of his own family members and those of his Cambridge classmates. His report in *Macmillan's Magazine* argued, "Talent is transmitted by inheritance to a very remarkable degree" (Galton, 1865). He found it not uncommon for many family members to be quite exceptional, not just a single son or daughter. He was convinced that both physical and psychological traits such as intelligence could be inherited. He also proposed,

"Everything we possess at birth is a heritage from our ancestors" (Galton, 1865). He felt that "the embryon [germinal material] of the next generation sprang forth from embryon of the previous generation." Such particles might segregate independently and were unaffected by the general state of the organism itself. In a preliminary sense, Galton described the continuity of germplasm and the segregation of unit factors for specific characters. He thus defined a "hard" concept of heredity, rather than the traditional "like begets like" of his predecessors (Olby, 1985a; Gillham, 2001a). If this were true, human nature was, therefore, much more important than human nurture. Once human heredity was understood, political and social ills could be corrected by encouraging the breeding of the best men and women. Galton came to believe that social progress then required good heredity. This would most likely foster a reformation of human society, even more than building more schools or improving housing for the poor (Cowan, 1972a).

In his 1869 book, *Hereditary Genius*, Galton attempted to apply statistics to human ability and heredity. He examined the lives of men adopted by different popes and given every advantage of wealth, and the natural sons born to eminent men. The latter were more likely to become eminent in their own right, implying the importance of heredity over acquired factors such as education or nutrition. In a similar fashion, he concluded that a close relative of an eminent man was more likely to become eminent than a more distant relative. He thought that the influence of an individual ancestor would diminish in geometrical progression as the generations passed (Galton, 1869a).

But children were not the same as their parents. Each human was considered "as a segregation of what clearly existed under a new shape, and as a regular consequence of previous conditions" (Galton, 1869b). Galton thought that acquired characters were unlikely to be transmitted to offspring. Variability certainly did occur, and two general types were evident in the human population. Slight variations among individuals were very common. Radical new types, outside the range of the general population, called "sports" were rare, but of more interest, because Galton thought that natural selection acted upon these and thus altered the species over subsequent generations (Smith, 1993). In this respect, Galton differed from his cousin, Darwin, who believed that evolution acted upon the minute variations among individuals rather than on the rare "sports."

Darwin's theory of Pangenesis proposed that each organ threw off microscopic particles called "gemmules" that circulated throughout the body to the generative organs and then formed egg and sperm which united to form a new organism. Galton proposed to test this hypothesis by transfusing blood from one breed of animal into another, and then looking for evidence of features of the transfusing parent's traits in the offspring. Galton also explained his reason for wanting to examine this issue: "To myself, as a student of heredity, it seemed of pressing importance that these postulates should be tested. If their truth could be established, the influence of Pangenesis, or the study of heredity would be increased..." (Robinson, 1979a).

Galton then solicited Darwin's help as he started a research program to test experimentally the predictions of the Pangenesis hypothesis. Galton sought different breeds of rabbits for transfusion studies in late 1869 (Galton, 1869c). He was able to transfuse between one-third and one-half of the blood from a white line into a dark line, and then bred the recipients. He reported that the first offspring of transfused rabbits showed nothing unusual (Galton, 1870). Several of the offspring did demonstrate a white star on the nose or a white forefoot, but Galton soon learned that these were common spontaneous variants among dark breeds of rabbits.

In 1871, Galton reported his breeding studies to the Royal Society. Thirteen litters after transfusion had produced 88 baby rabbits. If gemmules circulated in the blood, transfusion would have been expected to carry some white gemmules into the darker rabbits' circulation. But "in no single case has there been any evidence of alteration of breed." Galton was saddened to state, "the conclusion from this large series of experiments is not to be avoided, that the doctrine of Pangenesis, pure and simple, as I have interpreted it, is incorrect" (Galton, 1871a).

Darwin was not pleased with this attack on his position and noted that Galton had, in fact, misunderstood the theory of Pangenesis. Nowhere did Darwin state that gemmules circulated in the blood or any other bodily fluid. He did propose that the gemmules circulated from one cell to another, independent of circulation in vessels. Hence, Darwin did not believe that Pangenesis had "as yet received its death blow" (Darwin, 1871). Galton could only admit that he had indeed assumed that Darwin meant that gemmules circulated in the blood when he used the words in the original article "circulated freely" and by the "steady circulation of fluids." Such an assumption appears to have been a grave error (Galton, 1871b). Galton attempted several more transfusion experiments over the next three years, but found no positive results (Robinson, 1979a; Pearson, 1924b).

Because of all his disaffection with Pangenesis, Galton began to define his own theory of heredity. His 1872 article, "On blood relationships" presented his preliminary ideas on heredity before the Royal Society. He stated his purpose which would, in fact, occupy his attention to the rest of his life. It was to:

> analyze and describe the complicated connexion that binds the individual hereditarily, to his parents and to his brothers and sisters, and therefore by an extension of similar lines, to his more distant kinfolk. I hope by these means to set forth the doctrine of heredity in a more orderly and explicit manner than is otherwise practicable (Galton, 1872a).

He began with the fertilized ovum and argued that it contained all the hereditary elements that would create a new individual after gestation. But there were also latent elements which could be transmitted, but not immediately expressed until several generations later.

> From the well-known circumstance that an individual may transmit to his descendents ancestral qualities which he himself does not possess, we are assured that they could not have been altogether destroyed in him, but must have maintained their existence in a latent form. Therefore each individual may properly be conceived as consisting of two parts, one of which is latent and only known by its effect on his posterity, while the other is patent, and constitutes the person manifest to our senses (Galton, 1872a).

Galton recognized that there had to be a segregation of these hereditary elements. He thought this occurred randomly as the fertilized ovum formed. And not all the latent elements could be transmitted to each progeny generation. Some were lost over time, otherwise there would be, over many generations, far more than "could be packed into a single ovum" (Galton, 1872b). Galton also recognized the importance of reversions, the reappearance of a character seen in more distant generations. This implied that parents were, in fact, only partially "related to their own children." He thought that the large latent line from ancestral generations was more important from a hereditary point of view than the more direct patent line from the parents (Galton, 1872c). Unlike Darwin, Galton was also more convinced that external factors such as disease or nutrition had little effect on hereditary elements. His work in the future would continue to argue against the heredity of acquired features to any important degree. "The effects of use and disuse of limbs, and those of habits, are transmitted to posterity in only a very slight degree," he thought (Galton, 1872d).

At this point in his career, Galton began to focus on the broader human applications of heredity. Despite his training in medicine, he did not attend to individuals with specific characters or diseases that appeared to be transmitted from parent to children within specific families. Instead he looked at the implications of human heredity for society as a whole. The inheritance of human mental, physical and moral characters became "the fundamental concept of Galton's life and work" (Pearson, 1924b). He began to outline his ideas for society in an article titled "Hereditary Improvement" in *Fraser's Magazine* in 1873. He argued against the general opinion that encouraging healthy marriages for the good of society was a waste of time.

> It is objected that, philosophise as you will, men and women will continue to marry, as they have hitherto done, according to their personal liking; that any prospect of improving the race of man is absurd and chimerical, and that though inquiries into the laws of human heredity may be pursued for the satisfaction of a curious disposition, they can be of no real importance. In opposition to these objections, I maintain...that it is feasible to improve the race of man by a system which shall be perfectly in accordance with the moral sense of the present time (Galton, 1873a).

Galton again pointed out the fact that improved living conditions had not produced healthier citizens. The English upper classes possessed all the advantages of good nutrition, housing, and education, and yet continued to produce "narrow-chested men, delicate women and sickly children" (Pearson, 1924c). He argued that the good of the whole was more important than mere individual goals and aspirations.

> We must therefore try to render our individual aims subordinate to those which lead to the improvement of the race. The enthusiasm of humanity...has to be directed primarily to the future of our race, and only secondary to the well-being of our contemporaries (Galton, 1873b).

Galton certainly recognized the moral obligation to help the unfortunate in society:

> ...While helpfulness to the weak, and sympathy with the suffering, is the natural form of outpouring of a merciful and kind heart, yet that the highest action of all is to provide a vigorous national life, and that one practical and effective way of which individuals of feeble constitution can show mercy to their own kind is by celibacy, lest they should bring others into existence whose race is predoomed to destruction by the laws of Nature (Galton, 1873c).

He thus sought to improve the race in the future. He proposed to "anticipate the slow and stubborn process of natural selection, by endeavoring to breed out feeble constitutions, and petty and ignoble instincts, and to breed in those who are vigorous and noble and social" (Galton, 1873c). Galton initially called his concept of human selection "viriculture." Later he would coin the term "eugenics" to summarize his belief that the human race could be improved by encouraging reproduction of those fittest individuals in society.

Obtaining more data about heredity and families was necessary. Galton proposed to collect material on all aspects of human heredity using a series of Eugenics Record Society offices to be established around the country (Gillham, 2001b). After a time the information that was collected would help develop the science of human heredity to such a degree that Galton believed:

> ...When the truth of heredity as respects man shall have become firmly established and be clearly understood, that instead of the sluggish regard being shown towards a practical application of this knowledge, it is much more likely that a perfect enthusiasm for improving the race might develop itself among the educated classes (Galton, 1873c).

The leaders of society would then be expected to set an example for the social education of all classes by selecting their marriage partners based on fact and not merely on emotional attraction.

In December 1875, Galton composed a letter to Darwin in which he explained how offspring sometimes appeared to have characters intermediate between those of the two parents. For example, dark and light animals sometimes produced grey offspring. Galton thought that such individuals could be mosaic, a random mixture of cells expressing dark or white color, and producing en masse a grey appearance. He had also been applying his mathematical talent to postulate the segregation of different numbers of hereditary elements to produce such results:

> ...The number of units of each molecule may admit of being discovered by noting the relative number of cases of each grade of deviation from the main grayness. If there were two gemmules only, each of which might be either white or black, then in a large number of cases one-quarter would always be quite white, one-quarter quite black, and one-half would be grey. If there were three molecules, there should have been four grades of color (one quite white, three light grey, three dark gray, one quite black) and so on according to the successive lines of 'Pascal's triangle' (Galton, 1875a; Robinson, 1979b).

A vague blending of gemmules would not account for such specific numerical ratios. Galton was trying to convince Darwin that segregation occurred randomly as discrete elements were deposited in the fertilized ovum.

At this time, Galton had come to realize that "the laws of heredity are really concerned with deviations expressed in statistical units" (Cowan, 1972a). If gemmules were discrete physical entities, their random segregation from one generation to another could be expressed in mathematical formulae. Galton had read Prosper Lucas on human heredity and was convinced that the mere cataloguing of familial human characters really proved nothing about the hereditary mechanism. To understand how traits were inherited, statistics had to be applied to the pattern of segregation in human families (Galton, 1875b). He presented his ideas on heredity to the Anthropological Institute in 1876, and coined the word "stirp" to express the sum of gemmules in the fertilized ovum. The ovum appeared to be the only structure that carried such genealogical elements from parent to child. Many gemmules constituted the stirp, some developed into the fetus during pregnancy, and the majority remained latent and contributed to future generations. Among the patent gemmules, some were more potent than others. "Dominant germs" were those that eventually were expressed during embryonic development. He argued that approximately one-half of each person's heredity was derived from each parent, about one-fourth from each grandparent, one-eighth from each great-grandparent, and so on. This law of ancestral hereditary proposed a halving of contribution from each ancestor with each generation. The mean value of each trait, whether it be height, intelligence, or skin color tended to remain about the same from one generation to the next. Galton thought this law of regression explained the observed stability of such traits over time within a population (Galton, 1877).

Galton was convinced that only rarely would somatic gemmules change those in the sexual organs. Thus, somatic alterations were rarely inherited. He thought that the vast majority of alleged examples of the heredity of acquired features were a "collection of coincidences" (Galton, 1876). Because heredity counted much more than nurturing, Galton now proposed the term "eugenics" for the science which when applied would selectively encourage those who should reproduce to do so for the improvement of mankind in the future (Galton, 1876, 1883a). If such a science was to be developed and prove its worth to the educated public, Galton was convinced that he had to show that his theory worked with human data (Cowan, 1972a). The 1884 International Health Exhibition in South Kensington provided Galton the opportunity to establish an Anthropometric Laboratory. For three shillings each, 9337 people provided data as they were tested for height, weight, arm span, breathing power, strength of pulling and squeezing, hearing, vision and color sense. Galton was pleased with the mass of accumulating data and later moved the laboratory to the South Kensington Science Museum where it continued to collect more human data for another eight years (Cowan, 1972a; Forrest, 1974e).

Galton also recognized that physicians could be another important source of data on human heredity for his investigations. In 1883 he proposed "Medical Family Registers" in which a systematic collection of "hereditary peculiarities" could be amassed. He thought this would educate descendants as they became aware of any hereditary traits in their families and would, of course, expand the statistical research on human heredity (Pearson, 1924d). He discussed the idea with several prominent physicians as well as the British Medical Association (Forrest, 1974f). All endorsed the register as useful. Nonetheless, he recognized the sensitive nature of such family data.

> Most men and women should favor having their hereditary worth recorded. There may be family diseases of which they hardly dare to speak...It seems to me ignoble that a man should be such a coward as to hesitate to inform himself fully of his hereditary liabilities, and unfair that a parent should deliberately refuse to register such family hereditary facts as may serve to direct the future of his children; and which they may hereafter be very desirous of knowing. Parents may refrain from doing so through kind motives, but there is no real kindness in the end (Galton, 1883b).

Galton continued to work within the medical community and served as chairman of the Life History Sub-Committee of the Collective Investigation Committee of the British Medical Association. This group encouraged the collection and publication of quantitative data on human characteristics which could be used for statistical and hereditary research (Forrest, 1974g).

In the last decade of the century, Galton collected his opinions and statistical conclusions in two works that formed an "operational definition" of the term "hereditary." Rather than a vague "like begets like" concept as had been used earlier, he helped distinguish those characters that were in fact inherited from parents and other ancestors, and those factors acquired by life experience (Cowan, 1972b). The book *Natural Inheritance* in 1889 (Galton, 1889a), and the article "The average contribution of each of several ancestors to the total heritage of the offspring" in the *Proceedings of the Royal Society* in 1897 (Galton, 1897) brought together a lifetime of research experience. Galton recognized that his human data was still inadequate and that "by attempting to work with incomplete life histories the risk of serious error is incurred" (Galton, 1889b). His analysis of human height in parents and children did show statistical regression toward the population mean. He found that certain characters seemed to be inherited together. The stirp, Galton proposed, could be built of "minute particles of whose nature we know nothing...which are usually transmitted as aggregates" (Gillham, 2001c). And elsewhere he noted, "... in the process of transmission of inheritance, elements derived from the same ancestor are apt to appear in large groups, just as if they had clung together in the pre-embryonic stage, as perhaps they did" (Edwards, 1993).

All of the human characteristics he studied, when inherited, tended to revert to the population mean. Galton thought this meant that natural selection therefore had to operate on larger, discontinuous variations ["sports," or "saltations"] rather than on the continuous minute variations envisioned by Darwin. Variability between parent and child, and the occasional appearance of an ancestral trait [reversion] were not contradictory to heredity, but were common, and in fact, part and parcel of it. He thought, "The conditions that produce a general resemblance between the offspring and their parents must at the same time give rise to a considerable amount of individual differences" (Olby, 1985b). Galton concluded that a better understanding of human heredity would also be of service in throwing light on many questions connected with the theory of evolution (Galton, 1897).

Galton made pivotal observations toward the establishment of human heredity as a science. He attempted to define measurable characters such as height and talent and then statistically to correlate inheritance of such traits over several generations. Subsequent workers in the field of heredity such as J.A. Thomson of Edinburgh and William Bateson of Cambridge agreed that they were indebted to Galton for his concepts of inheritance, variance and reversion (Cowan, 1972b). Although his work was published widely in both popular magazines and scientific journals, it did not prove particularly interesting to the medical profession. When Galton began work on human talent in the 1860s, he collected dozens of family pedigrees and then divided them into different classes of ability. His attention then shifted from individual people and families to larger social units—classes and, indeed, society at large (Waller, 2001). His earlier work as a medical student had focused on individuals and their families. Later statistical studies required large masses of data from different social classes. His concern became not the health of individuals, but the eugenic health of society as a whole. Galton thus missed the statistic of one—the focus on an individual and on a family that formed the basis for the patient-physician relationship. Galton and many of his scientific colleagues, perhaps unconsciously, acted to replace the art of medicine with hard science. His definition of human heredity thus did not provide a working model that was particularly useful to medical practitioners in their daily professional lives.

Nine

Theories of Heredity and Medicine 1860-1900

The French physician Prosper Lucas described the development of schemes of heredity in the practice of medicine on the Continent and in England at this time. Doctors typically observed cases of illness that appeared in successive generations of a family, but it was not always easy to decide the question of how heredity related to human disease. His medical colleagues often asked Lucas, "Is it hereditary, or not?" (Lucas, P., 1847).

English physicians of the same era were also becoming more interested in heredity and disease, because it also appeared to them that many disorders did reappear in successive generations within specific families. The medical student guidebook on the patient history and physical examination from Guy's Hospital in 1851 noted that each medical history should "... give hereditary or acquired tendencies. Predisposing or exciting causes of disease should be investigated" (Newman, 1957). One physician noted in the mid-1860s, "The transmission of peculiarities of structure is a subject of considerable interest" within the medical profession (Harker, 1865).

Henry Maudsley was one of the first English alienists, physicians specializing in mental disorders. As the superintendent of the Manchester Royal Lunatic Hospital, he observed many examples of both familial physical and mental conditions in successive generations. He noted that while each person generally imitated his parents, deviations from the parental types occurred in many characteristics. The general family type produced similarities, but each individual was unique. He recognized that heredity thus produced both continuity and variety at the same time. Regarding the union of egg and sperm at reproduction, he noted, "We are ignorant of any single law of so-called vital combination...and we are totally ignorant in the present case of the element of the combining substance" (Maudlsey, 1862). His was no mere theoretical interest. "If we knew the laws of normal heredity, it might be possible with tolerable accuracy to predict the phenomena of [disease]" (Maudsley, 1863). Maudsley thought that physicians could use heredity, if it could be understood, in the guidance of patients and their families to forecast recurrence of disease in subsequent generations.

The London physician, William Sedgwick, had attempted to ascertain just such laws of heredity in a series of communications featured in the *British and Foreign Medico-Chirurgical Review* in the 1860s (Sedgwick, 1861, 1863a, b). His aim in this work was quite straightforward:

> The object of the present inquiry is to determine how far hereditary disease is subject to any rule or controlling influence capable of regulating its course and restricting its development, so as to produce some degree of order both in its appearance and transmission as opposed to the commonly accepted view that both its course and development are too uncertain and irregular for any controlling

> power to restrict the one or the other within certain and well-defined limits... (Sedgwick, 1863a).

The basic difficulty Sedgwick encountered in attempting to define such laws of inheritance was the limited family data on the occurrence of such supposedly hereditary diseases. Medical practitioners traditionally reported "rare" peculiarities, the "freaks of nature." Relatives in collateral or more remote branches of the family were often ignored (Sedgwick, 1863a). He urged physicians to take

> the history of all diseases, so as to determine how for not only the immediate parents or relations to the patient are similarly or not affected, but also the condition of the grandparents on both sides, and collateral relations in the order of their birth, [then] we shall possess a series of records of great practical value for determining the extent to which disease is liable to recur in successive generations, and also the probability of its affecting individual members of the same family (Sedgwick, 1863a).

Sedgwick clearly hoped hereditary laws would prove useful to physicians in understanding patterns of inheritance from one generation to the next and then in explaining to families the likelihood of such disease appearing in specific children born within affected families.

Given the limitations of the available data, Sedgwick was able to make some important observations that laid the foundation for work by subsequent medical practitioners in this area. Like Maudsley, he noted that while children tended to resemble their parents in many respects, each was a unique individual. "In the offspring of two dissimilar parents, there is never as a rule, complete fusion of the two parents, but a distribution of the characters peculiar to each..." The morbid character of one parent was either "completely repeated or completely absent, but not fused together in the offspring" (Sedgwick, 1863b). This important observation argued against a blending inheritance of factors from both parents, but rather the segregation of specific factors, and the frequent dominant expression of one parental type over that from the other parent.

Sedgwick also noted that certain disorders only appeared in offspring of one sex in affected families. Hemophilia was almost exclusively seen in male children born of unaffected mothers. The same pattern was observed for the skin condition ichthyosis. But in the case of cataract, some families demonstrated numerous females in successive generations with the eye defect while all the male offspring had perfect sight (Sedgwick, 1861, 1863a). More specific examples of his observations will be presented in subsequent sections of this chapter.

In some cases, a trait reappeared in a child that was totally absent in both parents, but had been present in a grandparent or prior ancestor. Families with color blindness and polydactyly were presented to illustrate this point. Such examples of atavism produced a more or less "perfect recollection of the disease itself" (Sedgwick, 1863b). This observation suggested the hereditary elements could be transmitted through subsequent generations, but not always expressed. Such "latent" hereditary elements, when expressed, increased variation within the population.

When a woman had several marriage partners, some physicians thought that the offspring of the subsequent marriages often resembled the first husband more than the current spouse. Sedgwick accepted this concept of telegony as a fact based upon studies in animals such as horses, and agreed that it also appeared to function in the human family as well (Sedgwick, 1863b).

However, progress in understanding the mechanism of human heredity was slow in coming. In 1880, one physician complained, "The study in detail of the laws governing heredity has been too much neglected" (Granville, 1880). William Aitkin, Professor of Pathology at the Army Medical School at Fort Pitt, commented to the British Medical Association that questions on human heredity were important, but "most obscure." He thought that current knowledge could not explain the role of heredity in either normal or disease states (Aitken, 1888).

This opinion would change dramatically during the decade of the 1880s in England. William Turner, Professor of Anatomy at the University of Edinburgh Medical School, commented before the B.A.A.S., "The object of heredity is, if I may say so, in the air at the present time. The journals and magazines, both scientific and literary, are continuously discussing it, and valuable treatises are appearing at frequent intervals" (Turner, 1889). Access to the expanding medical literature on heredity increased substantially after 1879 with the establishment of the *Index Medicus.* This monthly publication from the United States Surgeon General's Office contained a subject and author index of the world's medical literature. The Hereditary Disease Database (H.D.D.) used in this current work was prepared by reading the *Index* from 1879 and then compiling articles from the English medical literature (See Appendix for more details). Peak interest on the issue of heredity and disease occurred around 1890 as shown in Figure 9.1, substantiating Turner's impression. The medical historian Lopez-Beltran labeled the increasing interest on this topic in France as a "hereditarian wave" (Lopez-Beltran, 2003). The impressive rise in the number of British articles in the H.D.D. around 1890 certainly would qualify as a hereditarian tsunami.

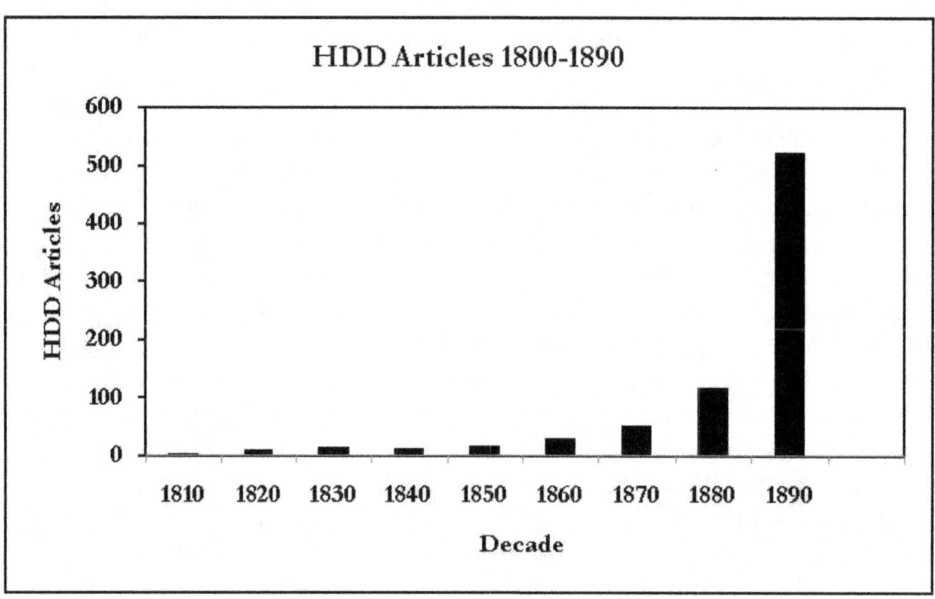

Figure 9.1

When Darwin discussed heredity during the 1860s, he expressed the opinion that the laws governing hereditary were obscure and poorly understood. The augmented interest in human heredity during the 1880s, however, raised the hope of some in the English medical community that this topic could be understood in more detail. The pathologist, Henry Campbell, thought the laws of heredity would undoubtedly be analyzed "just as Newton analyzed the complex movements of the heavenly bodies." This "second Newton" had not yet arrived on the scene, however, and heredity was still regarded as a "mysterious something" which molded the offspring into the likeness of the parents (Campbell, 1889).

The first necessary step to better understand human heredity clearly involved careful collection of data from families containing individuals with various diseases that appeared in successive generations. Horace Dobell, physician at the Royal Hospital for Diseases of the Chest, had corresponded with Darwin in 1863 regarding a standardized family history form he had devised to collect genealogical data on patients afflicted with respiratory diseases (Dobell, 1863). Darwin encouraged Dobell in his data collection efforts, because the "importance of hereditary transmission [of disease] can hardly be exaggerated..." (Darwin, 1863). The formal concept of a family tree or pedigree as a tool to trace disease from one generation to the next was outlined by C. Leslie at the Medico-Chirurgical Society of Edinburgh in 1881. Patterns of inheritance from parent to child could be systematically observed, showing both affected and unaffected persons over several generations (Leslie, 1881, 1882). The use of the pedigree to report human hereditary disease also increased dramatically during this decade. As the peak of H.D.D. references occurred around 1890, so also did the number of reports utilizing the pedigree to illustrate heredity of specific characters.

This type of graphic display of human hereditary data attracted the attention of practicing physicians because it seemed to correlate with specific patterns of disease heredity that had been noticed by the French physician Theodore Ribot. His work had been published in English in 1875 and was reviewed that same year in the British medical literature by Jonathan Hutchinson, prominent surgeon and dermatologist (Hutchinson, J., 1875). Ribot observed four basic patterns of inheritance:

1. Direct: from parent to child;
2. Indirect or reversional: an atavistic reappearance of the trait seen in any previous relative, such as a grandparent;
3. Collateral: the appearance of the trait found in another line of the family, such as an uncle or cousin;
4. Heredity of the influence—telegony: the appearance of a trait in the offspring of a subsequent marriage which was similar to that of the mother's first husband (Ribot, 1875).

Traditional inheritance meant the direct transmission of a trait from parent to child. But Ribot's patterns demonstrated that heredity could be revealed by a reversion or atavistic trait from a prior ancestor, and by the appearance of traits in collateral branches of a family. He also accepted that telogony, the heredity of influence, operated within the human community. Examples of the first three types of hereditary patterns defined by Ribot are presented in Figure 9.2. English physicians frequently mentioned Ribot's work after 1880 in describing the specific patterns of familial disease they reported in the burgeoning medical literature on heredity and disease.

Patterns of Heredity

Pedigree Charts	Ribot's Class	Clinical Examples
	Direct heredity	Ectopia lentis Huntington's chorea
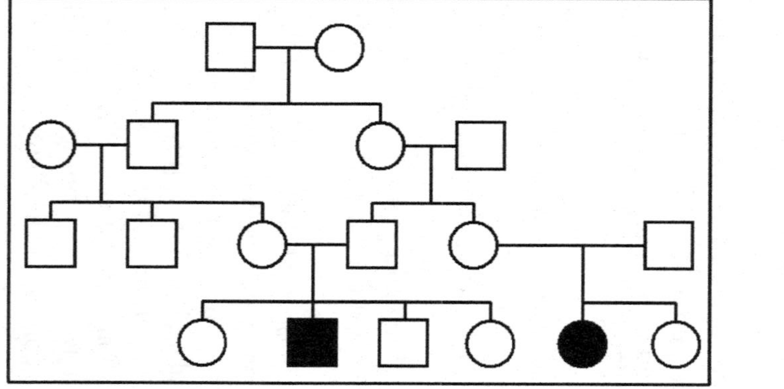	Indirect heredity	Optic atrophy Friedreich's ataxia

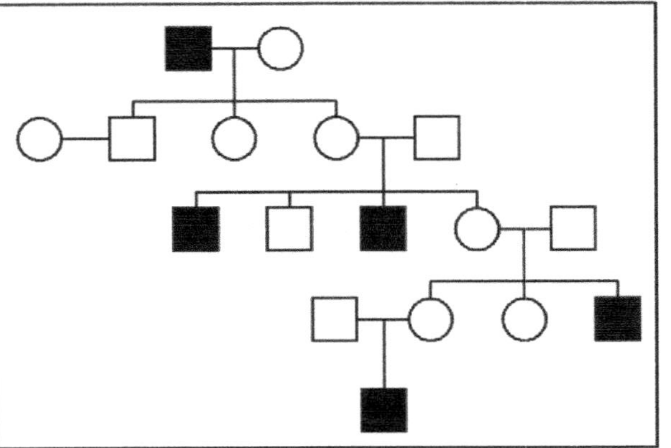

Sex-limited heredity

Colorblindness
Muscular dystrophy

Figure 9.2

MONOGRAPHS ON HEREDITY AND MEDICINE

The obstetrician R.A.O. Lithgow had become impressed with the progress that was being made toward understanding human heredity at this time. He commented at a medical society meeting, "The phenomena of inheritance are by degrees finding interpretation, and in all probability the grand law of heredity will one day be as well recognized and as firmly established as any of the so-called laws of the universe" (Lithgow, 1887). When that day came, heredity would become more than mere observation. Subsequently he noted, "[And] once the phenomenon of a natural field can be reduced to law, then that field truly becomes a science" (Lithgow, 1889c). Lithgow eventually published a monograph outlining his opinions called *Heredity* in 1889. He dedicated the work to Jonathan Hutchinson "who has strove perhaps more than any other leading authority to prove the influence of heredity in pathological processes..." The work was labeled as "the first systematic effort to trace the influence of heredity in all the main diseases which affect humanity" (Lithgow, 1889b). Lithgow believed that the germ cells held the key to the mysteries of generation and heredity. The molecules therein were the vehicles for heredity. He concluded, "All the elements and functions of the human body are subject to heredity...peculiarities, diseases and even acquired modifications" (Lithgow, 1887). Ribot had pointed out specific patterns of inheritance, and that heredity was not simply "like begetting like" (Lithgow, 1889c). A sampling of the diseases Lithgow examined to illustrate the role heredity played in causing important human diseases is presented in Table 9.1.

Another monograph entitled *Marriage and Disease* was published shortly thereafter by S.A.K. Strahan, physician and lawyer to the Middle Temple of London. His premise was "...much of disease, both physical and mental, which afflicts this and every other civilized people on the face of the Earth is to a large extent the result of hereditary transmission of a degenerate constitution or predisposition to disease" (Strahan, 1892a). While physicians were becoming more informed about heredity and disease, he observed the public was generally unaware of this important topic. As such, most people gave little attention to the inheritance of their children. Until public education was changed, the physician would "not be able to exercise to the full extent his highest function which is not to cure, but to prevent disease" (Strahan, 1892b). He also found the scheme proposed by Ribot "most useful" when analyzing the points of inheritance within specific families (Strahan, 1892c). Strahan's list of hereditary disease mirrored the one outlined by Lithgow. Evidence of asthma, hemophilia, color blindness, cataract and Bright's disease of the kidney often appeared in three to seven generations of specific families he had observed (Strahan, 1892d).

Table 9.1
Common Hereditary Diseases

Blood:
  gout, rheumatism, diabetes, scrofula, cancer, phthisis, rickets, syphilis
Nerves:
  epilepsy, chorea, insanity, hypochondriasis, neuralgia, apoplexy, paralysis
Senses:
  blindness, deafness
Degeneration:
  premature blindness, grayness, loss of teeth
Skin:
  psoriasis, leprosy
Asthma
Urinary calculi
Hemorrhoids
Albinism
Cretinism
Hernia
Icterus
Dropsy

Reference: (Lithgow, 1889a)

Public Discussions of Heredity and Disease

If physicians were hoping to alter the course of such hereditary diseases or even to prevent them, the public had to understand the role played by heredity in causing important human disease. One physician complained,

> The public, swayed by sentimental or religious influences, has compromised by acknowledging that certain terrible diseases 'run in families,' and at the same time showing no repugnance at intermarrying with such families, and no remorse at bringing into the world offspring who are deformed, diseased or depraved...It is hoped that ere long truer notions as to the inheritance of disease will filter through society and lead to practical results (Gubbin, 1894).

Bryce Duckworth, senior physician at St. Bart's Hospital, thought that for medical men,

> The study of hereditary tendency is of utmost value in clinical work, by knowledge of it, we have power to avert, not seldom, from individuals the malign evolutions of inherent potentiality. By variation of surroundings, we may accomplish much while the organism is young and plastic (Duckworth, 1889).

Both men agreed that knowledge about the mechanisms of heredity would empower physicians to diagnose and advise their patients on the best ways to ameliorate symptoms of potentially serious hereditary disease in young children.

W. Lauder utilized Ribot's patterns for hereditary disease to illustrate his Manchester "Health Lectures for the People" in 1886. He presented his findings before the public and observed that the relative proportion of a character often was derived mostly from only one parent. Less often, a true blending of parental features appeared in the offspring (Lauder, 1886). R.W. Felkin from the University of Edinburgh School of Medicine also examined examples of human heredity using Ribot's outline. He explored the topic in the public "Edinburgh Health Lectures." Felkin thought that such laws of heredity, though complex, had to consistently operate throughout the living kingdom in plants, animals and humans (Felkin, 1888).

Jonathan Hutchinson, one of the most prominent physicians of the day, had become interested in heredity and disease when he studied with Dr. Laycock at the York School of Medicine in the 1840s. After completing surgical training at St. Bart's Hospital, he then studied ophthalmology and dermatology at various London hospitals. He became a recognized consultant in these areas and continued to accumulate observations on heredity and human disease over many years (Hutchinson, H., 1946; "Jonathan Hutchinson," 1921). While the workings of inheritance sometimes "assume[d] the appearance of uncertainty and caprice," he agreed with Ribot that children received hereditary elements from both parents, and latent factors from more distant ancestors. Often a child resembled only one parent in a specific character. The reappearance of an atavistic trait from a grandparent certainly showed that hereditary elements could be latent at times and yet had passed unseen through several generations. Some hereditary tendencies might be "conditional," only appearing clinically when an exciting trigger such as an inadequate diet was present. Other hereditary characters were "unconditional," and appeared without any inciting factors. Hutchinson concluded that in his experience acquired characters could become hereditary and then reappear in subsequent generations. He believed that when acquired early in life or long ago in the history of the family, it was more likely that hereditary transmission of the trait would occur. Maternal impressions were different in his mind than other acquired characters. He concluded, "We are entitled to put aside the flimsy and often absurd statements by which the attempt is made, even by those who should know better, to bolster up such stories" (Hutchinson, J., 1890a). Hutchinson also believed that the first father continued to influence the offspring in subsequent pregnancies by a different father. He had observed the phenomenon of telegony in breeding of horses and other animals. He felt that the semen from the first father might alter the female ova which then would further influence the development of subsequent pregnancies by different fathers (Hutchinson, J., 1889b, 1890a, b). Hutchinson summarized his thoughts on heredity and human disease in an extensive series of lectures delivered before the Royal College of Surgeons in June 1881 (Hutchinson, J., 1881a, b).

John McKendrick from the University of Glasgow reviewed the current understanding of heredity at the cellular level in a discussion before the Philosophical Society of Glasgow in 1888. He presented recent microscopic observations from Germany on the behavior of nuclear chromatin during cell reproduction. W. Flemming had noted the longitudinal splitting of the chromatin during cell division. K. Rabl thought there were different sizes and shapes of chromatin threads characteristic of each cell. In 1888, Waldeyer labeled the nuclear chromatin threads as "chromosomes." During the 1890s, Theodor Boveri incorporated all of these observations to explain the duplication and segregation of specific chromosomes from one generation to the next in cell division (Stubbe, 1972). McKendrik stated that fertilization involved the fusion of one sperm cell with one egg. The number of "chromatin loops" [chromosomes] in each was identical. Daughter cells formed by subsequent division each received equal numbers of such chromatin loops, hence receiving elements from both male and female parents. He believed that all somatic cells then contained equal quantities of hereditary material from both parents (McKendrick, 1888). He cited work done by Strasburger in 1884 that developed the idea that the chromatin material, the nucleoplasm, regulated the cellular economy. He concluded that, "All metabolic changes in the cell substance are controlled and directed by the nucleoplasm" (McKendrick, 1888).

In the same year, J. Arthur Thomson, Professor of Natural History at the University of Aberdeen and Lecturer in Zoology at the University of Edinburgh Medical School, outlined the current understanding of the general laws of heredity in a presentation to the Royal Society of Edinburgh. He reviewed August Weissman's concept of the germplasm located within the cell nucleus and possessing a "definite chemical and special molecular constitution." The observation that both parents clearly contributed features to their offspring was mirrored in the cytological studies of Van Beneden and Boveri which demonstrated that both male and female nuclei contributed equally to the formation of the nucleus in the fertilized ovum. Therefore, variation occurred primarily by the "intermingling of the sex elements" at fertilization. Natural selection could then operate on such population variants. Both Weissman and Francis Galton argued that changes in the germplasm were the source of altered structure or function that then could become hereditary. If environmental factors did reach deeply into the ovum or sperm and changed the germplasm, rare examples of the inheritance of acquired characters might be explained (Thomson, 1888).

By the end of the nineteenth century, English physicians had been well informed about the novel ideas on heredity and disease. Three major presentations at that time summarized current thinking in this area. T.H. Bryce reviewed the topic at the opening of the new anatomy building at Queen Margaret College, University of Glasgow. He discussed how the germplasm was arranged into chromosomes that were the hereditary vehicles, carrying inheritance from one generation to the next. The meiotic reduction division of the chromosomes involved in the formation of egg and sperm was viewed as an important mechanism for segregating and assorting traits from both parents during sexual reproduction (Bryce, 1896). George Savage gave the Presidential Address to the Neurological Society in 1897 and emphasized the increasing interest in the field of heredity and nervous diseases. He also outlined the current views on the germplasm as the chemical substance that carried hereditary factors from parents to their children (Savage, 1897).

Finally, in March 1900, D.J. Hamilton, Professor of Pathology at the University of Aberdeen, summarized the state of human heredity and disease before the Edinburgh Medico-Chirurgical Society. His remarks and comments from the audience gave a good sense of physicians' opinions in this regard at that time. He reviewed the role of chromosomes in carrying hereditary material to successive generations. Hereditary traits only arose as variations within the germplasm, the hereditary material, of which chromosomes were comprised. There was no credible evidence that disease caused by external factors such as injury or infection could subsequently be transmitted from parent to child. And in a similar fashion, the notions that maternal impression and telegony could serve as sources of hereditary human disease simply did not occur (Hamilton, 1900). Despite the fact that they appreciated the science that been presented, the comments from the audience indicated that the majority of physicians, based upon clinical experience, still believed in the hereditary transmission of acquired characters (Hamilton, 1900). Another physician with an interest in heredity and disease, G. Archdall Reid, agreed that while the scientific community had concluded with Galton and Weismann that acquired characters were rarely, if ever, inherited, medical men had "curiously neglected consideration of this matter, assuming it was fact" (Reid, 1900).

On the heredity of acquired characters

At the beginning of this era in 1860, however, most medical men agreed with Darwin that the inheritance of acquired traits was a commonplace observation encountered in medical practice. Many physicians had seen or heard of a family in which a parent had been blinded in one eye and then produced a child also blind in the same eye. The experimental work of Brown-Sequard from 1850 to 1892 attempted to show in animals that inflicted injuries could indeed result in birth defects among offspring. He surgically severed the sciatic nerves or spinal cord tracts of guinea pigs. Offspring sometimes developed epileptic-like seizures or deformities of the ears, eyes or hind limb toes. Brown-Sequard regarded this as evidence for the inheritance of acquired traits (Brown-Sequard, 1875).

However, Francis Galton was not impressed. On the theory of pangenesis, such an injured part must throw off altered gemmules which then circulated to the sexual organs and subsequently resulted in altered egg or sperm. This seemed unlikely in his opinion (Galton, 1875). He noted that attempts to reproduce Brown-Sequard's work in France and Germany repeatedly failed. Morphological anomalies occurred in about 2% of all guinea pig offspring, which was about the frequency observed in this experimental series. Epilepsy was, in fact, a common finding in control animals that had never had a surgical operation. Emil Guyenot summarized such reports of acquired characters as "accidental coincidences mixed with fantasy" (Blacher, 1982a).

The German zoologist August Weismann accepted Darwin's theory of pangenesis, including the heredity of acquired characters, when he began his career in the 1870s. But by 1883 when he published *Essays on Heredity*, he had reconsidered his opinion:

> The inheritability of acquired changes is completely unsubstantiated either by simple observation or by experiment. The literature contains a number of instances which are claimed to prove that injuries—the loss of the finger, a scar, a wound received earlier, etc.—are inherited by the offspring, but in all of these instances the preceding history of like events is obscure, and therefore scientific criticism is impossible (Blacher, 1982b).

Weismann drew upon Galton's ideas on the continuity of the hereditary elements from one generation to the next. He coined the term "germplasm" for the vehicle of heredity. Regarding heredity of acquired traits he said:

> If the germplasm is not formed anew in each individual, but derived from that which preceded it, its structure, and above all its molecular constitution, cannot depend upon the individual...The tendencies of heredity, of which the germplasm

> is the bearer, depend upon this very molecular structure, and hence only those characters can be transmitted to successive generations which had been previously inherited, viz., those characters which are potentially contained in the germplasm. It also follows that those other characters which have been acquired by the influence of special external conditions, during the lifetime of the parent, cannot be transmitted at all (Blacher, 1982c).

Critics claimed that Weismann's concept of the stability of the germplasm was untenable because offspring never exactly duplicated their parents. Variation occurred, Weismann thought, by the mixture of hereditary elements from male and female parents during sexual reproduction. A less common source of change might occur by changes within the germplasm itself. He recognized, "... influences of different kinds might produce corresponding minute alterations in the molecular structure of the germplasm, and as the latter was, according to our supposition, transmitted from one generation to another, it follows that such changes would be hereditary" (Blacher, 1982d). Such changes in the molecular structure of the germplasm would be rare and not due to such factors as injuries acquired by a parent.

Weismann then began a long experiment over at least ten years that involved breeding white mice whose tails had been removed. After 22 generations, none of the 1,592 offspring demonstrated a tail that was any shorter than the original parental mice in the experimental series. He concluded:

> ... all permanent, i.e., hereditary variations of the body proceed from the primary modifications of the primary constituent of the germ; and that neither injuries, functional hypertrophy or atrophy, structural variations due to the effects of temperature or nutrition, nor any other influence of environment on the body, can be communicated to the germ cells, and so be transmissible (Blacher, 1982e).

Weismann thus argued that the germplasm was the source of variability through sexual reproduction, but varied little itself and remained in a state of "almost absolute constancy" over long periods of time. The germplasm was "at once readily variable and yet slow to vary" (Blacher, 1982f).

The controversy on the inheritance of acquired features was a frequent topic of discussion at professional science and medical meetings before 1900. J. Arthur Thomson could not accept the strict injunction against such inheritance. He reviewed opinions of Galton and Weismann before the Royal Society of Edinburgh in 1899 and argued that environmental factors must reach deeply into organisms and alter the germplasm, hence allowing the transmission of acquirements (Thomson, 1889). Jonathan Hutchinson labeled this dispute as a "logomachy," a battle only of words. He thought that the life experiences of parents clearly had an influence on the germ cells. Such tendencies could then be passed on to the offspring via sexual congress (Hutchinson, J., 1889a, 1896). H.C. Pope, President of the West London Medico-Chirurgical Society, was of the opinion that variation arose by the action of environmental factors during gestation itself (Pope, 1889). Richard C. Lucas, surgeon at Guy's Hospital, presented data showing that the modern fifth finger was becoming shortened and more crooked over time because of excessive writing which forced the digit into a cramped position. He thought the little finger was going the way of the little toe (Lucas, R.C., 1892). In a similar fashion, R.H. Charles examined the tibia, femur and astralagus bones in the Punjabi and European races. He explained the differences by the generation of constant pressure from squatting for long periods of time as was the Indian fashion (Charles, 1893). Clinical experience of the dentist E.S. Talbot and the obstetrician H. Barbour also favored the inheritance of acquired characters (Talbot, 1984; Barbour, 1894).

However, Thomas Oliver, physician to the Royal Victoria Infirmary at Newcastle, and Professor of Medicine at the University of Durham Medical School, agreed with Weismann that the cell nucleus carried the germplasm that produced "the tendency to variation." He thought this structure could not be influenced by "the character of the protoplasm that surrounds it" within the germ cell (Oliver, 1900). By the 1890s, more physicians came to see that there was little accurate evidence for the hypothesis that acquired characters could, in fact, be inherited. When W.C. Johnston discussed Darwin's and Weismann's views on this topic before the Medico-Chirurgical Society of Montreal, he noted that attempts to produce new varieties by altering the environment of experimental animals had consistently failed (Johnston, 1886). By 1897, Henry J. Campbell, anatomist and bacteriologist at Guy's Hospital, also concluded that sexual reproduction was the primary source of variation, and that injuries and other acquired characters had not been shown truly to be hereditary (Campbell, 1897).

MATERNAL IMPRESSIONS

A traditional explanation for birth defects had been that the mother was somehow frightened or stressed during pregnancy, and that this alteration in homeostasis was transmitted to the developing fetus and produced altered anatomy or function. Examples have been given in previous sections of cleft lip, abnormal hands and feet, blindness and a myriad of other birth defects that were believed to result from these so-called "maternal impressions."

During the period of 1860-1900, English physicians continued to explain birth defects by such a mechanism that was really a form of acquired abnormality. As one physician summarized the matter:

> Whatever be the explanation of the fact, it seems fairly proved to be by no means an infrequent occurrence that women who have, during pregnancy, been subject to some strong maternal impression, give birth to children with a deformity, in fact, which shows a marked likeness to the object which produced the impression (Liston, 1865).

For example, a woman in the third month of pregnancy was watching an organ grinder, when his monkey suddenly jumped on her back and frightened her badly. Her daughter was then born with the left arm and trunk looking like those parts of the monkey. The arm was "long, thin and withered looking...skin deeply stained with dark pigment and covered with an abundant crop of dark, tawny hair." In another case, a "nervous and very sensitive" woman shook hands with a man who had lost his third and fourth digits in an accident. When her child was born, it lacked middle digits of the hands and feet. She then had four normal children. During her last pregnancy, she again encountered the same man, again shook his hand, and subsequently delivered another child with the same abnormalities of the hands and feet (Liston, 1865).

A circus elephant frightened a mother of two healthy girls during her third pregnancy. A baby girl was born with double cleft lip. Three subsequent healthy children were then born. Another child was born with webbed fingers, and a final child had single cleft lip. Family history revealed a sibling of the father also had double cleft lip (Murray, 1860).

Another report analyzed five such cases. In one example, a woman at the fifth or six-month of pregnancy observed a child crying after he had smashed his fingers when a window closed on them. Her baby was then born with absent fingers. Two pregnant women saw a man having only one arm. Both women then bore children also having a single arm each. Another pregnant lady was bitten on the hand by a dog. Her baby was born lacking one hand. A scorpion stung another pregnant lady on the neck. Her baby was then born with a large mole on the same side of its neck. In a final case, a woman developed a boil on her chest during pregnancy and delivered a child with a boil on its chest as well (Whitfield, 1862).

The anatomist, John Struthers, from the University of Aberdeen Medical School recorded several series of hand malformations. In one instance, a child was born with syndactyly, the digits fused together making the baby's hands look like feet. No one else in the family had any hand abnormalities. The mother explained the cause as the result of a strange dream she had experienced during the third month of the pregnancy. She recalled that she imagined a man was murdered outside her home, and the perpetrator had then cut off the victim's fingers. The dream greatly troubled her throughout the rest of the pregnancy. She was not surprised when the baby was born with malformed hands (Struthers, 1863).

Another family was reported to have children in four subsequent generations affected with webbed fingers and triphalangeal thumbs [having two joints instead of the normal one]. Family tradition explained that the defect had appeared after a savage dog had attacked the great grandmother during her first pregnancy. In defending herself, her hands were badly torn. Her child was then born with the defects of his hands which passed on to subsequent generations (Barber, 1864). A similar dog attack that resulted in bitten hands of another pregnant woman produced a female child with webbed hands, polydactyly and malformed thumbs. The defect was subsequently transmitted through five generations (Morris, 1865).

Other abnormalities of the hands and feet continued to be attributed to maternal fright. Four generations of a family were affected by a disorder including absent thumbs, webbed fingers, absent second toes and webbed toes. The family explained the origin of the defects as the result of a fright suffered by the great-great-grandmother during her pregnancy (Montgomery-Smith, 1888). A report before the Clinical Society of London involved a family with 16 of 36 people in three generations affected by "lobster claw" deformity [ectrodactyly] in which the middle digits where absent. The great-grandmother was frightened when a beggar with deformed hands came to her door (Parker and Robinson, 1887a, b). The same anomaly in another family involving 24 of 36 members in three generations was attributed to the great-great-grandmother being frightened by an actual lobster during her pregnancy (Anderson, 1886).

During his studies in ophthalmology at the Royal London Ophthalmic Hospital, Jonathan Hutchinson had encountered many children born blind. He noted one family where the mother reported that she suffered from "great anxiety" during the pregnancy that her child would be born blind. Her fear was realized when the child was born and could not see (Hutchinson, J., 1866). Another eye disorder, retinitis pigmentosa, was sometimes associated with deafness. In one family of seven children, four were affected with the disorder. During the early phase of her third pregnancy, the mother was frightened by a robber, and fainted. Her child was subsequently born affected, as were three of four later children. The author of the note postulated, "It seems not improbable that the shock received by the mother when the susceptibility of her nervous system was exalted by pregnancy, was actually the origin of the family disorder that developed itself in the next generation" (Smith, 1882).

A large number of such reports claiming birth defects on the basis of maternal impression appeared during the 1880s. Robert Marcus Gunn, surgeon at the Royal London Ophthalmic Hospital, observed that mothers often attributed fright early in pregnancy as the cause of babies being born with all kinds of eye defects, including anophthalmia [absence of the eyeballs] (Gunn, 1889). In one family, a pregnant lady suffered a fright and her daughter was born with nystagmus, cataract and aniridia [absence of the iris]. The condition was subsequently transmitted to two of three children in the next generation (Lang, 1885). Francis Cross, surgeon at the Bristol Eye Hospital, reported the unfortunate case of the woman who had suffered two frightening episodes during her pregnancy. Not only did a dog bite her, but she had also witnessed her cook trying to stab another servant in her kitchen. The product of this pregnancy was a child with aniridia (Cross, 1885).

A series of 100 families with ichthyosis, a dry skin condition, was analyzed at this time. One mother explained the birth of her affected son by recalling that halfway through her pregnancy, she had developed a craving for table salt and consumed 1 oz. salt on bread several times each day. She believed this had caused a drying of the baby's skin to such an extent that the disease ichthyosis had developed after birth (Gaskoin, 1880).

The ear was also liable to malformation unless pregnancy was calm and relaxed. Simeon Snell, ophthalmic surgeon at the Royal Infirmary in Sheffield, noted a baby born with an absent left ear. The mother revealed that she had been severely frightened at the fifth month of pregnancy when an insect had landed on the side of her own face (Snell, 1887).

A circus in London had been exhibiting a two-headed nightingale. One pregnant woman was shown a picture of the unusual bird and began to worry that her baby would somehow look like this "freak of nature." At six months of gestation, she went into premature labor and delivered conjoined twins with two heads and one body. About the same time, another pregnant woman actually saw the bird at the circus and fainted. She also delivered conjoined twins. The author of this medical report stated, "It is difficult to escape the conclusion that there is a relation of cause and effect between this premonitory dread and its final fulfillment" (Clark, 1886).

The genitals too could be affected by events during pregnancy. A runaway horse frightened a woman in the third month of her pregnancy. Her daughter was subsequently born with a large clitoris. Four subsequent daughters also were born with a similar defect. All died shortly after birth. Post-mortem examination in one revealed adrenal cortical hyperplasia. The mother also had an inguinal hernia. The author proposed that the hernia acted as a predisposing cause in conjunction with the deep maternal impression altering the normal differentiation of the genital system (Phillips, 1887). Once acquired, the defect was then repeated in subsequent pregnancies.

Mental defect was also attributed to such maternal impressions as well. One mother experienced a bad dream at the fifth month of pregnancy. Her son was born an idiot. The physician author agreed that there was "no doubt that the explanation given by the parent was correct" (Lee, 1888). F.N. Manning, Inspector General of the Insane in New South Wales, Australia, reported a family in which three of the children were imbeciles. The mother reported problems with all three of those pregnancies. In one, she had suffered sunstroke, in another, she had fallen from a horse, and in the last, she had strained herself while cutting down a tree (Manning, 1886).

Certainly, the most famous of these maternal impression cases involved John Merrick. His story came to public attention in 1884 near London Hospital at a storefront that displayed a large sign with a hideous painting of a creature called "The Elephant Man." A traveling show had leased the storefront and charged admission for the public to gape at Merrick who was terribly deformed. Frederick Treves, a surgeon and lecturer in anatomy at the hospital, noticed the sign and paid the proprietor a shilling for a private viewing. He was both shocked and intrigued by what he saw that day, and arranged for Merrick to visit the hospital (Montagu, 1979a).

John Merrick explained that he had been born with a misshapen head and oddly proportioned limbs. Over time, large bony growths covered his eye and jaw. Huge sacks of dark skin covered his back. His right arm was swollen and stiff, but the other was finely formed. His legs looked like the right arm, and another ugly flap of dark skin protruded from his chest. He stated that his mother had been attacked and crippled by a circus elephant during the pregnancy. His deformities were, he believed, the result of that prenatal influence (Montagu, 1979b). Treves gave Merrick his business card. Merrick then returned to the public show again, not expecting to ever see the surgeon again. But, in fact, the two men developed a long-term relationship, and Treves presented detailed reports describing Merrick's condition to the Pathological Society of London in 1884 and 1885 (Treves, 1884, 1885a, b).

A short time later, the London police decided that the show was an outrage against public morals, and deported Merrick and his huckster. They toured Europe for several more years until 1886, when the Belgian authorities again banned the public exhibition. The showman decamped with all their funds and gave Merrick a one-way ticket to London. When he arrived at Liverpool Station, the public was again outraged, and the police escorted the unfortunate creature to an isolated waiting room in the station. Merrick then produced Treves's business card that suggested to the authorities that someone might come for him and solve the crisis at the train station. Treves did respond to the call from the police and took Merrick back to London Hospital. Clearly the man had no way to support himself. F.C. Carr Gavin of the hospital governing board arranged a public subscription to provide for his maintenance. Monies were provided to establish Merrick in two rooms of the hospital as a permanent guest (Montagu, 1979c).

Merrick became an object of curious interest for upper-class persons in London at that time. He was visited by many ladies in society and was flattered by their kindly attention to him. The Prince and Princess of Wales also came by. She presented him with her picture which he treasured for the rest of his short life (Montagu, 1979d). Merrick was happy at the hospital until the end came in 1890. His head had grown so large that he was required to sleep sitting upright, supporting it always on his knees. One night he appeared to lay down, but the massive skull fell backward, dislocating his neck and severing his spinal cord. His skeleton was subsequently presented to the Anatomical Museum at the London Hospital Medical College (Montagu, 1979e).

Over time, many physicians came to conclude that such explanations of birth defects supposedly resulting from "maternal impressions" were very "fanciful" (Manning, 1886). By 1890, physicians became even less convinced that such maternal impressions played any important role in causing birth defects. William Sym, ophthalmic surgeon at the Royal Infirmary in Edinburgh, reported a family with four albino children affected with decreased vision and nystagmus. In this instance, the mother could give no account "of those frights during pregnancy or maternal impressions to which patients so frequently attribute the peculiarities of their children" (Sym, 1890). In another family, the last of the children was born with cleft lip and palate, polydactyly and clubfeet. The parents could provide no history of "maternal impressions" (Marsh, 1889).

After the peak of activity in utilizing such maternal impressions to explain a host of birth defects, a marked decline in such reports occurred. The use of this explanation as a mechanism to explain birth defects essentially ceased after 1892. Relying on parents' account for the sudden appearance of unusual anomalies was no longer considered an adequate scientific interpretation of the facts. Theories in heredity and embryonic development were changing. British physicians were developing a more sophisticated understanding of hereditary defects that no longer could accept such traditional explanations.

Ten

Hereditary Disease in Medical Practice 1860-1900

During the latter half of the Victorian era, medical specialties began to evolve within the larger medical community in Britain. Traditionally, there had been a definite anti-specialty sentiment among medical men, as all physicians were expected to be competent generalists. One observer noted, "The narrowness of the mere specialist is to be guarded against in all departments of medicine" ("The narrowness of specialisation," 1870). By the 1880s, however, leaders in eye disease felt the time was right to plan an ophthalmological society. Because this specialty touched every branch of medicine and surgery, a broad membership could be useful to share information amongst all those who worked at "ophthalmic subjects." William Bowman and Jonathan Hutchinson from the Royal London Ophthalmic Hospital helped organize the Ophthalmological Society of the United Kingdom. The first meeting was held in June 1880 with 28 physicians in attendance. The Ninth International Conference of Ophthalmology was subsequently held in London the following year, further emphasizing the growing prominence of British eye disease specialists (Newell, 1980).

Eye Diseases

The Ophthalmological Society began publication of its *Transactions* in 1881 and reported many examples of the apparent role of heredity in diseases or malformations of the eye. H.R. Swanzy, ophthalmic surgeon at Adelaide Hospital and President of the Society, reported two families with ptosis, a congenital drooping of the eyelids. In one example, two brothers were affected; in the other, three brothers were affected, as were three children of one of these siblings, suggesting direct inheritance from parent to child (Swanzy, 1897). A similar direct pattern of inheritance was observed in a four-generation family with strabismus, a muscle imbalance causing the eyes to turn inward. The author noted, "Evidence seems fairly conclusive as to transmission" (Lang, 1888).

Myopia, or nearsightedness, was also commonly noted in parents and children of certain families. In one case, both parents were affected. All their children—four sons and four daughters—were similarly affected (MacLehose, 1897). Hyperopia, or far-sightedness, was likewise noted in a parent and a child (Sedgwick, 1863a). These conditions appeared to demonstrate direct inheritance.

D.C. Lloyd Owen, from the Birmingham and Midland Eye Hospital, reported a five-generation family with nystagmus, a rhythmic twitching of the eyes. Only the males were affected, and the trait appeared to be passed through unaffected females (Lloyd Owen, 1882). The same pattern of inheritance was observed in another four-generation family. M'gillivray felt that this was the same sex-limited pattern of heredity that had been seen in other families with hemophilia and pseudohypertrophic muscular paralysis (M'gillivray, 1895). Edward Nettleship from the Royal London Ophthalmic Hospital found another large family with nystagmus. Again, only males were affected and females were transmitters, but all the affected males also demonstrated amblyopia [decreased vision in one eye] and striking blue eye color. Unaffected males and females in the family all had brown eyes. This could be an example of the heredity of several traits in combination, later to be called linkage (Nettleship, 1886).

Several other families with nystagmus demonstrated a different pattern of heredity. F.W. Burton-Fanning of the Norfolk and Norwich Hospital observed a family in which males and females were affected in an equal number. Affected children were only born of affected parents (Burton-Fanning, 1895). Wood and Lawford reported similar families (Wood, 1896; Lawford, 1888). This was consistent with a direct form of heredity. Robert Doyne from the Oxford Eye Hospital commented that these findings might be explained by Weismann's theory, i.e., an external factor such as a failure of nutrition might have induced the "metaplasm" to reproduce a less fully developed type than was usually present in man, which resulted in a "partial reversion to a primitive condition" (Lawford, 1888).

Albinism was another familial eye condition associated with nystagmus. Affected children had very fair skin, light flaxen hair and absent pigment in the iris of the eyes. Lawford reported two families with dark parents and about half the children affected with albinism. In one example, a woman had married twice, but had affected children by only one partner (Lawford, 1889a). William G. Sym from the Royal Infirmary in Edinburgh reported another family with dark parents, and again about half the children affected (Sym, 1890a). Streatfield, from the Royal London Ophthalmic Hospital, observed three albino families. In one case, an unaffected woman had affected children in both her marriages to unaffected men (Streatfield, 1882).

Francis Galton examined the inheritance of eye color in three generations from 168 families. He calculated regressions from the data and concluded there was no change in the percentage of persons with different eye colors in the different generations. He argued that eye color did not produce "blended" offspring as height did. Eye color behaved as a discrete hereditary element (Galton, 1886). A confirmation of Galton's conclusion came from the inheritance pattern of the variation of eye color observed in a large family by William Sedgwick. The iris in these cases looked like the coat color of a tortoiseshell cat. Three generations of one family were affected. One affected parent passed the trait to 21 of his children—five females and 16 males. (Sedgwick, 1861a). This character acted like a discrete hereditary element and exhibited a direct pattern for inheritance.

The inability to recognize colors [color blindness] was also commonly observed in several generations of specific families. Population surveys found 3-4% of males affected, but only 0.1% of females with a similar disability (Bickerton, T.H., 1886; Bickerton, M.T., 1886). Lord Rayleigh, Cavendish Professor of Experimental Physics at Cambridge, chaired a research team that surveyed the incidence of color blindness among different classes of English society. This study found that overall about 4.2% of males and 0.4% of all females were affected. Different social groups, however, were found to have different rates of color blindness. Eton students had only 2.5% affected, while populations that tended to inbreed had higher frequencies. The Society of Friends (Quakers) had 5.9% affected males, Jews had 4.9% affected, while a deaf and dumb school had 13.7% colorblind males (Rayleigh, 1892; Carter, 1890). Red hair also seemed to be associated with the colorblind character. At Marlborough College, 9% of the boys had red hair, but of those with color blindness, 42% also had red hair. Other studies showed an association between red hair and color blindness in Jewish boys (Roberts, C., 1882). The inheritance pattern for the color blind trait was well known at the time. It usually was transmitted via unaffected woman and then affected only male children (Wolfe, 1879). Extensive pedigrees were reported reaching back several centuries showing the typical pattern of affected males born of unaffected daughters who were born of affected fathers (Legg, 1881; Pole, 1893). J.W. Legg had observed the same pattern of sex-limited inheritance for hemophilia.

In contrast, hereditary blindness did not follow one specific pattern for its inheritance in all families. William Sedgwick reported cases with direct inheritance in three successive generations, but only females appeared to be affected. In other families, an unaffected father had an affected brother, and then bore five affected sons of his own (Sedgwick, 1862, 1863a). Sym reported a family with direct heredity from an affected mother to three affected sons (Sym, 1890b). One particular type of hereditary blindness—Leber's disease—was believed to result from optic neuritis. Jonathan Hutchinson observed two affected daughters born of unaffected first cousin parents (Hutchinson, 1866). J.B. Story of St. Mark's Eye Hospital noted this indirect pattern of inheritance in two families with normal parents producing blind children of both sexes (Story, J.B., 1885; Story, J.A., 1885).

Malformations of the structures of the eyes were frequently observed to "run in families." Sedgwick reported direct transmission of coloboma irides [a wedge-shaped defect in the iris] through three generations (Sedgwick, 1861a). Complete absence of the iris [aniridia] could be passed from an affected parent to several offspring (Lang, 1885). Very small eyes [microphthalmia] often passed in a direct fashion from parent to child to grandchild over three generations in the families observed by Herbert Page of St. Mary's Hospital (Page, 1874).

Opacities of the lenses [cataracts] were common in certain families as well. In some examples, parents had normal eyes, but several children were born affected with cataracts (M'Hardy, 1879; Streatfield, 1882). More commonly, an affected parent transmitted the defect to several of the family's children (Bell, 1868; Solomon, 1885). C.S. Jeaffreson, from the Eye Infirmary in Newcastle on Tyne, reported such direct transmission as evidence for "strong hereditary tendencies" (Jeaffreson, 1886). G.A. Berry from the Royal Infirmary in Edinburgh reported cataracts in five generations of a family. Both sexes were affected; transmission was directly from parent to child in all cases. About half of the offspring were affected (Berry, 1888). Similar patterns for cataract inheritance were noted in several four-generation families (Thompson, T., 1889; Thompson, J.A., 1889). Equal numbers of males and females typically were affected. D. Gunn, from the Hospital for Sick Children at Great Ormond Street, observed cataract in three generations of a family, but in this case only males were affected (Gunn, D., 1898).

Cataracts frequently appeared in certain families in conjunction with ectopia lentis [dislocation of the lenses]. In some cases, parents were normal-sighted, but had several affected children (Hulme, 1862). In the majority of families, however, ectopia lentis was present in successive generations. A characteristic direct pattern of inheritance was typically noted. Wordsworth observed five affected generations in one family (Wordsworth, 1878), as did Morton in another family (Morton, S., 1879). Miles, from the Manchester Royal Eye Hospital, noted a family in which an affected father passed the trait to 8 of his 13 children. In another family, the mother had been married twice. By the first husband, she had three normal children. Her second husband had ectopia. Together they had ten children, and seven were affected, again supporting direct transmission of the trait from one parent only (Miles, 1883).

In other families, defects of the cornea seemed to be hereditary. The eye appeared normal at birth, but opacities developed. The trait appeared to be directly transmitted from one parent to the children (Oliver, C., 1892). Glaucoma [increased pressure within the globe] often followed a similar direct pattern for inheritance. Many families were described with an affected parent producing affected children of both sexes (Miles, 1883; Robertson, 1891; Smith, P., 1894).

Hereditary optic atrophy generally followed a rather different pattern for heredity. In rare families, an affected parent produced affected offspring (Batten, 1896; Suckling, 1887a). In the majority of cases, parents were unaffected and produced affected offspring of both sexes. The total number of affected children was generally less than the normal children in such families (Higgens, 1881; Ogilvie, 1896; Browne, A., 1888; Browne, E., 1888; Taylor, S.J., 1892; Taylor, J., 1891). One case had an affected woman whose unaffected sister then had an affected daughter in a collateral branch of the family (Suckling, 1887a). John Lawford noted another family in which three children and three first cousins were affected with optic atrophy. Such examples were not strictly "hereditary," meaning directly transmitted from parent to child (Lawford, 1889b). S.A. Habersham from the Marylebone General Dispensary observed the same character in first and second cousins of another family (Habershon, 1888), consistent with the pattern for indirect or collateral inheritance.

Ophthalmologists were particularly impressed with all the familial eye diseases they encountered in clinical practice. Numerous physicians collected pedigrees and then shared their findings in publications and at medical society presentations. Their work became more systematized as they began to identify characteristic patterns of inheritance for different disorders. Progressive vision loss due to deposition of a dark material in the retina of the eye [retinitis pigmentosa] has a striking clinical presentation. Jonathan Hutchinson recalled the case of a man who presented to the Royal London Ophthalmic Hospital in an agitated state. He cried, "I am going blind, Sir! You can do nothing for me, I know! It is in the family and has been for centuries, and at the present time I know more than thirty who are either blind or on their way to it. When once it begins it always goes on..." (Hutchinson, 1882). The inexorable progression of blindness certainly did appear to run in families and prompted Hutchinson to collect such histories in detail. In his own series of 23 families, he noted consanguinity in eight marriages (Hutchinson, 1869, 1882). Families were observed by other physicians in which unaffected parents who were first or second cousins also went on to produce affected children of both sexes (Davidson, 1886; Symonds, 1898). In other families, no bloodline connection was known between the unaffected parents, and yet a similar pattern of affected children was observed (Davidson, 1886; Simi, 1867; Snell, 1886; Cant, 1886). This was characteristic of the indirect form of inheritance. Edward Nettleship reported a different scheme for the inheritance of retinitis in a large family he examined. In this case, only males were affected. Unaffected females appeared to transmit the defect to their sons. Unaffected daughters then could transmit the defect to their sons in the subsequent generations. This appeared to be the same sex-limited pattern of inheritance noted for hemophilia (Nettleship, 1886). Other varieties of retinitis pigmentosa, such as choroiditis, were passed in a more direct fashion from parent to child (Gunn, R.M., 1882; Doyne, 1899;

Hutchinson, 1876). Here was an example of three types of one disease that could be classified by their specific hereditary pattern.

Certain people appeared to have better vision under specific light conditions. Individuals with night blindness cannot see well under low light intensity. This character can be directly transmitted from parent to child (Atwood, 1897). In other families, the same trait appeared to be transmitted only to male children through unaffected females, as in the example of hemophilia (Morton, A.S., 1892, 1893). And in a third example, the parents had normal vision and yet produced three affected children (Hutchinson, 1892a). Hence, different varieties of night blindness appeared to be inherited in three different ways.

Thomas Laycock, Professor of the Practice of Physic at the University of Edinburgh, observed a family with the opposite condition, day-blindness. Parents were normal-sighted, but five of ten children were affected (Laycock, 1866). H.R. Swanzy reported a similar family pedigree (Swanzy, 1873). Edward Nettleship collected a series of such family histories and noted that unaffected parents were often related [consanguineous]. The same defect often appeared in collateral branches of the extended families he investigated (Nettleship, 1880, 1886). This was consistent with the indirect or collateral pattern of inheritance.

Diseases of the Head and Neck

While ophthalmologists demonstrated a more sophisticated and systematic approach toward gathering data on heredity and eye disorders, other specialists also began to assemble similar family material. The formation of the ear appeared to be strongly influenced by heredity. Numerous families with direct transmission of deafness through four successive generations were noted at this time (Sedgwick, 1863a; Anderson, T., 1863; Love, 1896a). More frequently, parents had normal hearing and yet produced several affected children (Sedgwick, 1861a, b). More extensive pedigree analysis by H. Mitchell, Deputy Commissioner of Lunacy for Scotland, showed that collateral branches of such families often were affected as well, sometimes through four generations. This was another example of indirect heredity (Mitchell, 1863). W. Scott, from the Institution of the Deaf and Dumb at Exeter, observed deafness more commonly among people from isolated rural areas. He thought this might be the result of inbreeding [consanguinity]. For example, in Devonshire there was one deaf-mute per 1143 population, while in the more isolated Scilly Islands, the frequency was one per 446 people (Warden, 1887). C. Warden, from the Royal Institution for the Education of the Deaf and Dumb Children in Birmingham, examined the case records there and also found that consanguinity was an important factor in the etiology of deafness (Warden, 1887). James Love was an aural surgeon at the Glasgow Royal Infirmary. He examined several six-generation families and found deaf children born of normal parents in several collateral branches of such families. He was struck by the fact that the trait could re-appear in subsequent generations:

> Whether what is transmitted through the intervening apparently normal generations be a material substrate or not, it is not necessary to discuss, but that the character may disappear for one or many generations, and then reassert itself is an established fact (Love, 1896b).

Love also subscribed to a particulate model for heredity, rather than a blending of characters from both parents. He noted:

> If transmitted tendencies were simply diluted, the attenuation would, in time, become so great that they could be practically disregarded. But the qualities of the parents are not all passed on. Some are dropped, some are transmitted, and find expression in the children. Some are transmitted and remain latent for many generations. It is quite certain that some of the tendencies pass on undiluted... (Love, 1896c).

When parents were related but unaffected, they could carry these latent hereditary elements and then transmit them to their offspring and produce such disorders as hereditary deafness, again consistent with indirect inheritance.

Cleft lip and palate was another defect of the head region that was known to run in certain families. Horace Dobell, from the Royal Hospital for Diseases of the Chest, noted the defect in five successive generations of a family (Dobell, 1862). William Rose of the King's College Hospital noted an isolated cleft lip in four generations of another family (Rose, 1891). More commonly, an indirect pattern of inheritance was observed. In one example, a paternal aunt had cleft lip, as did one niece and one nephew (Murray, 1860). A father in another family was affected, as were three of his children. The father's niece, and first and second cousins were also affected (Sproule, 1863). Francis Mason from St. Thomas's Hospital collected a series of family histories showing direct transmission in some cases, but more commonly, several affected children were born of unaffected parents (Mason, 1877). Jonathan Hutchinson reported one such family with twenty children; half were born with cleft lip (Hutchinson, 1890b). W.A. Jamieson, Lecturer in Diseases of the Skin at the University of Edinburgh Medical School, observed a family also showing indirect inheritance. Cousins in several branches of the family were affected with cleft lip or palate (Jamieson, 1880). Richard Lucas, surgeon at Guy's Hospital collected a series of cleft cases. He did not see one particular pattern of heredity, either. He noted:

> When a large number of reliable cases are collected, it is probable that some general rule may be produced as to the relative frequency of its occurrence in males and females, and the reason a particular child should be selected to carry on the deformity may possibly be discovered (Lucas, 1888).

As was true in the example of night blindness, the inheritance of cleft lip and palate was different in different families. Lucas emphasized the importance of "reliable" family histories. It was hoped that more complete data from many families with different disorders would help elucidate a general theory for human heredity and disease.

Even the formation of the teeth appeared to be under hereditary control. Characteristic dental anomalies could be present in several generations. Hypolasia of the dental enamel was directly inherited from parent to child through three successive generations in several branches of a large family (Spokes, 1890).

Blood Diseases

The large number families with hemophilia reported in the medical literature at this time identified a pattern of inheritance peculiar to few human traits. As one mother noted, "...as far back as my own grandmother's generation, and from her downwards, the male children have been subject to great bleeding from slight causes" (Durham, 1868). The characteristic pattern of unaffected females transmitting the character to their sons, and their unaffected daughters then producing affected grandsons was observed in numerous families. Christopher Heath, surgeon at Westminster Hospital, also noted that uncles on the maternal side of the family could be bleeders as well as more direct descendants (Heath, 1868). J. Wickham Legg had been a medical attendant to the hemophiliac Prince Leopold and completed his *Treatise on Hemophilia* in 1872. His review of prior medical literature found an overwhelming majority of male to female affected individuals, often between 7 and 14 to 1 in various series of families. Affected females did occur, but tended to have milder bouts of bleeding (Legg, 1872a). By 1881, he was able to describe a six-generation family with the typical male predominance. At least 23 affected males occurred in the one specific family (Legg, 1881). William Osler subsequently described a family with 200 years of disease experience. He noted the disorder in male twins as well (Osler, 1885).

The great majority of hemophiliacs were male. Female bleeders did occur, but rarely. Thomas Oliver, Professor of Medicine at the University of Durham Medical School, described one such family in 1886. An unaffected man with affected brothers married a maternal cousin. He had three affected sons. One unaffected daughter had an affected daughter. Another unaffected daughter had three affected sons. One of them subsequently had an affected daughter (Oliver, T., 1886). Frederick Treves, surgeon at London Hospital, also described a large family with an affected female. Her father was affected, but her unaffected mother was his maternal first cousin. She came from a family of bleeders. This couple had an affected daughter (Treves, 1886). Herbert Page, surgeon at St. Mary's Hospital, examined a family with seven affected women in three generations. An affected woman had both affected male and female children. Her affected daughter subsequently had both affected male and female offspring herself (Page, 1887). But in a large five-generation family segregating hemophilia, the general rareness of affected females was well exemplified. Of twelve affected individuals in this case, only one was female (Wightman, 1894). The compiled cases in the Table 10.1 show male to female frequency of about 14 to 1.

Because hemophiliacs often bled into the large joints such as knees, hips, and elbows, the discovery of x-rays by William Roentgen in 1895 suggested another means to examine the structure of the bones affected. His work appeared in English translation in the science journal *Nature* early in 1896. Shortly thereafter the x-ray technique was used to locate a bullet lodged in the wrist bones of a patient (Jones, 1896). J.E. Shaw performed an x-ray study of the elbow of a hemophiliac the next year and found enlargement of the head of the radius and thinning of the articular cartilages due to recurrent bleeding and damage to the soft tissues of the joint (Shaw, 1897).

Hemophilia has been called "the most hereditary of hereditary diseases" (Graham, 1886). The general pattern of its inheritance of unaffected females transmitting disease to their sons was also recognized as the sex-limited type of collateral or indirect heredity observed in families with pseudohypertrophic muscular paralysis (Gower's disease), color blindness and diabetes insipidus (Legg, 1881; Sedgwick, 1882; "The hemorrhagic diathesis," 1884). No effective treatment existed for hemophilia at the time, and the painful episodes of bleeding and prolonged disability made for a miserable existence. Legg clearly recognized that prevention of disease transmission was the only management plan available. He stated that the male bleeder ought not to marry, "as his daughter's sons would almost certainly be affected." He also strongly recommended that unaffected children in bleeder families should remain unmarried because of the risks of transmitting disease to their offspring (Legg, 1872b). In the following decade, Osler made the same plea for marriage planning. He thought that daughters of bleeder families

Table 10.1
Families with Hemophilia
1860-1900

Generations Affected	Males Affected	Females Affected	References
4	10	0	Durham, 1868
5	11	0	Heath, 1868
1	2	0	Legg, 1871
3	7	0	Legg, 1871
2	3	0	Legg, 1871
2	5	0	Legg, 1871
1	4	0	Walker, 1872
1	3	0	Brigstocke, 1872
2	3	0	Legg, 1872a
3	2	3	Legg, 1876
3	7	0	Winter, 1880
6	23	0	Legg, 1881
3	9	0	Finlayson, 1882
4	3	0	Goodlee, 1884
2	3	0	Smith, J., 1884
2	4	0	Smith, J., 1884
3	14	0	Osler, 1885
4	9	2	Oliver, T., 1886
5	12	1	Treves, 1886
1	5	0	Moreton, 1886
3	3	0	M'caw, 1886
1	3	0	Graham, 1886
1	3	0	Skelton, 1887
2	5	0	Hope, 1887
2	5	1	Eve, 1889
3	5	0	Young, J., 1889
2	7	0	Sandler, 1898
2	16	0	Strahan, 1892
2	4	0	Shaw, 1897
3	3	7	Page, 1887
5	11	1	Wightman, 1894
Totals	204	15	

should not be permitted to marry, as it was through them that the tendency was propagated to their sons (Osler, 1885).

Other bleeding disorders appeared to have a decidedly different pattern for inheritance. Benjamin Babington at Guy's Hospital studied a family with hereditary epistaxis [nose bleeding]. Affected individuals did not develop joint hemorrhage. The example he observed was a five-generation family in which both males and females were affected: five males and seven females in all (Babington, 1865). Another family had three affected generations with seven males and four females affected (Radmore, 1884). In both instances, the character was transmitted directly from affected parent to child. Unaffected parents never produced affected offspring. This was consistent with the direct pattern of inheritance defined by Ribot.

Another unusual blood disorder appeared to be inherited by the same direct fashion. Hereditary splenic anemia produced episodic attacks of hemolysis that looked something like malaria. Breakdown of the red blood cells resulted in clinical jaundice. The spleen became enlarged. Direct transmission to both sexes through three generations was observed (Wilson, C., 1890; Wilson, C. and Stanley, 1892). This disorder was subsequently termed acholuric jaundice.

MUSCLE AND BONE DISEASES

The development of muscles and bones was also influenced by heredity. Edward Meryon of St. Thomas's Hospital described a familial disorder characterized by a normal nervous system with degeneration of muscles. The lower leg muscles tended to hypertrophy as they degenerated and were replaced by fat tissue (Meryon, 1866a). The disorder was most commonly seen in males, but did occasionally occur in females as well (Meryon, 1866b, 1870). William Gowers at the National Hospital for the Paralysed and Epileptic in London also collected extensive pedigrees of this disease. He observed, "...The disease is almost never to be heard of on the side of the father; when antecedent cases have occurred, they have almost invariably been on the side of the mother" (Gowers, 1879a). Gowers reported one family in which a woman had been married to two different men. Her brother had the disease, and she produced sons from both marriages also affected with this degenerative muscle disorder (Gowers, 1879b). In his compilation of 160 cases, there were six males for every one female example (Gowers, 1879a). W. Whitlaw, from the Belfast Royal Hospital, also reported a family in which a woman had affected sons in two different marriages. This "proves how strongly the hereditary influence is handed down by the female side," he thought (Whitlaw, 1885). Both Gowers and Whitlaw noted instances of twins born of a carrier mother. One twin was healthy and one affected (Gowers, 1879a; Whitlaw, 1885). F. Nicholson, from the Hull Royal Infirmary, on the other hand, observed a family in which both male twins were affected (Nicholson, 1889).

Table 10.2
Pseudohypertrophic Muscular Paralysis
(Meryon-Duchenne's Disease)
1860-1900

Generations Affected	Males affected	Females affected	References
1	1	1	Meryon, 1866b
2	4	0	Gowers, 1879b
1	2	0	Russell, J., 1869
3	5	0	Russell, J., 1869
2	4	1	Gowers, 1879c
1	4	0	Gowers, 1879a
1	2	0	Whitlaw, 1885
1	3	0	Moore, 1880
1	1	0	Fulton, 1881
2	3	0	Goodridge, 1882
1	4	0	Macphail, 1882
1	4	0	Nicholson, 1889
1	1	0	Pirie, 1892
2	5	1	Gowers, 1893b
3	5	1	Gowers, 1893b
1	5	0	Simpson, 1894
1	2	2	Coley, 1894
1	2	0	Hawkins, 1894
1	3	0	Taylor, J., 1894a
1	3	0	Little, 1896
Totals	73	6	

The findings for cases of pseudohypertrophic muscular paralysis reported in this era are summarized in Table 10.2. The ratio of affected males and females is 12 to 1. Affected females generally had a milder form of the disease than their affected brothers (Coley, 1894). Byram Bramwell, from the Royal Infirmary in Edinburgh, explained the characteristic pattern for inheritance of this disorder. The character came from the maternal side of family. Male offspring of unaffected sisters of male patients often were affected. Male children born of unaffected brothers were healthy (Bramwell, 1895). This was most consistent with the sex-limited pattern of collateral inheritance.

The German neurologist, A.J. Thomsen, observed an unusual inability to relax a contracted muscle in several members of his own family spread over four generations (Chapman, 1884). Thomas Buzzard, physician to the National Hospital in London, described the first cases of this myotonia disorder in England. That family had only two affected brothers (Buzzard, 1887). Subsequent families were found with affected parent and children, and often cousins were affected as well (White, 1889; Cook and Sweeten, 1890; Dreschfeld, A., 1890). One writer concluded that this characteristic pattern of illness made it "quite possible that the disease was really hereditary" (White, 1889). Larger pedigrees were then constructed to demonstrate the direct heredity of the character from parent to child through three or four successive generations (Clemesha, 1897; Gee, 1889).

Muscular atrophies appeared to be a separate form of hereditary degeneration, often involving specific muscle groups. Howard Tooth, from the National Hospital in London, first described peroneal muscle atrophy. The initial family histories he collected demonstrated more than one affected child in only about one-third of all cases (Tooth, 1886, 1889). Subsequent analyses found other more extensive pedigrees in which the inheritance pattern appeared to be sex-limited, like that of hemophilia. Wilmot Herringham, from St. Bart's Hospital, collected information from a large family with at least four affected generations. Females were unaffected, but could produce affected male children. Unaffected sons produced only normal children (Herringham, 1888). This writer could not explain his findings, which "makes one wonder what inheritance is." The daughters in the family clearly transmitted a form of weakness which they did not possess themselves. "It seems as if the daughter of the diseased father carried from the beginning of her life ova of two sexes, the female healthy, the male continuing in it the representation of the father's disease" (Herringham, 1888). This attempt at a mechanical explanation for such sex-limited heredity showed a prescient glimmer for the double mode of sex-linked inheritance for these traits that would be better understood in the following decades.

Joseph Ormerod, physician at the National Hospital, delineated another familial disorder involving generalized muscle atrophy that began in middle age. Direct heredity from a parent to two children was observed (Ormerod, J.A., 1885a). A similar family also showed direct parent to child transmission, but an uncle was also reportedly affected (Suckling, 1887b). The exact mode of inheritance for progressive muscle atrophy was clarified by an analysis of a large family from Nova Scotia. Four generations were involved; 27 people were affected. Males and females were equally afflicted. Direct heredity from parent to child was clearly demonstrated (Campbell, D.A., 1888).

The bony skeleton was involved in numerous families by hereditary variation as well. John Struthers, from the University of Aberdeen, noted a family with an unusual extra piece of bone above the elbow, termed a supracondylar process. The father and three of his sons had the same condition, while three other children were unaffected

(Struthers, 1873). Philip Pye-Smith at Guy's Hospital noted recurrent dislocation of the radial head in two brothers. The same condition recurred in their children (Pye-Smith, 1883). Another report from the Evelina Hospital for Sick Children demonstrated seven similar cases in four successive generations (Abbott, 1892). The Roentgen ray was used in 1899 to document another hereditary disorder of bony structure. The clavicles were lacking in a father and four of his children (Carpenter, 1899). All these examples demonstrated direct heredity from parent to child.

Exostoses are extra mounds of cartilage which can form anywhere on the bony skeleton. One large family was reported in 1863 with four generations of affected males (Price, 1863). Another family also showed four generations involved, but both sexes were affected (Poore, 1873). Similar direct examples of heredity were noted in multi-generation families (Hutchinson, 1880; Cotes, 1890, 1891; Griffiths, 1892; Eccles, 1896). In one case, an affected man had twice married normal women. He had affected offspring in both marriages. The reporting physician mused,

> One cannot resist the intellectual pleasure of wondering when and how and why this 'sport' was first started in a family. If we could answer this, then we should be able to unlock many a pathological mystery (Robinson, 1893).

A better understanding of how such mutations began certainly could, it was hoped, prove useful in the daily clinical practice of medicine.

Other hereditary defects of the skeleton did not appear to follow one particular pattern of inheritance. Reports from the Northeastern Hospital for Children observed a family with two of eight children affected with spina bifida. In another family, three normal siblings all produced children affected by clubfoot (Goodlee, 1884). Jonathan Hutchinson recorded another family with clubfoot in three successive generations with only affected male children (Hutchinson, 1890b).

Another "peculiar family history" involved the inheritance of fragilitas ossium [osteogenesis imperfecta]. Affected individuals had bones that often broke after minor trauma, or even spontaneously. One family had one affected boy, affected paternal uncles, and an affected paternal cousin (Pritchard, 1883). Larger pedigrees noted direct inheritance from parent to children of both sexes over three successive generations (Greenish, 1880; Atherton, 1894). One affected man had been married twice. He produced affected sons in both families (Spurway, 1896). The same family demonstrated heredity through four generations, clearly demonstrating a direct inheritance pattern for this character. Here again was a disorder with three different patterns of inheritance.

Malformations of the hands and feet such as shortened digits, extra or absent digits, and webbed fingers and toes, were observed in many different families during this period. The specific pattern of malformation was usually consistent among members of a particular family. The varieties of such malformations seemed to be quite expansive, but the pattern of inheritance almost always fit Ribot's direct form. John Struthers, from the University of Aberdeen, made an extensive study of such malformations. He reported several families with polydactyly in three and five successive generations (Struthers, 1863). Richard Lucas, surgeon at Guy's Hospital, noted a large five-generation family with polydactyly. Direct parent to child transmission was evident, affecting about 25 of 58 offspring (Lucas, 1881). The number of affected children born of one particular affected parent varied widely. In a second family, one polydactylous parent produced eight affected children, and his affected cousin produced four affected of eight total offspring (Muir, 1884). In another pedigree, both parents were affected. All of their children and grandchildren were born with polydactyly. Drake-Brockman wondered whether "the dichotomy of the cells of the ovum" could explain the duplication of the digits (Drake-Brockman, 1892). Another case report in December 1896 used the new X-ray to show that polydactyly could be the result of bifurcation of the fifth metacarpal in the hand and the analogous metatarsal in the foot to produce the extra digit (Morgan, G., 1896).

The hereditary character for polydactyly could also remain latent, although transmitted through several generations. Sedgwick reported a five-generation family in which two generations had no affected individuals. The fourth and fifth generations then redemonstrated the character that had been evident in their great-grandfather and great-great-grandfather, respectively (Sedgwick, 1863b). In an extensive six-generation pedigree, Wilson observed direct inheritance in most lines of the family. But, in one branch, two generations were skipped before producing another affected child. In two other lines, one generation was unaffected, and yet affected children appeared in the subsequent generation (Wilson, G., 1896).

Shortening and inward curving of the fifth digit [clinodactyly] also was clearly hereditary. One affected parent produced four affected children, including a set of male twins (Sedgwick, 1863a). Brachydactyly involved the shortening of one or more digits and was noted to be hereditary in many families. William Turner, Professor of Anatomy at the University of Edinburgh, reported several families with shortened fourth metacarpals in the hands. He had evidence of such defects in between five and seven generations of different families with typical direct heredity from parent to child. He called this a "striking instance of hereditary transmission" (Turner, 1883, 1889). Another variety of brachydactyly had a somewhat less apparent pattern of inheritance. J.A. Ogle of St. George's Hospital reported a large family in which affected people had two phalanges in digits one and two, and only one phalanx in digits three and four. Finger and toe nails were also absent. Typical direct inheritance was evident in several families, but as with polydactyly, the character could remain latent and then reappear in subsequent offspring (Ogle, 1872).

Thomas Annandale, surgeon at the Edinburgh Royal Infirmary, collected a large number of familial examples of hand malformations in his monograph *The Malformations, Diseases and Injuries of the Fingers and Toes* published in 1866. He cited cases of more complex hand malformations involving polysyndactyly [extra digits combined with webbing of the digits]. One affected family demonstrated direct transmission of the character from parent to children through four successive generations (Annandale, 1866). Similar examples were observed in 3-5 successive generations in other cases. No examples of skipped generations were reported in this series (Barber, 1864; Harker, 1865; Morris, 1865; Hutchinson, 1890b). However, one other family had 21 affected individuals over five generations. There was one example of an unaffected woman transmitting the character to five of her children (Smith, W.R. and Norwell, 1894).

In yet other families, the digital joints were fused [ankylosis]. Horace Dobell reported several families where the defect was evident in four and five generations. Direct heredity was the rule in these cases (Dobell, 1862, 1863). In another family, a double thumb was associated with ankylosis in four successive generations (Young, D., 1898). Such examples were consistent with the direct pattern of inheritance.

The suppression of digits [adactyly] also produced a broad range of different hand and foot malformations. Hutchinson noted several families with absent digits four and five. The character was passed in a direct fashion from parent to child over three generations (Hutchinson, 1892b). Another family demonstrated the absence of thumbs, webbed fingers, absent second toes, and webbing of the other toes. Direct heredity through three generations was evident (Montgomery-Smith, 1888).

H.A. Fotherby reported a characteristic pattern of digit suppression that he labeled the "lobster claw deformity." Individuals with ectrodactyly had absent middle digits of the hands and feet. The hands looked like the pincers of a lobster. Such a striking malformation was not rare, and large families were investigated. Fotherby's cases encompassed five generations and demonstrated direct inheritance (Fotherby, 1886). Another large family demonstrated 16 of 36 descendants affected over three generations. Male and female twins with the deformity also were present. A second large family revealed 24 of 36 descendents affected through four generations (Anderson, W., 1886). Another four-generation family history showed 13 of 18 affected individuals (Tubby, 1894). Ectrodactyly was not confined to the United Kingdom. An affected three-generation family from China was also observed (Thomson, 1892). In all cases, direct heredity was evident. Approximately half of all children (56 of 97 total) in affected lineages had inherited the character from an affected parent.

Diseases of Metabolism

It became evident at this time that maintenance of normal body chemistry was also influenced by heredity. Thomas Brunton studied pharmacology and human physiology at St. Bart's Hospital in the 1880s. His experience there indicated that diabetes mellitus [the inability to regulate blood sugar] could sometimes appear in brothers and sisters of a family, but was not frequently "hereditarily transmitted," i.e, transmitted from parent to children (Brunton, 1880). Frederick Pavy had studied diabetes mellitus with Claude Bernard in Paris in the 1850s and developed his expertise with such endocrine diseases at Guy's Hospital in London. He described 11 families with diabetes in a presentation before the British Medical Association. The disease often affected siblings with normal parents. In one such family, five of twelve were affected. However, he was able to demonstrate direct heredity of the character from parent to children over three successive generations in one family. Another three-generation family showed that latent transmission of the character could happen as well (Pavy, 1885). Subsequent study showed repeated examples of the disorder in 2-4 generations of affected families (Campbell, H.J., 1887; Frew, 1887; Given, 1896; Oliver, T., 1900).

Diabetes insipidus is another defect of body chemistry in which water regulation is affected. Affected individuals must drink constantly to avoid dehydration. Typically 2-3 quarts of water are consumed at one sitting. One man was reported to drink two gallons overnight every day of the week. If he could not quench his thirst, he became faint. Samuel Gee of St. Bart's Hospital noted a large family with this unusual character. Nine males and two females were affected over four generations. Unaffected females appeared to transmit the character from their affected fathers to their own sons (Gee, 1877). The same pattern of inheritance was noted in other families (Clay, R.H., 1889; McIlraith, 1892). Although females could be affected, their degree of disability appeared slight compared to their brothers (McIlraith, 1892). This special form of indirect heredity was consistent with the sex-limited pattern of inheritance.

HEART AND LUNG DISEASES

Disorders of the lung and heart often appeared among several members of particular families. One study of asthma found examples of 14 families with more than one affected person. In eight cases, direct heredity was noted from parent to child. In other cases, more distant relatives were affected (Salter, 1860). Serious heart disease was well known to affect one generation after another in certain unfortunate families. William Gairdner, Professor of Medicine at the University of Glasgow, noted: "Sudden death from heart disease is frequently hereditary...[as a] characteristic [in] certain families sometimes for several generations" (Gairdner, 1880). The family of the author Matthew Arnold provided an example of such familial heart disease. Men over three generations were afflicted with valvular disease and angina pectoris, resulting in sudden cardiac death ("The late Mr. Matthew Arnold," 1888; Osler, 1896). The development of aneurysms[7] that could rupture, resulting in sudden demise, was also noted to be directly transmitted from parent to child in examples of two and three generation families (Powell, 1880).

NEUROLOGICAL DISEASES

The specialty of neurology developed in the latter half of the nineteenth-century as well. The journal *Brain* was begun in 1876 to report findings related to neurologic diseases and became the official publication of the Neurological Society of London after its first meeting in 1888 (Schurr, 1985). Henry Maudsley was a leader in this field and believed strongly in the influence of heredity on the nervous system. He thought that a hereditary predisposition in the nervous organization of specific people could be triggered by stress, malnutrition or another disease and result in seizures, insanity or other neurologic conditions (Maudsley, 1870). Francis Anstie of the Westminster Hospital argued that the transmission of an enfeebled nervous organization to children would "render them peculiarly liable to the severe neuroses" (Anstie, 1880). Samuel Gee gave an example of one such fragile family with a predisposition to nervous disease. A parent had defective vision in one eye and produced two children with seizures, two with night terrors and two more with migraine headaches (Gee, 1884).

Migraine headaches were often reported by sufferers to have been in their families for generations. Sedgwick reported three generations affected with direct parent to child transmission (Sedgwick, 1863a). Edward Liveing at King's College Hospital studied 26 affected families and demonstrated direct heredity (Liveing, 1873). The general consensus within the neurologic community was that migraine typically followed the direct pattern of heredity, from parent to child, often affecting several members of the same family (Drysdale, 1885; Gowers, 1893a).

Huntington's chorea had been observed on Long Island in the United States since the late 1700s. George Huntington came from a family of physicians that had cared for patients with this unusual disorder for three generations. Affected individuals had no symptoms until age 30 or 40, and then began a gradual progressive course with spasmodic grimaces of the face and twisting of the extremities. The course was always inexorable, resulting in insanity and an unpleasant death later in life (Huntington, 1872, 1910). The same disorder came to be recognized in English families as well. One family recorded in 1880 had at least five generations and 27 persons affected. Direct parent to child heredity was evident (Harbinson, 1880). Another family demonstrated the character in six successive generations with 25 affected persons (Menzies, 1892). The rule of heredity was quite rigid in such cases. According to Suckling, this disease "could not skip a generation; if a member of an affected family escaped, then the inheritance in his or her case ceased" (Suckling, 1889c). Statistics reported from choreic families in this era are presented in Table 10.3. Approximately half of the offspring of affected parents were also affected; the sexes were about equally affected, as well. Direct heredity was the rule. One physician called Huntington's chorea one of the most hereditary of all diseases (Menzies, 1893).

Table 10.3
Huntington's Chorea
1860-1899

Generations Affected	Total Affected	Males Affected	Females Affected	References
5	27	8	12	Harbinson, 1880
2	5	3	2	MacLeod, 1882
1	2	2	0	West, 1884
3	4	1	3	Suckling, 1889b, c
6	25			Menzies, 1892
3	13			Menzies, 1892
2	6	3	3	Russell, J.W., 1894
2	6	6	0	Clarke, 1897
2	4	2	2	Clarke, 1897
3	8	3	5	Stewart, 1899
Totals	96	28	27	

Warren Tay from the Royal London Ophthalmic Hospital reported another unusual degenerative neurologic disorder. A child developed a large white patch near the macula of the retina in the eye. Seizures, nervous degeneration and death occurred before age two years. The neurologists Jonathan Hutchinson and Hughlings Jackson examined the child, but could reach no diagnosis (Tay, 1884). Three years later, two more affected children had been born to the same parents. Clearly a hereditary disorder was developing in such cases (Tay, 1884). Tay collected several more cases from other families, noting in one instance, the parents were first cousins and had two of six children affected (Tay, 1892a). E. Kingdon, an ophthalmologist from the Children's Hospital in Nottingham, observed that such cases often occurred in Jewish families, from a community in which consanguineous marriages were common (Kingdon, 1892). Tay later found evidence of consanguinity in many of his families as well (Tay, 1892b). As larger pedigrees were examined, it became clear that affected families could produce as many as five children with this disorder, all of them dying in infancy (Kingdon, 1894; Kingdon and Russell, 1897). This disorder was labeled amaurotic family idiocy and followed the indirect pattern of inheritance.

A similar pattern of familial occurrence was observed in another degenerative neurologic disorder termed Friedreich's ataxia. Tremors of the arms and legs and nystagmus characteristically developed in childhood and became progressively worse in adult years. Julius Dreschfeld at the Manchester Royal Infirmary described one of the earliest English families, including three brothers and two sisters affected; the parents were normal (Dreschfeld, J., 1876). Larger pedigrees revealed that several collateral branches of the families could demonstrate the same disease. Affected cousins were noted in one instance (Brock, 1893). Joseph Ormerod, of the National Hospital in London, described four branches of one family affected with this disorder (Ormerod, J.A., 1885b). He discovered another family in which a man, his daughter and two of her children appeared to have the same condition (Ormerod, J.A., 1887). This apparent direct inheritance was decidedly unusual, however.

Information on the families reported in the English literature with Friedreich's ataxia is presented in Table 10.4. The published pedigrees did not always include all unaffected offspring. In aggregate, the total affected children were about 50 percent of the unaffected offspring. Consanguinity was evident in certain families. Goodhart reported one family with five affected children. The parents and maternal grandparents were first cousins (Goodhart and Carpenter, 1888). Hodge noted another family with three affected children in which the parents were first cousins (Hodge, 1897). The hereditary factor for ataxia could remain latent and yet reappear in a subsequent generation. In one family, an unaffected female had two affected brothers. She married twice. By one husband, only normal children were born. By her second husband, she bore a son affected with ataxia (Taylor, J., 1894b). No evidence of consanguinity was noted in this case.

William Gowers, a neurologist from The National Hospital, summarized the general pattern for inheritance of Friedreich's ataxia. Children of both sexes could be affected; consanguinity was not infrequently evident, and collateral relatives such as aunts, uncles and cousins were also often affected (Gowers, 1893c). This was considered quite compatible with the indirect pattern of inheritance.

In a similar fashion, other neurologic diseases also appeared to follow the indirect pattern for inheritance. In such examples, several children in one family and their cousins in collateral branches of the same family typically were affected. A family with microcephaly in three of nine children born of normal parents also demonstrated consanguinity, another feature that was often recognized in such indirect inheritance. Both paternal grandparents of the affected children in this case were first cousins (Sankey, 1878). George Shuttleworth was the Medical Superintendent at the Royal Albert Asylum in Lancaster. He recalled that Darwin had noted that such consanguinity intensified hereditary tendencies already latent in both parents. The births of abnormal offspring were therefore not surprising in such marriages (Shuttleworth, 1886).

Table 10.4
Friedreich's Disease
1860-1899

Males Affected	Females Affected	Unspecified	Unaffected	References
3	2		10	Dreschfeld, J., 1876
4	1		4	Gowers, 1881
2	1		7	Power, 1882
2	2		15	Ormerod, J.A., 1887
3	2		2	Goodhart and Carpenter, 1888
1	1		1	Ormerod, M., 1888
2	0			Suckling, 1889a
1	1			Suckling, 1889a
2	1		11	Clarke, 1889
1			3	Hinshelwood, 1889
3	1		15	Brock, 1893
1	2			Tressiden, 1893
1	1		1	Anderson, J.W., 1893
1	1			Morton, J., 1894
3		2	22	Taylor, J., 1894b
3	1		9	Clarke, 1894
2	1		5	Nolan, 1895
2			5	Stawell, 1895
1	2		5	Hodge, 1897
1	2		5	Whyte, 1898
40	22	5	124	Totals

Epilepsy frequently appeared to affect several members of certain families. A.H. Bennett from the National Hospital reported a series of 100 seizure cases and found that 26% had other affected family members (Bennett, 1879). Gowers reviewed 1250 of his patients and reported 36% with a positive family history for epilepsy (Gowers,1880). Males and females were equally affected, and no consanguinity was found in this group of families (Gowers, 1885). But, J. Russell Reynolds from University College Hospital found only 12% of his epileptics had affected family members (Reynolds, 1880). Another author labeled epilepsy "eminently a hereditary disease" (Bennett, 1879). Gowers noted, "There are few diseases in which heredity is a more important etiological condition" (Gowers, 1880). Nevertheless, Reynolds was not so certain and advised against assigning heredity as the cause of seizures in any particular case without investigating the possibility of other contributing factors (Reynolds, 1880).

The heredity of epilepsy was, however, quite irregular. Several affected children might be born of normal parents (Sedgwick, 1863a). The character could also be latent, skipping a generation only to reappear again (Oliver, J., 1886). One Irish family had affected siblings in both the maternal and paternal lines, although the parents themselves were normal. Subsequently, three of their sons were born with epilepsy, while three daughters were normal (Russell, W., 1889). J. Oliver from the Medical College at Newcastle on Tyne argued that heredity then played "an all important role in the production and reappearance of the disease in families" (Oliver, J., 1886), but no specific pattern of inheritance was evident.

M.G. Echeverri, from the City Asylum in New York City, investigated the development of epilepsy in the offspring of affected parents and reported his findings in the British medical literature in 1880. He collected data on 553 children born of 136 epileptic parents. A total of 275 children (49.7%) developed seizures: 195 died of convulsions in infancy, and 78 went on to develop epilepsy as older children. Such data convinced him that the direct heredity of epilepsy did exist, and that epileptics should not marry because of their likelihood of producing affected children. He also mentioned the traditional Scottish method for preventing the birth of epileptics in the clans. If a man produced an epileptic child, he was gelded. Women who had the "falling sickness" were banished from the community. If one should become pregnant, she was buried alive. These tactics were developed to preserve "the common good," lest the whole nation "should be injured or corrupted" (Echeverri, 1880).

Kidney Diseases

Diseases of the urinary system were frequently observed to recur in several members of certain families. In one example, four children born of first cousin normal parents developed nephritis, excessive loss of the protein albumin in the urine, that resulted in accumulation of fluid in body tissues (Benson, 1893). This was consistent with the indirect pattern of inheritance. The same observation was made in a family in which several children with multiple cysts in the kidneys [polycystic disease] were born to parents who appeared to be normal (Roberts, F.T., 1880; Forbes, 1897). In other families with the same disorder, however, one parent and several children were affected, suggesting direct inheritance (Newman, 1897). Bladder and kidney stones frequently recurred in several members of affected families. In one family, normal parents had a son affected with bladder stone. The mother came from an area in which bladder stones were common. Her brother and his children also were afflicted (Teevan, 1863). In other examples, direct heredity was clearly evident. Three successive generations of people with bladder stones were evident in another large family tree (Clubbe, 1872).

Weakness of the inguinal rings, resulting in hernias, was evident in three and four successive generations of certain families (Sedgwick, 1863b; Couch, 1895). Formation of the urethral opening on the underside of the penis [hypospadius] was sometimes observed in several children born of normal parents (Lindsay, 1893). In other large pedigrees spanning six generations, direct father to son heredity of the trait was evident (Lingard, 1884).

SKIN DISEASES

Dermatology was another of the earliest specialties to develop in Britain during the nineteenth-century. Thomas Bateman and Anthony Thomson established the first hospital devoted to skin diseases in 1819, called the London and Westminster Infirmary for the Treatment of Diseases of the Skin. Blackfriar's Hospital was established in 1841 and became the leading center for teaching and research on skin diseases at that time. The Dermatological Society of London was initiated in 1882 as a locale for the presentation of instructive cases (Rook, 1979). In 1895, the Dermatological Society of Great Britain and Ireland was formed to facilitate communication between all physicians and surgeons interested in diseases of the skin.

Jonathan Hutchinson established himself as a leader in dermatology and told the British Medical Association that the laws of human heredity could be exemplified by a study of skin diseases (Hutchinson, 1890a). He commented, "We cannot afford...in investigating the very difficult subject of hereditary transmission to neglect any hint which the facts of pathology may offer" (Hutchinson, 1886).

As one example, the development and maintenance of the hair seemed to have hereditary components. Premature hair loss [alopecia] was noted in a mother and her son (Hutchinson, 1886). H. Radcliffe Crocker from the Skin Department at University College Hospital reported direct heredity of this character through three successive generations (Crocker, 1893). Unusually fine, fragile hair [trichorexis nodosa] also appeared to be a hereditary condition. One family demonstrated the trait in three successive generations (Steven, 1889). Thomas Anderson, Professor of Clinical Medicine at the University of Glasgow, noted direct parent to child transmission of the same character in a five-generation pedigree (Anderson, T.M., 1883, 1887). Macular xanthelasma palpebrum, a rare disease of the eyebrows, was evident in one mother and her daughter (Fagge, 1868). A larger pedigree investigated by William Church from St. Bart's Hospital showed several instances of such direct heredity in different branches of another family (Church, 1874).

The color of the hair often appeared to be controlled by hereditary factors. White forelock was observed in three and four successive generations of two different families (Morgan, J.H., 1890; Goodlee, 1884). The transmission of hair color itself, however, did not appear so simple. In one family, a red-haired parent married to a dark-haired spouse produced dark-haired children. When these then married, the atavistic, latent character of the red hair was evidenced by the fact that four of seven grandchildren again demonstrated red hair (Sedgwick, 1863a).

Persons with albinism had almost no pigment in their skin and eyes. The sudden appearance of such individuals in a family has always raised questions about the origin of such changes in coloration. In Ceylon (now Sri Lanka), the typical native has dark hair and dark-colored eyes. Several families with dark parents produced albino children: four in one family, and three in another. Local wise men concluded that the white races had originated from just such "accidents of nature" (Davy, 1861). Larger pedigrees of affected families often showed albinism in collateral branches, and the presence of consanguinity, as well. In one example, two brothers who had an albino cousin married two sisters. One couple produced three albino children. The other couple produced eight normal children. One of them later married and produced four albinos among twelve children in the next generation (Sedgwick, 1861a). A Negro family from St. Kitts in the British Leeward Islands demonstrated albino children in two branches. The unaffected parents were cousins in one lineage and second cousins in the other (Boon, 1892). Consanguinity is common in small isolated island populations and may well have played a role in the development of albinism in such cases. The family histories in all these cases were consistent with the indirect pattern for inheritance.

Direct heredity of other skin diseases also was evident. Epithelioma adenoides cystica was a skin disorder in which the face and trunk were covered with white papules containing black points beneath the surface of the skin. A mother and two of her daughters were affected (Brooke, 1893). Keratosis palmaris et plantaris produced dry patches on the palms of the hands and the soles of the feet. Direct inheritance through five subsequent generations was reported in a large pedigree (Pendred, 1898).

But, in other examples of skin disorders, different forms of heredity appeared evident. A rare ulcerating skin condition termed xeroderma pigmentosum was first described in a family having two sisters and one brother affected. Parents and other relatives in the family were normal (Crocker, 1883, 1884). The disorder was termed familial, but not hereditary because it did not appear in successive generations (Crocker, 1887). Other affected families were collected in subsequent years, each showing affected siblings but normal parents (Reid, 1887; Hunter, 1889; Anderson, T.M., 1892). Thomas Anderson summarized data from 26 cases found in nine families, and found "In no instance has the disease been hereditary" (Anderson, T.M., 1889). However, one potential clue to the hereditary nature of xeroderma was presented in another family where unaffected parents were, in fact, first cousins (Phillips, 1895). The presence of the disease in collateral branches of the family would likewise suggest the indirect pattern for heredity.

SUMMARY

British physicians at this time were intensely interested in the heredity of human disease. Before 1890 they were convinced that heredity was a very important factor in the etiology of much human disease. The Hereditary Disease Database graph (Figure 9.1) shows the dramatic increase in the number of articles reporting such hereditary disorders in the decades before 1900.

The patterns of heredity outlined by Ribot proved useful to physicians as a means of organizing their thoughts about human inheritance. The increasing use of pedigrees to summarize the presence of affected and normal individuals in different generations of families was also seen to correlate with the characteristic direct, indirect and sex-limited patterns for inheritance already described in the previous chapter. While the use of the pedigree and the total number of articles on hereditary disease peaked in 1890, a decline occurred thereafter until the end of the century.

The attention of the medical profession at this time was beginning to turn away from heredity as a major cause of human disease. In 1878 Louis Pasteur published his ideas that much of human disease was, in fact due to contagion, to germs passed from one person to another. The rapid discoveries in the field of bacteriology appeared to indicate that most, if not all, disease could be due to "offending microbes" (Beecher, 1960). Opinions within the medical profession on the causes of diseases were shifting rapidly. Before 1870, the prominent dermatologist, Erasmus Wilson, could confidently state that the skin condition eczema occurred because of hereditary weakness of the constitution of the patient. Parents and children were often affected (Wilson, E., 1869). However, by 1900, the cause of eczema was believed to be the result of a parasitic infection possibly involving the "macrocossus of Una" (Freeman, 1900). R. Smith from the Bristol Medical School acknowledged that specific germs had been identified as the cause of syphilis, tuberculosis, typhoid and leprosy (Smith, R., 1888). Walter G. Smith, Professor at Trinity College Medical School in Dublin, felt that a revolution was happening in the 1890s within dermatology and other medical specialties. He quoted the German dermatologist Kaposi as stating, "There is no single disease, whether warts, eczema, psoriasis, pruritis cutaneous, inflammation, erysipelas, etc. which would not be attributed to a fungus." There was a real concern that dermatology, and by extension, the other branches of clinical medicine would become mere sub-sections of bacteriology (Smith, W.G., 1892).

As the nineteenth-century came to a close, the relative importance of heredity and infection in the causality of human disease remained uncertain. Heredity was on the decline; infection was ascending rapidly. Opinions on the causes of several important human diseases will be considered next in the following chapter.

Eleven

Does Heredity Really Account for the Causation of any Important Human Diseases?

The previous chapter has demonstrated the understanding of physicians that certain human diseases, often rare, were the result of hereditary influence. But what about the causes of more common disorders that afflicted thousands of people? By 1850, half the English population had become urban. The growth of industrial cities provided a living environment that was decidedly less healthy than the bucolic countryside. Crowded houses with poor ventilation coupled with polluted air from the burning of coal fostered the spread of airborne contagions. Impure water and food were also important sources of intestinal infections (Woods and Woodward, 1961).

Clinical observations of the era suggested the contagious nature of many of these diseases that caused significant human mortality. In one instance, within ten days over one summer, seven children in one family were affected by infantile paralysis [polio]. This observation was believed to "strongly confirm the growing belief that infantile paralysis is an acute infective disease" (Pasteur, 1897). Between 1873 and 1900, the causative microbes of most important infectious diseases were elucidated using techniques of microscopy and bacteriology. Public health officials at the local government level and physicians in daily practice came to accept the fact that such recent discoveries in basic biology would eventually be applied to human medicine and result in improved well-being for the patients. The historian P. Weindling characterized this opinion as a "critically utopian belief in the power of scientific usefulness" (Weindling, 1992). If specific bacteria caused specific human diseases, public health measures then logically should focus on case identification, isolation to prevent further spread to close contacts, and disinfection of the environment to inhibit public dissemination. The Sanitary Act of 1866 required local governments to standardize criteria for cleaner water and living conditions for the public. Local Boards of Health employed physicians to find those affected by contagious diseases and then to utilize modern scientific techniques in order to prevent further spread throughout the populace (Fee and Porter, 1992).

In general, a healthier British public resulted more from improved sanitation and living conditions rather than from specific medicines provided by the doctors. Tuberculosis, whooping cough, cholera, scarlet fever and typhoid fever all became less important by the end of the nineteenth-century, despite the lack of any specific medical intervention. The dramatic decline of smallpox, however, did coincide with mass vaccination of the public during the Victorian era (Woodward, 1961). Improvements in public health did eventually occur, mostly due to an enhanced general standard of living with cleaner air, water and food. By 1900, mortality from airborne disease had declined by 44%, while food and water-borne illnesses decreased by 33%. Life expectancy during the 1800s rose from 36 to 50 years in Britain (Woods and Woodward, 1961).

William Cheyne was a pathologist at King's College London and taught the first English medical school course on bacteriology in the 1880s. Within three weeks of Koch's announcement that he had isolated the microbe that caused tuberculosis, Cheyne was demonstrating the bacillus to his students in London (Worboys, 2000a). One important public health fact emerged from his studies: although everyone was exposed to germs in the air, water and food, not all became ill. Infection clearly involved both an infectious germ, and also an abnormal response of the human body to the invasion by the germ. Both aspects of infection had variability. Some types of germs were more virulent than others; some humans had stronger or weaker tissues, and hence could better resist or fall ill under the influence of the infective microbe. British physicians working in the field of bacteriology came to appreciate the importance of both aspects of infectious disease. A metaphor developed to conceptualize this notion of the bacterium as the "seed" and the tissues of the human body as the "soil." Both were necessary for actual clinical infection to develop. One surgeon noted, "It was necessary to add to the bare and naked germ theory the hypothesis that there is a varying resisting power in living tissue, and that germs do not always find it a fit nidus for their development and multiplication" (Worboys, 2000a).

Long years of clinical experience of physicians throughout the Empire had also demonstrated that different human races had different susceptibility to contagious diseases. Europeans were sensitive to malaria, while Africans in general were resistant. The reverse was true for smallpox infections. G.S. Woodhead, from the Laboratory at the Royal College of Physicians, thought that such differences in constitution could be hereditary. He thought "long-continued...acclimitisation through successive generations" (Woodhead, 1892) changed humans in such a way that resistance eventually became hereditary and was passed to successive generations. Within a single population, individual variability to infection was evident as well. Clearly, each person had different living soil. Other diseases, poor diet, drugs or alcohol abuse could weaken the constitution. Predisposition to infection then constituted all the strengths and weaknesses of the individual tissues as they confronted the onslaught of infectious microbes (Lithgow, 1889). If the hereditary soil was enfeebled, local infection could establish itself. Multiplication of the germs could then result in clinical disease (Oliver, 1900).

Diathesis

The predisposition to disease, or "diathesis," was a traditional concept that attempted to explain why disease developed in certain individuals. The term meant "that state of the body which makes it acquire certain diseases" (Ackerknecht, 1982). Physicians in the nineteenth century assumed that many human disorders were the result of diathesis, or predisposition to disease, which was often hereditary. Mental illness, cancer, gout, rheumatism, leprosy, rickets and tuberculosis were all considered to be diathetic because they frequently recurred within certain families and often in successive generations. Clinical observations over the years, rather than arithmetic compilations of numbers, carried considerable weight. One anonymous physician commented in 1846 on the "extensive instances of the law of hereditary predisposition...[that]...were occasionally under the notice of most practitioners" certainly convinced them that the 'dogma' on the heredity of diseases had to be correct ("Book Review," 1846). Alexander Tweedie summarized the general medical opinion that "the hereditary predisposition to scrofula, consumption, gout and insanity" was a "part of the medical creed" (Waller, 2002). Not only the general appearance of each individual, but specific variations in both tissue structure and function were believed to be hereditary, making each person uniquely resistant or susceptible to the various agents which could result in human disease (Coats, 1889).

Rheumatism and Gout

Rheumatic fever was believed to result from a sudden chilling of the skin. High fever and inflammation of the joints and the heart muscle then ensued (Osler, 1892a). In 1888, Archibald Garrod surveyed 500 general medical patients at St. Bart's Hospital and found a 20% incidence of rheumatic fever in immediate family members. Among the individuals who had suffered from rheumatic fever themselves, 30-35% identified other family members who had also had the same disease (Garrod, A.E. and Cooke, 1888).

Rheumatoid arthritis was a chronic disease characterized by stiffness and thickening of the joints in the hands, knees and feet (Osler, 1892b). Alfred Garrod of King's College Hospital investigated 80 cases in 1880 and found a positive family history in 25-30%, implying a hereditary predisposition (Garrod, A.B., 1880a). Numerous pedigrees were available which demonstrated the familial recurrence of the disorder in two and three generations, typically passed directly from one parent to several offspring (Sedgwick, 1863a; Hutchinson, 1896a).

Gout also had long been considered to be hereditary. As early as 1772, James Jay had observed, "Gout must be looked upon as a hereditary disease" (Waller, 2002). In the nineteenth century, William Gairdner in his treatise *On Gout* noted, "Gout is not always descended from father to son in an uninterrupted succession, but after passage over a generation or two...It rarely fails to resume its dominion even in a third or fourth generation" (Waller, 2002). Archibald Garrod also investigated the underlying causes of gout. Recurrent episodes of fever with severe pain and swelling of the joint of the great toe made life miserable for many sufferers. He found elevated levels of uric acid in the blood of individuals during gouty attacks, which seemed to be triggered by rich food and alcohol consumption (Osler, 1892c). Gout was more common in men, and often passed directly from father to son in several successive generations (Sedgwick, 1863a). A predisposition or peculiarity of the organs involving digestion and excretion of specific food or drink appeared necessary for disease symptoms to develop (Lithgow, 1887).

Garrod discovered families with four affected successive generations. Although the disease could occur as a single case, at least 50% of his examples had a positive family history. Symptoms of the disease could sometimes be avoided or at least ameliorated by careful living: avoiding beer, wine and excessive meat, coupled with vigorous exercise (Lauder, 1886). But nonetheless, the offspring of those with the gouty predisposition might produce children "fully under the hereditary influence of their grandparents and liable to development of the malady from the ordinary exciting causes" (Garrod, A.B., 1880b). The disease might be avoided by conservative living, but the diathesis was still present and could be passed along to the next generation.

Leprosy

The ancient disease leprosy had been assumed to be contagious for centuries. Lepers were routinely confined to isolated colonies and prevented from daily commerce with the rest of the population. However, as early as 1842, James Simpson began revising these long-held opinions in his study of leper hospitals throughout Europe. Familial cases seemed to be very frequent. The existence of the dread disease in a parent and several children suggested the inheritance of a predisposition to the disease. In isolated regions he thought, "The malady seems to be transmitted through an old hereditary taint in particular families" (Simpson, 1842). Everyday experience also argued against the contagious nature of leprosy. A wife caring for an affected husband did not readily acquire the disease (Adams, 1814). Nursing sisters who cared for lepers in hospitals for more than forty years never developed any symptoms of the disease (Osler, 1892d).

However, Sedgwick found families in which leprosy was common in collateral branches among uncles, aunts and cousins. Although the trait could skip generations, he found examples of direct transmission from father to son (Sedgwick, 1863b). An expert committee from the Royal College of Physicians examined the evidence for the contagious nature of leprosy and concluded in 1867 that, in fact, the disorder was hereditary in nature. The isolation of lepers in closed colonies was no longer felt to be necessary, but prohibition of marriage to prevent further spread of the character was believed to be an appropriate public health measure (Worboys, 2000b; Squire, A.B., 1880).

Microscopic examination of lymph nodes from patients with leprosy subsequently revealed the existence of characteristic bacteria which were presumed to be the cause of the disease itself. Gerhard Hansen from Norway first reported these findings in the English literature in 1875 (Hansen, 1875). Within ten years, leprosy was once again viewed as an infectious disease, but one which required a specific constitution or soil before it could develop (Osler, 1892e). Along these lines, George Thin analyzed the development of leprosy in the town of Parcent in the Spanish province of Aliconte. A leper moved to the area in 1850; leprosy had been unknown there in prior years. Over the next few decades, his children and grandchildren developed the disease, simulating hereditary transmission of the affliction. The familial nature of the disease could have reflected a hereditary predisposition, but Thin argued that leprosy was, in fact, an infection transmitted by intimate contact between parent and child over many years (Thin, 1892).

Tuberculosis

Tuberculosis was a major public health hazard in the late Victorian era, producing about 70,000 deaths each year. One in forty adults between 20 and 60 years was afflicted and had symptoms at any one time (Alborn, 2001a; Worboys, 2000a). Phthisis [pulmonary tuberculosis] was traditionally assumed to be hereditary in nature because so many family histories revealed the disease in a parent which then reappeared in subsequent offspring. Family pedigrees frequently revealed disease in grandparents, parents and children in successive generations (Sedgwick, 1863a). H. Hartshorne accepted the opinion, "Hereditary predisposition is universally believed to be a principal factor in the production of all forms of scrofula. Every physician must know instances of its recurring in several members of one family in successive generations" (Hartshorne, 1880). James

Clark summarized the general opinion of the day in his 1834 *Treatise on Tubercular Phthisis*. He thought, "That pulmonary consumption is a hereditary disease—in other words, that the tuberculous constitution is transmitted from parent to child, is a fact not to be controverted" (Waller, 2002). When both parents were affected, the risk that the children would be affected was increased by four-fold (Hartshorne, 1880). Symptoms of the disease also developed in these families at an unusually young age (Williams, C.J.B. and Williams, 1887). The marriage of related individuals also increased the risk for hereditary transmission of disease. Such consanguineous marriages from scrofulous stock were clearly recognized as factors increasing the likelihood that children would be affected (Greenhow, 1862; Hartshorne, 1880). As one author noted, "Marriages of consanguinity when there is a family tendency to phthisis...are obviously most hurtful..."(James, 1888). James Clark agreed that careful choice of marriage partners could affect the next generation. "The predisposition which is often entailed on...offspring might be checked, and even extinguished," he thought. But, such a change in inheritance might require "a few generations" to remove the taint from the family (Waller, 2002).

British physicians of the nineteenth century were concerned that heredity strongly predisposed individuals to the development of tuberculosis. One noted, "In no disease is hereditary predisposition more evident..." (Thomas, 1888). Daily contact with affected persons did not appear to spread the disease. A 21-year review of infection among the medical staff at Brompton Hospital for Diseases of the Chest in London in 1879 revealed only two individuals affected with tuberculosis (Bennett, 1880). At the same time several reviews of thousands of patients from the same hospital reported a positive family history for tuberculosis in 48-66% of all cases (Alborn, 2001b). In 1865 James Pollock from the Brompton Hospital argued, "The phthisical should not marry, those strongly predisposed by family inheritance of the disease should not marry; near relatives also predisposed should not marry" (Alborn, 2001c). Other surveys also revealed the frequent occurrence of affected children born of affected parents (Table 11.1).

Not all English physicians accepted the popular notion on the hereditary nature of consumption at this time. By the middle of the nineteenth century, Henry Ancell was able to state in a *Treatise on Tuberculosis*:

> So large a proportion of the population is affected with the tuberculous state of the blood...that in individual cases, and in masses of cases, it is very frequently difficult, and sometimes impossible to determine when disease is transmitted hereditarily and when it has been acquired (Waller, 2002b).

In 1846, Benjamin Phillips collected statistics on the family history of 2023 children with scrofula. When one parent was affected, the offspring had only 4% greater risk of developing the same disease than those born of unaffected parents (Waller, 2002c). Francis Galton later examined the question of heredity and tuberculosis and found 26% of the children were affected when one parent was also affected. When both parents were healthy, only 18% of the offspring were affected. He concluded that tuberculosis was partly hereditary and also due to some other exciting cause (Galton, 1889). J.E. Squire from the North London Hospital for Consumption collected 1000 clinic patients and found an incidence of 24.9% when parents were healthy. When one parent was affected, 33.7% of the children were also affected. When both parents had tuberculosis, 39.5% of the offspring were diseased. In his 1897 report, Squire agreed with Galton that a hereditary predisposition in such families did exist, but could account only for the 9% difference in disease frequency between offspring of affected and unaffected parents (Squire, J.E., 1897). Further analysis of the data from private patients, a more well-to-do clientele, revealed the startling fact that only 12% of children born of an affected parent in that family setting developed symptoms of tuberculosis. Such data suggested that familial cases more likely reflected the effects of close living in crowded quarters and suggested that tuberculosis might, in fact, be a contagious disease (Squire, J.E., 1897; Steven, 1892). J.H. Bennett from the Royal Infirmary in Edinburgh observed as early as 1879:

> We have seen the children in many families become phthisical, in whom no hereditary taint could be traced...among the six or eight cases of phthisis [there], not one could be traced to hereditary causes. Although, therefore, there can be no doubt that weakness in parents is a cause of weakness in the offspring, it is by no means as general or influential a source of phthisis as is usually supposed (Bennett, 1880).

A summary of findings on heredity and tuberculosis is presented in Table 11.1.

Table 11.1
Tuberculosis and Heredity
1860-1899

Family History	Percent Children Affected	References
One Parent Affected		
Hospital Patients	26	Galton, 1889
	34	Squire, J.E., 1894, 1895
	37	Williams, C.J.B. 1887
	30	Williams, C.J.B. 1887
	24	Williams, C.J.B.1887
Private Patients	12	Squire, J.E., 1897
Both Parents Affected	40	Squire, J.E., 1894
Unaffected Parents	25	Squire, J.E., 1894
	18	Galton, 1889

Jean Villemin determined the underlying infectious cause of tuberculosis in work with experimental animals during the 1860s. He was able to transmit the disorder from one animal to another with inoculation, and could postulate that close habitation facilitated transmission of the disease as an infection from parent to offspring (Vellemin, 1862). Similar results were duplicated shortly thereafter in England (Worboys, 2000c). However, medical experts in consumption such as Richard Cotton at the Brompton and Samuel Wilkins at Guy's Hospital continued to deny the contagion of this affliction (Worboys, 2000d).

Robert Koch announced his claim in 1882 to have found characteristic bacteria within the human tubercle, the lesion in the lung found in those with tuberculosis. British reaction was not immediately in agreement. Julius Dreschfeld, Professor of Pathology at Owen's College in Manchester, did not deny the existence of the tubercle bacillus. He continued to argue that human tuberculosis was hereditary. Clinical evidence had shown that it was not easily transmitted from person-to-person, and the demonstration of infection in experimental animals meant nothing in terms of understanding the cause of human disease, in his opinion (Worboys, 2000e).

Over the next decade, however, the tide of British opinion turned toward accepting the infectious nature of tuberculosis (Robertson, 1882; Andrew, 1884; Marsh, 1886; Elsner, 1886). G. Barling, Professor of Pathology at Queen's College in Birmingham, stated "without hesitation" that the bacillus was the cause of tuberculosis (Barling, 1891). William Osler noted that Koch's identification of the tubercule bacillus was "one of the most masterly demonstrations of modern medicine" (Osler, 1892f).

Nonetheless, James Pollock claimed in his 1883 Croonian Lecture that there must exist a hereditary predisposition to tuberculosis because although all were exposed to the bacillus, only a few actually developed the disease (Pollock, 1883a, b). In the following year, T.H. Green reflected the opinion of many physicians at the time that two elements were required to produce phthisis: first the bacillus, and then an abnormal state of the pulmonary tissue in which it lodged (Worboys, 2000f). C.T. Williams from the Brompton came to a similar conclusion:

> If we are to accept the bacillary theory at all, we must suppose that the various and well-known predisposing causes of phthisis such as dampness, soil, bad ventilation, bad confinements, and other debilitating conditions must act by preparing a fit soil for the bacillus either by bringing about some low inflammatory conditions or by weakening the resisting powers of the constitution (Worboys, 2000g).

The "seed and soil" metaphor for tuberculosis became widely accepted before 1900 in Britain. Clearly the disease was an infection, but there was also a hereditary predisposition that provided "enfeebled lungs for the bacillus to grow" (Green, 1883). The predisposition resulted when "the epithelial protective covering of the lungs [became] too little resistant...too readily penetrated by the parasite of the disease" (Hamilton, 1900). Such predisposition did appear to have a hereditary basis. C.A. Davies examined the frequency of tuberculosis in the small villages that dotted the Isle of Man in the south of England. The climate was generally mild, and there were no cities with air pollution and crowded living conditions. However, the incidence of disease was twice that in the mainland population. The frequency of tuberculosis was correlated with the degree of inbreeding in the more isolated villages of the island, suggesting the importance of transmitted hereditary predisposition to develop the actual disease (Davies, 1900).

It had long been believed that the predisposition in lung tissue also produced a characteristic phthisical appearance with an elongated face, narrow chest, bushy eyebrows and long eyelashes (Strahan, 1892a; Hamilton, 1900). Francis Galton collaborated with Frederick Mahomed, surgeon at Guy's Hospital, in an attempt to identify individuals with the predisposition to tuberculosis. They photographed patients with phthisis and those with other medical conditions from the general hospital wards. Composite pictures were prepared of the two groups. No characteristic phthisical facies could be identified. They concluded that the predisposition to disease might well exist, but did not result in any specific outward manifestation which could be readily recognized by a trained clinician (Mahomed and Galton, 1882).

Treatment options for such tuberculous diseases were typically limited. Horatio Prater thought that one should try to keep the patient comfortable. James Whitehead suggested, "When the disease, the elements of which were identified, has once developed its probable form, all efforts at what is termed a radical cure will be unsuccessful" (Waller, 2002d). Because the disease was part of one's constitution, which was more or less fixed at birth, altering the somatic environment with medication, bleeding or diet could not really change the constitution and cure the patient or his family of the hereditary disease. Hence, therapy was often frustrating and useless (Waller, 2002e).

However, if both the infectious seed and the predisposed soil in the lungs were required before actual disease developed, the fate of patients with tuberculosis no longer seemed absolutely helpless. A person was not necessarily the victim of his own heredity. As early as 1869, Pollock had recommended techniques for improving "the soil." If the general health of the individual could be improved, it was hoped that the body would then repair the lung damage and suppress the development of further disease symptoms (Worboys, 2000h). Forty years later, the importance of the diathesis had lessened, and tuberculosis became "...a disease one may hope to see exterminated" by better housing and sanitation (Alborn, 2001). T.J. Perkins from the Brompton noted, "The adverse influence of heredity may be kept in check by a healthy life and removal from tuberculous surroundings" (Alborn, 2001d). Public health measures to decrease the spread of contagion by banning public expectoration, and to enhance the general health of those infected by developing sanitaria with fresh air, high-quality food and exercise seemed good general policies (Worboys, 2000h). As a disease resulting from the interaction of the tubercle bacillus and a suitable pulmonary nidus for infection, public health measures which limited "close living, unsanitary homes...changeable climate, dusty occupations and ill-assorted marriages" would hopefully lead to an attenuation of the tubercular taint in English society (Oliver, 1900).

CANCER

Both tuberculosis and cancers were diseases rather commonly encountered in clinical practice. It would not be too surprising then to note a family with cancer in three successive generations where many individuals also were afflicted with tuberculosis (Blake, 1891). Williams also surveyed families afflicted with both types of illnesses. He found among 134 families with breast cancer, 55% of relatives also had tuberculosis. When 129 families with uterine cancer were examined, 46% of the relatives had tuberculosis, and among 53 families with cancer of the tongue, 42% of relatives also had tuberculosis (Williams, W.R., 1887). If phthisis had a hereditary predisposition, an analogous diathesis could well exist for cancer.

Analysis of population studies reported in previous chapters found the common recurrence of cancer in the offspring of affected parents. The results of hereditary cancer surveys from this era are summarized in Table 11.2. Uterine cancer recurred in 8-24% of cases, while breast cancer reappeared in 13-24% of all cases. Tumors of the skin structures were less frequent, appearing in 3-15% of offspring. Like tuberculosis, cancer also was more common in certain ethnic groups. The virtual absence of cancer in primitive tribes was particularly notable (Dunn, 1886). E.A. Howlett from the Hull Royal Infirmary used a familiar analogy to express the importance of heredity in cancer. It meant "a certain peculiarity of soil which favors development of some specific germ; and applied to cancer we must admit that a certain peculiarity or predisposition may exist, which is capable of being transmitted from parent to child" (Howlett, 1893). Jonathan Hutchinson served as President of the International Congress on Dermatology held in London during 1896. He thought that heredity played an important role in predisposing children to cancer. The occurrence of the same type of cancer in parent and child suggested that, "germinal matter must have been transmitted" (Hutchinson, 1896b).

The overall importance of hereditary predisposition in the etiology of cancer remained in dispute. Herbert Snow, surgeon at the Cancer Hospital in London, collected data from several large populations of cancer patients. He also surveyed the medical staff and general medical patients from the hospital wards and found approximately the same percentage of those with a family history of cancer as that noted from cancer patients. He believed that only a small percentage of cancer cases truly had a hereditary predisposition. There were specific families, however, in which cancer recurred repeatedly from one generation to the next. In those families a diathesis might well have existed (Snow, 1880, 1883, 1885, 1891, 1893a).

By 1890, John Simon, surgeon at St. Thomas's Hospital, was convinced that cancer was much like tuberculosis. Cancer involved unusual growth of tissues on a predisposed soil that was prepared by heredity. Some factor, perhaps a microbe, irritated the tissues which then began to grow abnormally. Such a working hypothesis had proved successful in understanding the nature of tuberculosis and could guide future research on the etiology of cancers (Simon, 1892). Strahan also thought the same seed and soil model could be useful in the study of cancer (Strahan, 1892b).

While the existence of such "cancer" families was real, they were rare in clinical practice. In one case, a grandfather had eye cancer, his son and daughter had tongue cancer, and a granddaughter had lymph node and breast tumors (McAldowie, 1879). In another example, a grandfather had cancer of the lip, one daughter had rib sarcoma, another had gastric cancer, and a granddaughter had breast cancer (Cameron, 1886). And breast cancer appeared in a man who fathered six daughters with the same tumor, a son with throat cancer and another son with epithelial cancer of the arm (Power, 1898). Another large family documented the existence of various cancers through five successive generations (Hardman, 1894). In other cases, it appeared that a specific type of tumor was transmitted directly from one generation to the next. A father, two sons and one daughter had the benign facial tumor adenoma sebaceum (Taylor and Barendt, 1893). The pigmented tumor melanotic sarcoma of the choroid [lining of the eyeball] appeared in a mother and her daughter (Silcock, 1891). Sebaceous tumors of the skeleton appeared repeatedly in several families spanning from two to seven generations. Direct transmission from parent to child was evident in all cases (Hutchinson, 1891; Barrett and Webster, 1891, 1892). Cancer of the stomach also recurred in successive generations. The example of Napoleon Boneparte's family was a well-known instance (Fox, 1880). H.T. Butlin, surgeon at St. Bart's Hospital, collected 24 family pedigrees demonstrating recurrent breast cancer. Nineteen families had two cases, three families had three cases, and two families had four cases. In almost all instances, the predisposition to cancer appeared to be directly transmitted from mother to daughter (Butlin, 1895).

Table 11.2
Family History and Cancer
1860-1899

Type of Cancer	Positive Family History	References
Uterus	8%	Darwin, 1893
	8	Snow, 1880
	8	Snow, 1883
	13	Snow, 1885
	24	Williams, W.R., 1884
	10	Williams, W.R., 1886
	20	Williams, W.R., 1895
Breast	13	Snow, 1880
	15	Snow, 1883
	18	Snow, 1885
	24	Williams, W.R., 1884
	13	Williams, W.R., 1886
	24	Williams, W.R., 1895
Epithelioma	3	Snow, 1883
	14	Snow, 1885
Sarcoma	10	Snow, 1883
	11	Snow, 1885
Healthy Physicians	19	Snow, 1885
Chest Disease Patients	11	Snow, 1885
General Medical Patients	26	Snow, 1885

In contrast, the possible contagious nature of cancer was supported by several observations at this time. One man had cancer of the lip. His dog licked the man's lip and subsequently developed cancer of the tongue. A hospital nurse washed the bandages from a woman with uterine cancer. She then developed cancer on her arm. In one small town, five surgeons from one hospital all developed cancer within a brief period of time (Budd, 1887).

During the 1890s, several pathologists reported the microscopic appearance of various organisms that were associated with cancerous tissues and could be the infectious agents responsible for initiating tumor growth. William Russell, from the Royal Infirmary in Edinburgh, noted a budding organism in several cancer tissues. He thought it was a yeast and might be the causative factor in such cancers (Russell, W., 1890). M. Ruffer from the Royal College of Physicians Laboratory then reported the association of a protozoan with breast cancer tissues. The nucleus of the parasite had different staining characteristics that clearly differentiated it from the nuclei of the cancer cells. Division of the nucleus was also observed, suggesting reproduction of the protozoa within the malignant tissues. Fifty cases were studied, and the protozoan was observed in all examples of tumor (Ruffer and Plimmer, 1893). Subsequent work examined 1278 cancer samples and found the "parasitic protozoa" in 1190 examples. Normal tissues never had the characteristic organism. J. Buchanan sought the cancer parasite in examples of breast, bladder, gallbladder, tongue, palate, bowel, ovary, testis, vocal cord, stomach and uterine tissues. The same parasite was consistently found in the cancerous material (Buchanan, 1900).

Evidence also accumulated that cancer acted like an infection because it could at times be transmitted from one experimental animal to another (Buchanan, 1900; Smith, 1900; Monsaurat, 1900). In the tissues of these animals, intracellular organisms were observed resembling protozoa or yeast (Smith, 1900; Monsaurat, 1900; Parsons, 1900). The similarity between cancer and tuberculosis was stunning. Heredity appeared to play some role in tissue susceptibility to what appeared to be a local infection. Subsequent unregulated tumor growth then produced symptoms of disease. A.T. Brand summarized the excitement in the field of cancer research of the 1890s when he stated that he was convinced a microorganism causing cancer would soon be identified and then shown to fulfill Koch's postulates for infection (Brand, 1903). If this were true, then public health measures conceivably could likewise decrease the risk for both tuberculosis and cancer.

The association of the microorganisms with various types of cancer was clear, but were these really infectious particles, and if so, did they really cause cancer? (Galloway, 1893). George Dean, pathologist at the Royal Hospital for Sick Children in London, re-examined some of the tissues in which Russell had claimed to find microbes associated with cancer. He had worked at the Pathological Institute in Berlin in conjunction with Rudolf Virchow. Careful examination of the tissues by these men noted staining bodies in and around both cancerous and normal tissues. The microscopic entities appeared to be hyaline, a protein product of tissue degeneration. Such artifacts were not really microbes, and thus could not be the alleged infectious cause of different cancers (Dean, 1891). By 1900, Herbert Snow and other leading cancer experts agreed that the evidence of pathologic fungi or protozoa was still lacking. No organisms had been isolated in pure culture or consistently transmitted experimentally in animal studies (Snow, 1893b; Kanthrack, 1891; Barwell, 1894).

Other work suggested that non-infectious environmental factors also might contribute to the development of cancer. People living in certain houses with polluted water over many years often developed cancer (Haviland, 1895). Persons living in old houses with damp climates also had an increased risk for cancer (Russell, A., 1900a, b, c).

While the search for the germ causing cancer continued, analysis of the cancer cells suggested that the disease process resulting in cancer began as a reversion of the cells to a more primitive and unregulated state, almost like an ameba. Cell division ensued in an aberrant fashion, producing abnormal tissues that acted as malignant structures to damage and destroy normal organs (Snow, 1893c, 1898). G.R. Williams observed that each cancer type had a characteristic microscopic anatomy that was distinct from the general inflammatory response seen in most true infections. In this respect, cancer could be seen as a defect in cell development (Williams, G.R., 1891). As early as 1889, John Marshall suggested that such regulation of cellular growth must originate within the nucleus of the cell. He observed that the hereditary properties had been associated with structures [chromosomes] within the cell nucleus. Microscopic examination showed alterations in these structures during tumor development. There were "remarkable movements and changes of form in the core of this little bit of nucleus, most wonderfully tufted arrangements, feathering themselves out this way and that...We must endeavor to search out this mystery, to look at the minute anatomy of the nucleus of the cancer cell" (Marshall, 1889). His comments argued that the cell nucleus, therefore, contained the hereditary elements that predisposed to the abnormal cell replication and growth that characterized malignant tissue transformation.

Conclusion

By 1900, sufficient evidence had accumulated to conclude that many rare disorders involving different body systems clearly had an important hereditary causality and thus reappeared in successive generations of particular families. Characteristic patterns of inheritance defined by Ribot were identified and associated with specific disorders. Ectopia lentis, for example, demonstrated direct heredity, Friedreich's ataxia had indirect heredity, while hemophilia demonstrated the sex-limited pattern for its heredity.

More common diseases, such as cancer and gout, were well known throughout the general population. Frequently, several people in one family were similarly affected, but in general, heredity did not appear to play the deciding role in causing such diseases. The "seed and soil" model argued that a predisposition was necessary for many diseases, including those associated with an identifiable pathogenic microorganism. Such a predisposition seemed to have a hereditary basis as well. During the late nineteenth and early twentieth centuries, the precise diagnosis and actual treatment of these infectious scourges became a triumph of modern medicine.

By the end of the nineteenth-century, the relative importance of heredity in causing important human diseases was becoming more questionable (Wilson, 2003). The historian H.K. Beecher noted that the rapid discoveries in the realm of bacteriology suggested that all diseases might be the result of such "offending microbes." The importance of hereditary predisposition to disease in general suffered a great blow. In his opinion, "The contemplation of the place of hereditary factors in disease became unfashionable and even somewhat disreputable" (Beecher, 1960).

For the medical man of this era, however, heredity still remained an important factor in human disease. He saw the recurrence of specific characters, both normal and abnormal, in parent and child, one generation after the next. If a better understanding of how human heredity actually worked could be had, a more precise comprehension of its role in producing such diseases could conceivably guide each physician in his care of affected families. J.K. Love, from the Glasgow Royal Infirmary, observed:

> ...but in every case where well-defined [hereditary] tendencies can be dealt with, the result is as inevitable as that of an equation, and would be definitely predictive if we knew the powers of all the forces as formally as we do those of the figures in an equation (Love, 1896).

The dawn of the twentieth century would be accompanied by the development of just such a theory of heredity having the precision, just like an equation, to predict the results of offspring from specific parents. The influence of heredity on the transmission of both normal and disease characters would be abundantly elucidated in the first decade of the new millennium.

Part IV
Twentieth Century Medicine and Genetics

Twelve

The Decade of Discovery 1900-1910

THE ENGLISH SCHOOLS OF HEREDITY

In 1889, Francis Galton presented his theory of heredity in the book titled *Natural Inheritance*. He was the first scientist to apply modern statistical theory to analyze how human children varied from their parents in both physical and psychological traits (Galton, 1889). His work stimulated a generation of young biologists to further investigate questions of inheritance, reversion and variation in plants and animals, as well as in human beings. Comments from this younger group of scientists generally credited Galton with opening the entire field of human heredity to scientific investigation. They agreed that they owed a great deal to him for his efforts (Cowan, 1972).

One of the rising stars in the field of heredity and variation was W. Frank Raphael Weldon (b 1860). He had originally intended to become a physician, but became fascinated with the study of zoology at St. John's College Cambridge. He received a First Class Natural Sciences Tripos in 1881 and focused his subsequent work on invertebrate morphology, performing field studies on marine life in the Bahamas and at the Marine Biological Association Laboratory located in Plymouth.

Weldon read Galton's book as soon as it was published and began to study morphological variation in marine invertebrates. He discovered that measurements of several features appeared to follow a Gaussian natural distribution. This application of statistics to physical characteristics from nature marked the beginning of the science of biometrics (Gillham, 2001a). Further development of this new science advanced as Weldon was appointed Jodrell Professor of Zoology at University College London in 1891. There he began a collaboration with the statistics professor Karl Pearson. Weldon provided the raw data from field measurements, and Pearson then developed statistical tests to analyze the variations found in nature. Pearson admitted that he had initially known little about variation and evolution, and credited his own interest in biometry solely due to Weldon's suggestions. Pearson recalled later that without Weldon's "inspiration and enthusiasm" he would never have begun investigations in the realm of biology (Froggatt and Nevin, 1971).

Much of the data Weldon collected from marine invertebrates did fit a normal curve. He noted though, that the ratio of forehead breadth to body length in the Naples crab in particular appeared to be bimodal (Weldon, 1893). Pearson interpreted the data as showing two overlapping normal curves, suggesting two distinct groups within the crab species. Weldon and Pearson thought this finding indicated evidence of natural selection resulting in two distinct populations, and possibly a second incipient species of crab evolving at that time. Weldon was convinced that he had discovered a tool for the study of biologic evolution in action. He urged, "The problem of animal evolution is essentially a statistical problem...These [problems] are all questions of arithmetic, and when we know the numerical answers to these questions for a number of species, we shall know the direction and the rate of change in these species..." The method to be used for the analysis of such evolutionary problems was to be "statistical." This meant that "accurate measurements of several factors needed to be done, including abnormality of offspring in terms of abnormality of parents and vice versa," reflecting the importance of understanding ancestral heredity as outlined earlier by his mentor, Francis Galton (Weldon, 1893; Provine, 1971a).

The second collaborator in this quest, Karl Pearson, was another rising young man in the British academic world. He began his career at King's College Cambridge and worked intensely in the humanities as well as in mathematics. He studied widely in philosophy and religion while preparing for the Mathematical Tripos. He eventually was named only Third Wrangler and became despondent. However, this performance did eventually earn him a fellowship that allowed time in Heidelberg to investigate German philosophy and literature, physics and the law. Pearson returned to King's College in 1880 and read widely in the same areas. Although he qualified as a barrister, he never practiced law and focused his immense energies on mathematics and engineering. He then accepted a position as Professor of Applied Mathematics at University College London in 1884, and several years later became Professor of Geometry at Gresham College as well. He developed statistical tools to analyze graphical representations of data from diverse fields of human endeavor: engineering, economic output and other characteristics of society. He thought that scientific knowledge would become the source of shared values that defined and expanded modern culture (Porter, 2004a).

Pearson had also read Galton's 1889 book *Natural Inheritance* and thought that such nascent ideas on variation could be given a solid mathematical basis. His work with Weldon at University College London after 1891 explored a broad range of data on natural variation in living populations. He became convinced that deviations from the normal curve showed that natural selection was at work. He told his Gresham students: "For the first time in the history of biology, there is a chance of the science of life becoming an exact, mathematical science. Men are approaching the questions of heredity and evolution from a new standpoint" (Porter, 2004b). When Pearson analyzed raw biologic data, he functioned as a pure mathematician and sought evidence of skews in the curves he generated. He tended to ignore other possible causes of population variation, and just focused on an investigation of the numbers as a reflection of what he perceived to be evolution at work (Porter, 2004c). Over the next few years, Pearson became convinced that statistics could unify biology and the other sciences as well. He thought that this "new tool in science...would give certainty where all was obscurity and hypothesis before" (Porter, 2004d). In the field of natural history, he predicted:

> The loose quantitative or descriptive reasoning of the older biologists must give way to an accurate mathematico-statistical logic. The trained biologist may discover and tabulate facts, much as the physicist does today, but it will need the mathematician to reason upon them. The great biologist of the future...will be a mathematician trained and bred (Porter, 2004e).

Pearson continued to refine the mathematical basis for Galton's law of ancestral heredity and was able to summarize it by the end of the decade. He thought, "It seems to me that the law of ancestral heredity is highly probably...the simple descriptive statement which brings into a single focus all the complexities of hereditary influence" (Pearson, K., 1898).

But Galton and Pearson differed in their interpretations of how evolution actually worked. Galton had long believed that natural selection primarily worked on "sports," the sudden and spontaneous appearance of significant variants within a population. Pearson's correlations of numerous minor variations convinced him that selection operated in a more gradual scheme as first described by Darwin (Porter, 2004f). In any event, Pearson concluded that no particular theory of heredity was necessary to explain how characteristics were transmitted by the egg and sperm from one generation to another. Such formulations in biology might develop in the future, however. He proposed in 1900:

> Till we know what class of characters blend and what class of characters is mutually exclusive, we have not within our cognizance the veriest outlines of the phenomena which the inventors of plasmic mechanisms are in such haste to account for...The numerical laws for the intensity of inheritance must first be discovered from wide observations before plasmic mechanisms can be anything but the purest hypothetical speculation (Pearson, K., 1900).

For Pearson, the study of evolution implied a study of change in human society as well as in the natural world. He sought to take a larger view on the importance of his work in biometry. He surmised,

> Here for the first time was a possibility—I will not say a certainty—of reaching knowledge as valid as physical knowledge was then thought to be, in the field of living forms and above all in the field of human conduct (Greenwood, 1940).

He was a socialist and hoped the application of his science would benefit the broader populace (Porter, 2004g).

At Weldon's suggestion, the Royal Society founded a Committee for Conducting Statistical Enquiries into the Measurable Characteristics of Plants and Animals. The first meeting was held in January 1894 with Galton as chairman and Weldon as secretary. This organization provided a forum for the discussion and application of statistical models to questions of evolution and heredity (Froggatt and Nevin, 1971). Controversies developed among the committee members from its inception. Galton thought evolution was discontinuous, operating on large variants, while Weldon and Pearson thought a continuous process operating on numerous small variations was more likely (Provine, 1971b). The controversy became more heated in 1895 when Weldon prepared a report for the committee correlating the death rate of a type of crab with a measurable shell dimension. Biologists such as William Bateson who reviewed the material did not understand the mathematical biometric analysis of the evolutionary process and sent inflammatory letters to Galton as chairman (Froggatt and Nevin, 1971; Provine, 1971a). Attempts were made to ameliorate the conflict by appointing Bateson to the committee to lend his biologic knowledge to the analysis of the evolutionary data (Froggatt and Nevin, 1971). The original members did not like this idea either, fearing the work of the group would become bogged down in further controversy.

After one meeting when Bateson was present, Pearson was not at all pleased. He wrote to Galton in 1897:

> I felt sadly out of place in such a gathering of biologists...The Committee you have got together is entirely unsuited...It is far too large, contains far too many of the old biologists type...The older school of biologists cannot be expected to appreciate these [statistical] methods...[The Committee] is far too unconscious of the fact that the solutions of these problems are in the first place statistical, and the second place statistical, and only in the third place biological (Pearson, K., 1897).

Over the next few years, the focus of the group gradually did shift from statistics to experimental breeding, much to the dismay of the founders. By 1900 the friction between the members had become so great that Galton, Pearson and Weldon all resigned in disgust (Froggatt and Nevin, 1971; Kim, 1994a; Provine, 1971a). The organization was then renamed the Evolution Committee of the Royal Society. Conflict in this new realm of biometry continued as the proponents of continuous vs. discontinuous variation marshaled their evidence (Eisenhart, 1970; Provine, 1971a). By the start of the new century, Pearson and his colleagues had reported many examples of continuous variation of characters in natural populations. Likewise, Bateson and his co-workers had found extensive evidence of discontinuous variation among different biologic species.

William Bateson had been a student with Weldon at St. John's College Cambridge. He focused his studies on vertebrate embryology and did field studies sponsored by Johns Hopkins University in the United States. He had little training in chemistry and physics, and "knew virtually no mathematics" (Coleman, 1970). He was appointed Fellow at St. John's in 1887 and began a study of the origins of variations that acted in natural selection. Bateson summarized his work in an 1894 book titled *Materials for the Study of Evolution.* Using examples from plants, animals and humans, he argued that discontinuous variation rather than minute continuous variation was the rule in nature and provided the grist for the process of natural selection. He became familiar with the medical literature on human variation and found numerous examples of such "sports" in humans involving alterations in ribs, vertebrae, fingers, toes and branchial cleft remnants. Bateson was convinced that, "The discontinuity of the species results from the discontinuity of variation" (Bateson, W., 1894a). He was not certain of the origin of such variants, but felt that there had to be some hereditary mechanism to transmit them to subsequent generations. His research in the late 1890s then focused on how such variation could be transmitted, as elucidated in a series of "systematic experiments in breeding" (Bateson, W., 1894b). In 1899 Bateson was appointed deputy to Alfred Newton, Professor of Zoology, and began regular teaching responsibilities. He was able to gather a group of young students to assist in his studies on breeding of peas, poppies and poultry (Bateson, B., 1928a).

The application of mathematics and statistics to breeding studies was being investigated throughout Europe at this time. Pehr Bohlin studied crossbreeding of various peas, cereals and barley. He reported to the 1897 Agricultural Congress in Stockholm:

> ...in the F1 [first generation] there was no variation, while the forms appearing in the F2 [second generation] and subsequent generations represented all possible combinations of the parental characteristics and could be predicted with almost mathematical accuracy (Von Tschermak-Seysenegg, 1951; Stubbe, 1972a).

Hugo de Vries, from the University of Amsterdam, had extensive experience as a plant breeder and collected data on crosses from eleven different species. He treated each character individually and examined their transmission independently. Before 1900 he also detected characteristic ratios in the offspring for many such characters (Stubbe, 1972b; Zirkle, 1964). Carl Correns, at the University of Tubingen, had studied crosses of maize and peas beginning in 1892. He too found one class of F1 offspring, and the reappearance of all the parental types in the F2 generation with characteristic ratios (Von Tschermak-Seysenegg, 1951; Stubbe, 1972c). Erich von Tschermak was another plant breeder who studied in both Austria and Belgium in the late 1890s. His analysis of segregation likewise showed characteristic ratios of both one and two characters in subsequent generations (Von Tschermak-Seysenegg, 1951; Stubbe, 1972d). Bateson summarized his appreciation of how statistics should be applied to such breeding experiments in a discussion before the Royal Horticultural Society in 1899. His own observations had convinced him that variants in plants typically appeared suddenly as "sports." He thought these nascent varieties could potentially become separate species over time. Bateson's study in plants argued that evolution was not slow and gradual, but could, in fact, "proceed at a gallop." He urged the plant breeders to collect statistics on the frequencies of different offspring of different parental crosses, because he was sure that crossbreeding studies would help unravel the mysteries of evolution—how varieties arose and then how they were transmitted to offspring (Bateson, W., 1899).

An 1894 book called *Plant Breeding* by C.H. Bailey referenced an 1865 work "Versuchen uber Pflanzhybriden" that had been published by an Austrian monk, Gregor Mendel (Mendel, 1865). Correns read Mendel's paper in April 1896 but did not appreciate its relevance to his own plant breeding studies until he began to collate his data in late 1899. De Vries became aware of Mendel's work about the same time. Both he and Correns published brief reports in early 1900 on Mendel's work in plant breeding as a means of interpreting the hereditary segregation of characters from parent to offspring in fixed numerical ratios (Olby, 1987). Von Tschermak read the de Vries paper and immediately recognized its relevance to his own breeding studies. He prepared a detailed summary of his breeding data in the new Mendelian light. It was published in the summer of 1900 (Olby, 1987).

Although Bateson had accumulated a large body of breeding data himself showing the transmission of characters, he did not have a satisfactory theory of heredity to predict accurately the results of specific parental crosses. He presented a lecture course titled "Practical Study of Evolution" during the 1899-1900 academic year at Cambridge. His notes commented, on "Heredity: No glimmering of an idea on what kind of process it is" (Cock and Forsdyke, 2008a). Bateson's need was suddenly met in the summer of 1900 when he read the reports of the three continental plant breeders explaining the Mendelian theory of heredity (Olby, 1987). He understood immediately the importance of these new concepts in elucidating his own work. Previously he had no "principle" of heredity; now, he felt he possessed a "law" that could be validated experimentally. He realized that hereditary transmission of variants could occur in a predictable fashion and not necessarily be lost in the population by interbreeding (Darden, 1977), providing "the theoretical foundation for discontinuous evolution" (Kim, 1994a). Bateson became the "most ardent advocate of the new view on heredity in England." He believed that Mendel's work was as fundamental to biology as the atomic theory was to chemistry (Dunn, 1991).

The Biometric-Mendelian Controversy

One of the reasons Weldon and Pearson left the Evolution Committee in 1900 was because they believed the Royal Society would not welcome future publications on statistics, heredity and evolution. With Galton's financial support, they established a new journal *Biometrika* with Pearson and Weldon as co-editors (Kim, 1994b). But the new serial was not designed to be parochial. Pearson noted to Bateson in February 1901:

> [*Biometrika*] was not intended to be exclusive—nothing will be foreign to us. So that if you do not aid us, we at least may find room to print and meet your future criticisms (Provine, 1971c).

The first issue of the journal appeared in December 1901 and was anything but non-controversial. Weldon presented a 27-page long critique of the basic elements of Mendel's analysis of hereditary mechanisms. He reviewed the raw data from Mendel's original report and argued that statistically the results did not agree with the predictions of the laws. He presented some of his own data on human eye color and showed that the percentage of brown or blue eyes in children could in no way be predicted based on application of Mendel's concepts. He concluded that the Mendelian pattern might hold in a few specific cases only and was not a general hereditary "law." He noted also that Mendel's work might apply only to the inheritance of alternative characters such as hair color rather than to continuous characters such as stature or intelligence.

> The fundamental mistake which vitiates all work based upon Mendel's method is the neglect of ancestry and the attempt to regard the whole effect upon offspring, produced by a particular parent, as due to the existence in the parent of particular structural characters...(Weldon, 1901).

Weldon thought that the application of biometric principles, specifically analyzing the ancestry of each cross, had to be considered before any general rules for heredity could be derived.

Bateson hurriedly prepared a book-length response to Weldon's criticisms. His *Mendel's Principles of Heredity—a Defence* appeared in 1902 and answered these points one by one. He thought, "It is scarcely possible to over-rate the importance of this discovery...Previous ideas of heredity and variation...must be reconsidered, and in great measure modified" (Bateson, W., 1902c). Wilmot Herringham from St. Bart's Hospital complimented Bateson, calling the book a "most fascinating and exciting thing." The main points were "clear and intelligible," and Bateson did not "in the least exaggerate their immense importance" (Herringham, W.P., 1902). In the same work, Bateson also began to develop the notion that continuous and discontinuous variation were both explicable in Mendelian terms. He presented all of Mendel's publications in English translation, and noted that Mendel himself had addressed the heredity of continuous variation. For example, Mendel reported the results of petal color in crosses of white and purple *Phaseolus* [beans]. The offspring presented a continuum of colors from purple red to pale violet to white. Mendel proposed that the petal color could be due to the combination of two or more entirely independent factors, which individually segregated during reproduction like any other character in the plants (Bateson, W., 1902d; Provine, 1971d). Bateson then applied the same notion to other graded characters:

> In the case of a population presenting continuous variation, in regard to, say, stature, it might be easy to see how purity of the gametes...might not in ordinary circumstances be capable of detection. There are doubtless more than two pure gametic forms of this character, but there may quite conceivably be six or eight. When it is remembered that each heterozygous combination of any two may have its own appropriate stature, and that such a character was distinctly dependent on external conditions, the mere fact that the observed curves of stature gave 'chance distributions' is not surprising...(Bateson, W., 1902e)

What Bateson meant by "chance distributions" was clarified in a report to the Evolution Committee that same year. He further expanded his intuitive notion of heredity and statistics.

> Continuous characters, such as human height, must be the result of more than one such pair of possible allelomorphs...If there were as few as, say four or five pairs of possible allelomorphs, the various homo- and heterozygous combinations might, as seriation, give so near an approach to a continuous curve, that the purity of the elements would be unsuspected, and their detection practically impossible (Bateson, W., 1902a).

Despite the fact that the two schools of thought on heredity appeared to be approaching problems from a similar vantage point, in fact, their paths began to diverge more widely after 1902. The historians Froggat and Nevin have outlined the courses the scientists took. The biologists tried to explain the inheritance of specific characters in particular cases with mathematical ratios. The biometricians were more interested in calculating the likelihood that a character would appear in the offspring of lineages with the character in measurable proportions. The biologists hoped to explain breeding results with a hereditary theory based on the physiology of reproduction involving egg and sperm. The biometricians proposed strictly empirical models that fit the numerical observations without postulating any physiological mechanisms at all (Froggatt and Nevin, 1971).

Bateson and Weldon had been students together at Cambridge but the heredity-evolution debate had driven them far apart. Weldon and his colleagues sought experimental breeding data that would refute the general applicability of Mendel's laws for inheritance in plants and animals (Kim, 1994c). Bateson noted to Pearson early in 1902 that he and Weldon could not collaborate on these issues. He lamented that "...all partnership between us was at an end..." But Bateson continued to appreciate Pearson's sincere scientific curiosity:

> I respect you as an honest man, and perhaps the ablest and hardest worker I have met, and I am determined not to take up a quarrel with you if I can help it. I have thought for a long time that you are probably the only Englishman that I know at this moment whose first thought is to get at the truth in these [the inheritance] problems...(Provine, 1971e; Pearson, E.S., 1936).

Pearson seemed to appreciate Bateson's trust in his intellectual pursuit and offered his opponent an opportunity to explain his point of view in *Biometrika* (Provine, 1971e).

Nevertheless, behind the scenes the interaction between these principal players was more emotional and less intellectual than it would appear in these references. In May 1902, Bateson wrote to Pearson asking for "a couple of lines" in the journal to express his interpretation of the recent articles on Mendelism (Bateson, W., 1902b). Pearson responded positively, observing that his publication was "open to anyone," but he would "under no circumstances pay for publication of a paper in which the tone in the least resembles that of your book on Mendel's principles." Pearson attached a note to Weldon on the back of this letter indicating his opinion of Bateson's arguments. He noted that Bateson "may say what he likes about my or your logic, but he is not going to befoul the pages of *Biometrika*, which has *permanent value*" [emphasis added] (Pearson, K., 1902b). Pearson, as the editor, thereafter planned to carefully regulate exactly what material was allowed to see the light of day in <u>his</u> journal.

By the following spring, Bateson had prepared an article that was acceptable to Pearson for publication in the journal, but it was becoming evident that the editor was tiring of the animosity between the two factions. He agreed to publish Bateson's response, limiting him to six pages of text, and he hoped "this controversy must cease..." The issue was really the clash between the two theories of heredity. Pearson began to realize that such contention was distracting him from the development of the science of biometry.

> Personally I think it very advisable that all parties both to this and the other controversies should return for a time to the collection of new observations, and facts, and after a year or two's material it will then be possible to return, perhaps in a less heated manner, to the consideration of the bearing of these facts upon theories (Pearson, K., 1903a).

For the maturation of this new science, he believed more data on heredity was needed before one could usefully evaluate the merits of one theory over another.

Nonetheless, the intellectual sparring continued in the journal over the next several years as each side attempted to present examples supporting the relevance of the biometric or the Mendelian theories for heredity. Pearson examined the inheritance of human eye color. The children of dark or light-eyed parents were also dark or light, respectively. No eye color bred true. When the grand parental ancestry was considered, however, more accurate predictions could be made. Blue-eyed grandparents always had blue-eyed grandchildren; brown-eyed grandparents always produced brown-eyed grandchildren. These results fit the expectations of the biometric theory (Pearson, K., 1902a). Another study reached opposite conclusions. A physician, F.A. Woods, studied the inheritance of rabbit coat color in 350 animals over three or four generations. He found that albino animals with dark ancestors only produced albino offspring. This would not have been predicted with Galton's biometric law, but did fit the behavior of a Mendelian recessive character (Woods, 1902).

The interpretation of the data sometimes hinged not just on theory, but also on the quality of the data itself. Weldon reviewed material on the inheritance of albinism, the absence of skin pigment in humans. G. Arcoleo had collected the statistics on the incidence of albinos in Sicily. When parents were apparent heterozygotes, too many albino offspring were born. When both parents were albino, children with normal skin pigment were also born. Both of these observations would not have been expected under Mendel's laws. He concluded:

> ...These results show how necessary it is that the phenomenon of alternative inheritance should be studied in the light of fuller experimental knowledge concerning the correlation between cross-bred individuals and their ancestors; they show the futility of attempting to express such phenomena in terms of formulae based on the unproved hypothesis of gametic purity [Mendel's laws] (Weldon, 1904).

Bateson responded with a note to correct an error in translation of the original report that, in fact, showed that there were no cases of pigmented offspring born of two albino parents. Hence, in his opinion, the results were quite consistent with the Mendelian hypothesis of albinism as a recessive trait (Bateson, W., 1905a).

But were the two theories of heredity mutually exclusive? As early as 1902, one of Pearson's colleagues thought they might be compatible. George Udny Yule had been Pearson's demonstrator at University College London and was appointed Assistant Professor of Applied Mathematics there in 1896. He examined the statistical aspects of variation in a randomly breeding population. He noted: "...discontinuous variation must merge insensibly into continuous variation simply owing to the compound nature of the majority of characters with which one deals." He expanded upon the observation on just this point that Bateson had made in *Defence* that same year. Yule also wrote prophetically:

> It was essential if progress is to be made, that biologists—statistical or otherwise—should recognize that Mendel's laws and the law of ancestral heredity are not necessarily contradictory statements...but one perfectly consistent the one with the other, and may quite form parts of one homogeneous theory of heredity (Yule, 1902).

Subsequently, Pearson himself analyzed the segregation of characters in a large population. He demonstrated that Mendelian ratios for a single character would be stable in a randomly breeding population over time. He finally concluded in a 1904 paper titled "On a generalized theory of alternative inheritance with special reference to Mendel's laws," that, in fact, the two theories were compatible and not mutually exclusive (Pearson, K., 1903b, 1904e).

Weldon, on the other hand, refused to accept the usefulness of Mendel's work for anything in the realm of heredity. He assigned several of his zoology students to begin breeding experiments with mice to test the validity of the Mendelian hypotheses. Arthur Darbshire had graduated from Balliol College at Oxford and was demonstrator in comparative anatomy at University College London. His breeding experiments involved crosses between albino and Japanese waltzing mice. His first *Biometrika* paper reported the heredity of four different coat colors in the offspring. He also noted different frequencies of albino mice for parents with different ancestry. Both these points, he thought, argued against the validity of Mendel's laws to explain the results and were more consistent with the biometric approach (Darbshire, 1902).

Bateson followed this work with interest and wrote to Darbshire early in 1903. The two began a protracted correspondence over the next three years. Darbshire declared, "I am absolutely unbiased about Mendel and am keen to come to an unprejudiced conclusion on it" (Kim, 1994d). Darbshire published three other papers in *Biometrika* over the next two years on his breeding studies. Each one claimed that the ancestry of specific lines predicted results in the offspring, all in agreement with the biometric expectations. Bateson enumerated 28 errors in Darbshire's analysis of the breeding results and patiently explained to the young scientist how Mendelism could be used to interpret the data.

By 1904 Darbshire found himself in a quandary. He had initially tried to "refute what Mendelian theory really was..." (Kim, 1994e). But, he was instead forced to conclude that the characters he had studied in mice did, in fact, segregate in accordance with Mendelian expectations. Weldon and Pearson were not at all pleased with this outcome. Pearson thought that the young student had been seduced by that "dominant anaesthetist [Bateson] from Cambridge" (Provine, 1971f). Darbshire subsequently noted that this experience had convinced him that there should be no warring parties in science, but rather the triumph of truth (Darbshire, 1907).

Weldon then set another student to work on the mouse breeding issue. Edgar Schuster had graduated from New College Oxford in 1901. He worked with Weldon in the Department of Comparative Anatomy on the breeding of the Oxford house mouse, not the "fancy" breeds used by Darbshire. He performed the breeding experiments for three years but did not publish any findings until 1905. He first met Bateson in 1904 and clearly utilized Mendelian theory to explain his findings. The outcome of his work did not please his mentors at all. He noted:

> ...It is hardly necessary to point out that with regard to characters, color-productiveness and albinism, the mice under consideration here behave in complete accordance with Mendel's laws, both with regard to dominance and segregation (Schuster, 1905).

He would later echo the words of his colleague Darbshire that, "People who are studying the same problems by different methods should work in sympathy with one another" (Schuster, 1909), and not remain locked in perpetual conflict.

Such sympathy was not evident at the August 1904 meeting of the British Association for the Advancement of Science in Cambridge. Bateson was President of the Zoological Section. He introduced a series of papers on breeding in plants and animals that he was convinced documented the truth of the Mendelian theory of heredity. He claimed that this theory "had begun to coordinate the facts of heredity, until then utterly incoherent and contradictory" (Bateson, W., 1904). The biometric approach used a "gross statistical method [as] a misleading instrument; and applied to these intricate discriminations, the imposing correlation table into which the biometric Procrustes fits his arrays of unanalysed data, is still no substitute for the common sense of trained judgement" [in biology] (Provine, 1971g).

Weldon and Pearson then countered with criticisms of these data and provided their own results that appeared to contradict those expected using the Mendelian approach to heredity. Weldon concluded, "until further experiments and more careful description of the results are available, it was better to use the purely descriptive statements of Galton and Pearson than to involve the cumbrous and undemonstrable gametic mechanisms on which Mendel's hypotheses rested" (Provine, 1971h). Bateson responded and claimed he had "no doubt of the result" of this debate in the future (Froggatt and Nevin, 1971). Pearson thought that the excitement of the controversy drove Weldon to even greater intellectual activity after this battle (Provine, 1971i).

Pearson subsequently blamed the controversy for over-working his friend Weldon and contributing to his untimely death in 1906. The Cambridge biologist C.C. Hurst had examined the breeding records from the *General Stud Book for Race Horses*, and concluded that chestnut coat color was a Mendelian recessive to bay and brown. He prepared a short paper on the topic and asked Bateson to submit it to the Royal Society for publication. Weldon reviewed the report and refused to believe it. He threw himself into a furious study of the 20 volumes of the *Stud Book* and found several apparently contradictory results that were inconsistent with such a Mendelian interpretation. He was deeply involved in this aspect of the controversy when he developed influenza and died of pneumonia (Provine, 1971j). Bateson sent his condolences to Pearson who was embittered by the loss of his friend and colleague. Pearson replied:

> Only a few days before his death he condemned in stronger language than I have ever heard him use of any individual the tone and contents [of your work]. It is a judgment in which I believe every man who has the interests of science in heart will concur (Provine, 1971k).

Pearson pointed out to Bateson, "It is not a question of comparing theory with theory, but of trying to understand different aspects of the problem of inheritance and putting them into a harmonious whole" (Pearson, K., 1906b). In a lecture titled "Nature and Nurture," he argued, "We need to observe, measure and record, to analyze by the methods of exact science" (Porter, 2004h). The reason for this attempt was clearly for the betterment of society. Pearson was convinced that the physical, moral and "psychical" characters in humans were all inherited to approximately the same extent. A healthy environment was certainly necessary for a fulfilling life. But the future of the population more importantly required good heredity, he thought. "You may improve your environment and your nurture, but no improvement will make the dull or feeble-minded sharp-witted or the weak in body the parents of stout children." Hospitals and charities of the time kept alive the weakest who, in the past, would have died and failed to reproduce. The future health of society therefore required the prevention of reproduction by those unfit to become competent parents (Pearson, K., 1906c).

Historians have proposed a number of reasons for the continuation of the biometric-Mendelian debate long after the major actors began to see the possibility of the united theory for heredity. There were differences in social status. Both Weldon and Pearson were professors at leading universities, well positioned within the English academic community. Bateson, on the other hand, was an assistant at Cambridge. His breeding work was considered unorthodox, and he was nearly an academic outsider (Olby, 1988).

After 1900, all three men were attempting to define new academic disciplines and sought institutional support for their research plans. Although Weldon had been appointed Professor of Zoology at Merton College Oxford, he could not convince the administration to budget money for experimental research. Pearson, at University College London, carried a heavy teaching load and was supplemented by grants from the Draper's Company and from Galton himself after 1904. Bateson was steward at St. John's College Cambridge and supported his research by small grants from the Royal Society and private individuals (Kevles, 1980, 1985a; Herringham, C.J., 1903, 1906). The historian Lyndsay Farrall has characterized all three as acting as if each was in a state of siege, fighting for his academic life (Farrall, 1975).

Pearson had become a socialist as a young man and tended to view the world in collective terms (Porter, 2004g). The biometric theory that focused on populations thus appealed to him. Bateson was more conservative and analyzed particular cases. The fact that Mendelian heredity focused on individuals within specific families made more sense to him (Kevles, 1980). The scientific methods used by the two camps also differed. Bateson tended to function like a field biologist, collecting many different facts and attempting to draw general principles from the data. This was primarily an inductive or Baconian method. Pearson was trained as a mathematician and functioned in a more deductive fashion. Early in the new century, he argued for a preliminary theory to guide the collection of facts, followed by an empirical test of the theory using the information available (Cock, 1973).

It also became clear during this controversy that the two sides did not communicate well. The biometricians had been trained in mathematics and claimed that the Mendelians were inept and could not understand the statistical treatment of the biologic data. Pearson did not mince words in his criticism: "One can only hope that the persistent exposure of the blunders made by non-statistically trained biologists when they test problems of heredity may ultimately produce some effect" (Pearson, K., 1904f). He continued, "It has been absolutely necessary to point out one after another of Bateson's blunders" (Pearson, K., 1904b). On the other hand, the Mendelians were trained in biology and argued that the biometricians could not adequately follow the experimental methods they used to study heredity (Kim, 1994a). Pearson admitted, "As far as I appreciate Mr. Bateson's position it is to be unintelligible" (Pearson, K., 1904b). The American biologist Raymond Pearl (who had worked with Galton at University

College London) commented that Pearson often missed biological points as much as Bateson missed mathematical points:

> I think the impression among biologists that biometry is proving rather a sterile field comes from the unfortunate fact that 1) Pearson who has grounded the subject mathematically hasn't at all the biologists' point of view, and 2) that most of the biologists who have taken it up haven't gone to the trouble (or have been constitutionally unable) to work up through the mathematical side...(Kevles, 1980).

There is no question that the debate involved the two distinct ideologies proposed to explain the facts of heredity. But the biologist William Provine has argued convincingly that much of the controversy involved clashes between personalities (Provine, 1971a). Both Pearson and Bateson had strong egos. Pearson could be dominating. He was a skillful writer and lecturer, and gave clear expositions of his ideas. But his style could be "bitter and contemptuously controversial." He was "apt to attribute intellectual differences of opinion to stupidity or even moral obliquity" (Greenwood, 1940). George Yule observed:

> Those who left him and began to think for themselves were apt, as happened painfully in more instances than one, to find that after divergence of opinion, the maintenance of friendly relations became difficult, after expressed criticism, impossible (Yule, 1995).

Bateson likewise rarely minced words in his responses to those who disagreed with his ideas. His attacks on Weldon and Pearson were called "bombastic" and even "grossly and gratuitously offensive" (Kevles, 1980). His research had been viewed by many of his contemporaries as rather unorthodox. His opinion in this regard was, "The term 'controversial' is conveniently used by those who are wrong to apply to the persons who correct them" (Cock, 1973). Personal animosity continued even after Weldon's death in 1906. Two years later, Pearson and Bateson were seated next to each other at an awards dinner. Pearson claimed later that Bateson had refused his greeting and turned his chair sideways to avoid contact with Pearson throughout the entire evening (Froggatt and Nevin, 1971).

The sociologist Kyung-Ma Kim has argued that physicians at this time were not involved in the personal conflicts of the biometricians and the Mendelians and therefore formed, in a sense, a "neutral jury" which could validate the usefulness of the divergent hereditary hypotheses (Kim, 1994f). The next section will examine the relative importance of the biometric and Mendelian models for heredity as applied to English medicine of the period.

HEREDITY AND HUMAN DISEASE

Physicians daily encountered disorders that appeared to be hereditary, to run in the family from one generation to the next, while others clearly had an environmental cause, from toxins or contagions found in food, drink or other people. Each physician was therefore in a unique position to observe firsthand the "effect of both environment and of heredity in the etiology of disease" ("An investigation," 1900). The explosion of knowledge regarding infectious disease after 1880 tended to submerge the fact that hereditary factors also could result in human disease. George Archdall Reid lamented early in the new century, "the professional neglect of the study of heredity. The subject [could be] peculiarly our own" (Reid, 1902).

A better understanding of infectious disease certainly was a fact of medical life after 1900. The number of diseases previously thought to be hereditary was decreasing each year as scientific discoveries revealed their true etiology. Disorders such as tuberculosis, leprosy, syphilis, and pityriasis rosea all appeared to run in families, and therefore were traditionally believed to be hereditary in origin. But all of them had recently been shown to result from infection by specific microorganisms (Lucas, 1904). One medical commentator noted, "Heredity in disease is year to year growing more and more discredited. Its decline has coincided with, and is consequent upon, the rise of bacteriology" (Oliver, C., 1892).

Most physicians of the day were not ready to completely discount the existence of hereditary disease. T. Oliver, Professor of Physiology at the College of Medicine in New Castle on Tyne, pointed out that there appeared to be an inherited susceptibility to acquiring even infectious diseases in humans. Many persons were exposed to germs, but only some became infected and demonstrated signs of the disease in question (Oliver, T., 1900). Byram Bramwell from the Edinburgh Royal Infirmary agreed. Pulmonary tuberculosis [phthisis] was due to infection by the tubercle bacillus. However, certain families seemed to be unusually susceptible to this common infection (Bramwell, 1902). Frederick Burton-Fanning of Norwich noted that 54% of his tuberculosis patients had positive family histories for the same disease. He also thought that heredity played a predisposing role in those families. He observed many children affected even when parents had no clinical signs of infection themselves (Burton-Fanning, 1902). W.A. Rees told the Middlesex Hospital Medical Society that predisposition to certain diseases such as gout and rheumatism also appeared to be inherited (Rees, 1903). R.C. Lucas of Guy's Hospital summarized the general opinion that certain rare human disorders did have a hereditary basis in 1904, when he spoke at the Society for the Study of Diseases in Children. The human conditions he thought were hereditary in origin are listed in Table 12.1.

Reid had also complained that no medical school provided any systematic study in the area of human heredity and disease (Reid, 1902). No textbook on the subject existed until he prepared the *Laws of Heredity* in 1905. The book was specifically addressed to medical practitioners because he viewed them as "the largest body of scientific workers" in the population (Reid, 1905a). The daily observations of physicians could expand the knowledge base for the new science of medical heredity. Reid was convinced that "Heredity concerns medical men more nearly than any other body of scientific workers...One day, a systematic knowledge of the laws which control the reproduction of living things will be considered as necessary a part of the equipment for the struggle against disease as anatomy or physiology" (Reid, 1905b). For this reason, Reid urged that medical colleges should now offer a course on heredity for medical students (Reid, 1905c). J. Arthur Thomson, Regius Professor of Natural History at the University of Aberdeen, reviewed this first text for medical men on heredity and disease. He too agreed on the potential importance of this field of study, and believed an understanding of human heredity should become a part of the "professional equipment of the physician" (Thomson and Washburn, 1905).

While the medical school curriculum offered little opportunity to learn about heredity, the British medical literature carefully reported new developments in this field. A somewhat unlikely orator, William Turner, surgeon and Professor of Anatomy at the University of Edinburgh, delivered the Presidential Address to the 1900 British Association for the Advancement of Science meeting. His description of chromosome motion during cell division was as illustrative as anything written, even a century later. In his opinion, the formation of two daughter cells, each containing the same number of chromosomes as the parental cell, formed the basis for hereditary transmission of characters from one generation to the next (Turner, W., 1900).

Table 12.1
Hereditary Human Disease 1904

Peroneal atrophy	Dayblindness
Deaf Mutism	Nightblindness
Hemophilia	Ichthyosis
Colorblindness	Psoriasis
Polydipsia	Polydactyly
Coloboma iridea	Lobster claw deformity
Aniridia	Congenital hip dislocation
Amaurosis	Clubfoot
Cataract	Cleft lip
Strabismus	Cleft palate
Myopia	

Reference: Lucas, 1904

At this time, other physicians had begun to think creatively about the nature of the hereditary elements. John G. Adami had been a college friend with Bateson at Cambridge (Adami, M., 1930). He emigrated to Canada and became Professor of Pathology at McGill University. In May 1901, he outlined a physical model for the hereditary material when he spoke before the Brooklyn Medical Club in New York. He showed that the formation of egg and sperm in the process of meiosis halved the hereditary material. Their union to form the zygote [fertilized egg] returned the total amount of hereditary material to the amount characteristic of the species. Individual variation then resulted from such "fortuitous comingling" of chromatin during sexual reproduction. He asked, "Can we imagine a chemical substance so constituted as to be capable of modification in its molecular constitution...without undergoing complete change and without other properties being lost." The physical structure of each individual then was reflected by the "outcome of the structure and properties" of the hereditary material. He was certain that the visible chromosomes and the hereditary material he proposed were identical. He envisioned this material as having a central ring to which side chains could be added or subtracted. Different side chains then would control different features of the cell. Adami also proposed that environmental factors could alter specific side chains, allowing for the inheritance of acquired characters (Adami, J.G., 1901a, b, c).

Subsequent study appeared to confirm that the chromosomes were the bearers of hereditary material. Mitosis involved the duplication of "a definite number of rod-like bodies known as chromosomes," which then split longitudinally to form two daughter chromosomes. These traveled into two daughter cells, maintaining a constant number through successive generations. Reproduction of gametes involved a different process termed meiosis. Each egg or sperm contained only half the chromosomes of its parental cell type. Fusion of the egg and sperm thus restored the number of chromosomes (Walker, 1904). An estimation of the number of chromosomes in human cells was obtained at this time by studying several malignant tumors. The most commonly noted number was 32 in the nucleus of these human cells (Farmer, Moore and Walker, 1906).

Adami re-addressed his physical model for inheritance at the 1906 British Medical Association meeting held in Toronto. He was convinced that the chromosomes did convey the hereditary material from one generation to the next. Variations among the "loops" of the chromosomes might determine particular characters of the cells (Adami, J.G., 1906). Each parent supplied an equal number of chromosomes in the egg or sperm, which fused to form a fertilized egg. But recent work had shown two types of sperm—one produced male and the second female offspring. The difference in the two types of sperm appeared to result from an "accessory chromosome," implying that human sex also was controlled by chromosome constitution. Adami noted that cellular physiology, to a large extent, relied on the action of specific ferments or "enzymes." These appeared to be formed in the cell nucleus and were transported to the cytoplasm for their action in the cellular economy (Adami, J.G., 1906, 1907). The concept that the chromosomes were the bearers of hereditary material that controlled the production of enzymes would be expanded over the next several decades, as the interaction between genetic material and enzyme proteins became better understood.

The first careful exploration of chromosomes and Mendelian theory to appear in the British medical literature was included in the summaries of eight lectures held at University College London in November 1904. The biometrician W.F.R. Weldon discussed "Current Theories of the Hereditary Process" and agreed that the chromosomes did appear to be the physical bearers of heredity during cell division. He argued that the biometric theory he had proposed with Pearson fit breeding data from plant and animal studies better than the Mendelian theory outlined by Bateson and his colleagues. He did acknowledge that a general theory for heredity would someday develop by combining ideas from both the competing schools of thought (Weldon, 1905a, b). Pearson and Bateson both attended the lectures and took careful notes of the speaker's contrasting remarks between the two theories of heredity (Pearson, K., 1904a; Cock and Forsdyke, 2008b).

British physicians now began to discuss the contemporary theories of heredity at their own society meetings. The biologist J. Beard from the University of Edinburgh appeared before the Section on Psychological Medicine of the British Medical Association in July 1904. He described the mechanism of meiosis and thought that this "coincides with but is possibly not identical with the reduction of chromosomes." He noted the segregation of dominant and recessive characters that could eventually provide "mathematical laws to explain heredity" (Beard, 1904).

The Pathology Section of the British Medical Association also examined the connection of heredity and disease at its July 1905 meeting. Frederick W. Mott, pathologist at Maudsley Hospital in London, presented several family trees illustrating the heredity of color blindness and hemophilia. He also reported cases of Friedreich's ataxia affecting three children born of healthy parents who happened to be first cousins. He thought, "Convergent heredity may have been the cause of focusing a disease strain of remote ancestral origin." Such an event was "suggestive of the Mendelian doctrine."

Charles Bond, surgeon to Leicester Royal Infirmary, then discussed diseases affecting only one sex such as hemophilia in males. If sex was a Mendelian character, other human traits could be associated with one sex or the other during meiosis, and result in human diseases affecting only one sex of the offspring. The biologist C.C. Hurst of Cambridge commented that medical men should start to collect careful pedigrees from families that appeared to have such hereditary diseases. While Mendel's laws seemed to hold for the inheritance of simple characters in plants and animals, their application to more complex human traits would require much more factual data in the future (Mott, 1905; Bond, 1905).

Whether Mendelism applied to humans was quite controversial. Reid noted that most human children were a blending of characters from their parents. With the exception of eye color and perhaps a few other traits such as the Mongolian eyelid, human hybrids appeared to blend every character as exemplified by skin color in children of dark and light parents (Reid, 1907). G.P. Mudge from the London Hospital Medical School countered with observations he had made of crosses between Canadian red Indians and white Europeans. He identified six features of the Native Americans that distinguished them from the Europeans: nature of hair, eye color, skin tone, cheekbone and nose structure, and facial hair pattern. All combinations of these features were found in the children of such crosses. The grandchildren, however, demonstrated the reappearance of latent European traits. This pattern of segregation of characters was consistent with Mendelism (Mudge, 1907).

The Harveian Oration at the Royal College of Physicians in November 1908 was titled "On Heredity in Relation to Disease." Joseph Ormerod, physician at St. Bart's Hospital, discussed the competing theories in this area. He commended Galton and Pearson for their hard work, but admitted, "It may be that statistics do not appeal so forcibly as they ought to do to the medical man, because he has principally to deal with individuals." It was evident that studying human heredity in particular families was difficult. One could not control breeding, and at least three generations of accurate family history was necessary. Interpretation of the patterns for inheritance could also prove difficult. He suggested, "It may be necessary to refer it for its interpretation to someone who knows the business well." But the question remained of how far the Mendelian theory could be applied to human data. Eye color, hemophilia, albinism and certain skin diseases had been interpreted as following Mendelian patterns for inheritance. He thought, "It would appear in some cases the Mendelian proportions work out—in enough, perhaps to encourage further research, but I do not know whether more can definitely be said" (Ormerod, 1908a, b). The usefulness of Mendelism to medical practice still appeared quite tentative.

R.H. Firth discussed heredity and disease before the Aldershot Military Medical Society in 1909 and outlined different recessive, dominant and sex-limited human characters. He also suggested that medical men should collect disease pedigrees. He believed within twenty years enough data would accumulate to answer important questions on "deformity, color and constitutional tendencies to special diseases" (Firth, 1909). W. Bevan Lewis discussed the role of Mendelism and disease at the Medico-Psychological Association in the same year. In his opinion, the "data obtained from the minute analysis of their compounded factors in carefully studied pedigrees, and their accordance with Mendelian principles, would prove of enormous importance in our studies of the heritage of disease" (Bevan-Lewis, 1909).

The Glasgow Southern Medical Society also sponsored a discussion of the impact heredity might have on human diseases. T.K. Monro from the Glasgow Royal Infirmary was not certain of the ultimate answer to how heredity worked in man, but thought, even in 1906, that Mendelism provided "the best modern teaching" on the subject (Monro, 1906). Because of their continued interest in heredity and disease, British physicians sought to learn from both the biometric and the Mendelian schools of hereditary thought. Their imagination had been captured.

Pearson and the Doctors I

In 1904, University College London provided space for Galton to establish the Eugenics Record Office (E.R.O.) and then to begin the collection of data on human heredity. The Draper's Company funded the Biometric Laboratory at the college that same year and appointed Pearson as director. Primary areas of research were to involve the heredity of tuberculosis and insanity, and the effects of heredity and environment on the educational progress of English schoolchildren (Farrall, 1985a). Galton died in 1911, and his estate established the Galton Professorship of Eugenics with Pearson as the first appointee. The College then established a Department of Applied Statistics that incorporated both existing laboratories. The E.R.O. was then renamed the Galton Laboratory for National Eugenics (Jones, 1993). Pearson believed the unit should apply statistical results to inform social issues and hence improve the welfare of the entire nation (Farrall, 1985a).

Physicians were involved in the early work of both these institutions. The University Senate appointed an advisory board; four of the seven members were physicians: J. McPherson, F.W. Mott, E. Nettleship, and J.S. Simpson. However, the board did not play an active role in the daily activity of the research units or of its journal *Biometrika*, leaving Pearson in control of virtually every aspect of the organization (Farrall, 1985a). Pearson had mixed feelings toward the medical profession. Because physicians were not trained in statistics, they did not really understand the biometric approach to heredity. As early as 1896, he noted, "...medical men [had not] yet fully appreciated that he [had] really shown how many of the problems which perplex them may receive a partial answer," (Magnello, 1998) regarding questions of heredity in human disease. He thought that medical science of the day was too quick to prescribe treatment for patients or define public health policy based on clinical wisdom rather than on a solid statistical basis. As such, he held little respect for most physicians (Porter, 2004j). On the other hand, his research units were not affiliated with a medical school, and he needed a source of pedigree data on human characters and disease. He noted that the production of such material "lies outside the qualifications of the present staff of the laboratory" (Pearson, K., 1909a). Pearson encouraged physicians to collaborate with the laboratory when questions of heredity arose. A memorandum reported, "Already the laboratory is consulted very largely by medical officers of health, by school medical officers and by independent medical men engaged in statistical problems who have not a staff adequate in numbers and training to deal with these matters" (Farrall, 1985b).

Several studies were published at this time that resulted from cooperation between Pearson and the doctors. Cancer was a common human ill of great social concern, and it often appeared to run in families. W.T. Hillier collected data from 3000 cases of carcinomas among patients at the Middlesex Hospital in London. He believed that hereditary predisposition could be an important factor in causing such cancers. Of 2368 female cancer patients, the family history was positive in 14.6% of cases. In 632 male patients, relatives were affected in 7.8% (Hillier and Tritsch, 1904). Pearson later examined the statistical correlation of family history seen in the same cancer patients and those from the general hospital wards. He concluded that the correlation of cancer and family history was so slight as to be within the sampling error, suggesting that in the main, heredity had little or no effect in causing cancer (Pearson, K., 1904g).

Pulmonary tuberculosis [phthisis] was another chronic disease with great social morbidity at this time. W.C. Rivers from the Mount Vernon Hospital for Consumption and Diseases of the Chest in Middlesex, consulted Pearson on family history forms that could be used to analyze hereditary predisposition to this disease (Rivers, 1908). He also submitted 50 pedigrees of consumptive families as part of a larger study of heredity and this disease (Rivers, 1907a, b). Rivers noted that the family predisposition to consumption could be found to be closely connected with the family incidence of "nasal, nasopharyngeal and dental abnormality" which might allow easy entry of the tubercle bacillus into the victims' lungs (Rivers, 1908).

Pearson's journal *Biometrika* was another vehicle for reporting work on heredity performed by English physicians. F.A. Woods studied the inheritance of coat color in rabbits over 3-4 generations. He noted that albino animals, born of dark parents, always produced albino offspring. This was not expected under the biometric theory, but certainly did fit the behavior of a Mendelian recessive character (Woods, 1902). J.E. Adler and J. McIntosh reported a human family with two albino children born of first cousin parents. Prior family history was unremarkable for four generations. They commented, "From a Mendelian view, both parents might be considered as carrying recessive albinism" (Adler and McIntosh, 1909).

However, examples of what might be considered Mendelian "dominant" characters did not so easily fit that model. T. Lewis and D. Embleton from University College Hospital London analyzed the family history of ectrodactyly—"lobster claw deformity"—with split hands and feet. The trait was generally directly transmitted from parent to child, and there was some variation in degree of the disorder in the offspring. There were 44 affected and 32 normal people in this family, an excess of "dominant" type. Under Mendelian law, an equal number of normal and affected persons were expected (Lewis and Embleton, 1908). Their results did not therefore fit the proportions expected.

Physicians such as Lewis and Embleton clearly exhibited more than a passing interest in human heredity. When reviewing his files on ectrodactyly, Lewis noted to Pearson that he also found pedigrees of cataract, polydactyly, ichthyosis, hemophilia and optic atrophy. He said he was intensely attracted to the notion of heredity and human disease. "So large a field is open, and such an interesting one, that one only regrets that time is nowadays such a tyrant"[8] (Lewis, 1906).

Pearson himself then examined another family with ectrodactyly. This Scottish pedigree had 25 affected and 14 normal persons. He investigated this instance because:

> I wanted to ascertain independently to what extent simple Mendelism really applied to an obviously inherited and fairly simple human deformity. I wanted to convince myself that Mendelism does or does not apply to such cases by handling the data myself.

The excess of affected persons did not make sense from a Mendelian point of view (Pearson, K., 1908e). Lewis concurred with this interpretation.

> It may be...the case that Mendelism applied to certain human deformities, but the conclusions which are being drawn, or implied, conclusions having a serious sociological aspect, are at present ahead of the facts at our disposal (Lewis, 1908).

Other physicians attempted to utilize Pearson's approach to study human heredity in the world. John Macpherson was Commissioner in Lunacy for Scotland and investigated family histories of insanity and other neuroses. He presented a lecture on the topic before the Royal College of Physicians in Edinburgh in 1904. The *Edinburgh Medical Journal* planned to publish this report. The physician asked Pearson if he could borrow some figures illustrating the mechanism for heredity that Pearson had used in his publications (Macpherson, 1904). Several years later, the Science Committee of the British Medical Association encouraged Macpherson to investigate heredity and human ability by examining family histories of members of the Royal Society of Edinburgh. MacPherson noted to Pearson that this might also provide evidence for the usefulness of the biometric theory of heredity (Macpherson, 1908).

In 1902, Edward Nettleship, one of the leading ophthalmologists in England, decided to retire from clinical practice. In his extensive experience at the Royal London Ophthalmic Hospital, he had encountered many eye diseases that reappeared in successive generations. He decided to focus his retirement energies on collecting data from such families to better understand the role heredity might play in the etiology of specific eye disorders (Lawford, 1922; Rushton, 2000). Over the next few years, Nettleship did collect family histories showing inheritance of color blindness, cataract, albinism and retinitis pigmentosa. He was not well read in the science of heredity and was unable to analyze the data he had in-hand. Nettleship contacted Pearson at the Galton Laboratory in 1904 and asked about terminology to be used to designate offspring of the same parents. Pearson suggested the use of the term "siblings" (Pearson, K., 1904d). Nettleship also asked about how one interpreted the family data he had been accumulating. "I am, as you know, not a reader, and am ashamed to confess that I do not know whether you have formulated any theory of heredity. If you have please give me a reference." This physician was of the opinion that Pearson's position was "a modified Galtonism" (Nettleship, 1906b). Pearson did not wish to discuss diverse theories of inheritance. Instead, he suggested that if Nettleship was interested in questions about the theories on heredity he should consult his colleague Weldon (Pearson, K., 1905b). Pearson then "turned the tables" by asking Nettleship if he had any clinical experience with albinism (Pearson, K., 1904c). Nettleship replied that he had been collecting pedigrees on such cases and had data on 60 albinos from 23 families. He asked whether Pearson had formulated any further "scheme for collecting cases of family albinism" and suggested sending a letter to other physicians asking for information on affected families (Nettleship, 1904a). He already knew that Edward Stainer, from the Skin Department of St. Thomas's Hospital, had been studying material on human heredity for many years and had several extensive pedigrees with albinism spanning several generations (Nettleship, 1904b). Stainer was eager to collaborate on this project, noting, "I am greatly interested in hereditary defects and have collected many facts dealing with malformations and diseases" (Stainer, 1905a, b). The dermatologist Jonathan Hutchinson was also known to have extensive experience on heredity and albinism (Nettleship, 1905c).

The two men thus began their collaborative effort to gather information on the heredity of human albinism. Nettleship authorized Pearson to use his name in a letter asking for information on albinism that was then sent to the 350 members of the

Ophthalmological Society. Nettleship also sent letters outlining the scheme of the proposed research project to leading British medical journals (Nettleship, 1905b). The circular brought responses from many physicians with new pedigrees on albinism. Nettleship was beginning to think of heredity in quantitative terms, suggesting that all these families would prove useful in "giving proportions affected with albinism" (Nettleship, 1905d). Physicians from many disciplines contributed material from all over the Empire. Jonathan Hutchinson offered to send some of the family data he had accumulated over more than fifty years of clinical experience (Hutchinson, 1905). William Bulloch from the London Hospital Medical College contributed several albino pedigrees (Bulloch, 1909). Another physician from the Gilbert Islands in the Western Pacific noted an albino family with affected collateral branches. On these isolated islands consanguinity and polygamy were commonly practiced (Murdoch, 1908). The Scottish ophthalmologist, C.H. Usher, became an active collaborator in this endeavor as he investigated the inheritance of albinism in the family of Lord Sherbrooke (Pearson, K., 1905a). Several other families were noted in different locales around Scotland. An Edinburgh lawyer was affected (Usher, 1908a), as was another family located in Glasgow (Usher, 1908b). More isolated areas also had albino families. One was noted from the Barrow Islands, and another from Skye recorded affected relatives four generations back in time (Usher, 1909a, b).

Nettleship had also begun to make preliminary steps at a hereditary explanation of his own, using other pedigrees. He observed:

> The degree of heritability (if that is a word) of different conditions...seems to vary so much that at first sight one is tempted to believe in different laws for different conditions. Probably however it is a matter of degree, rather than of kind. If the liability to transmission is very slight, intensification by consanguineous union may bring it out to increase the probability of its appearing; and such apparently isolated cases have lead to the belief in consanguinity being per se the cause of certain peculiarities and congenital diseases. When the disease or liability to it is much more transmissible, being passed down continuously from one generation to the next and the next after, the added help of consanguinity is not needed and but little attention is paid to it. The latter is true for cataract it seems; the former in some degree for retinitis pigmentosa, and still more for albinism which, in man, seems to be the least easily transmissible of any I know (Nettleship, 1906c).

By September 1907, the project on albinism had advanced to the point where Pearson proposed that they write a book on the subject. He wanted it to be a "classic," but admitted that he could not do it by himself. Pearson seemed curiously uninformed about the known scientific data on albinism. He mentioned to Nettleship, "I have a sort of idea of somebody experimenting with transfusions of blood into albino rabbits, but I cannot remember the paper" (Pearson, K., 1905c). The work he could not remember was, in fact, the transfusion experiments by his mentor Francis Galton in the 1870s, attempting to prove Darwin's theory of pangenesis. Nonetheless, Pearson suggested that each should write individual parts for the book and then he would review the whole for "homogeneity" (Pearson, K., 1906a). Nettleship agreed that this was a good idea and contributed 81 pedigrees of albinism, with consanguinity demonstrated in 30% of all families (Nettleship, 1906d). The project of collecting pedigrees and detailed medical histories continued for several more years. Nettleship mentioned the "forthcoming monograph on albinism by Pearson and Nettleship" in a lecture at the Ophthalmological Society in June 1909 (Nettleship, 1909).

The work finally appeared as a *Monograph on Albinism in Man*, as a part of the *Draper's Company Research Memoirs* from the Galton Laboratory. Pearson thanked the physicians from around the world who had submitted clinical material for the book. He was the general editor, and Nettleship and Usher contributed clinical material on animal and human cases. Part I was published in 1911 and included a detailed description of the different types of albinism found in different human races. Part II appeared in 1913 and included anatomical studies of the eye, skin and hair from albino humans and animals. Part IV appeared next in the same year and presented over 600 pedigrees of albinism and 700 references from the medical literature. The introduction to Part IV indicated that Part III was intended to statistically analyze all the family data on albinism (Pearson, K., Nettleship and Usher, 1911).

But the project on albinism also became mired in the Pearson-Bateson controversy. Nettleship mentioned to Pearson that he had corresponded with Bateson in late 1905, sending him pedigrees on several eye diseases and the circular recruiting new cases of albinism. He noted, "I do not suppose you will have any objection to this." But he was, in fact, already aware of the controversy between the two men and wished to avoid involvement. He wrote to Pearson:

> I am entirely with you in working to keep clear of controversy, if only for the reason that I myself am in no position to hold views of any kind. It seems to me what we want now and for sometime is facts—not only on albinism but most of the other human pathological and developmental heredity. This is really an expression of my ignorance of the various controversial questions...(Nettleship, 1905b).

He assured Pearson that he would not "show him [Bateson] any of our material collected for the albinism project" (Nettleship, 1905a).

Pearson was very protective of the data and did not want to share it with Mendelians of any stripe. The physician George Mudge, from the London Hospital Medical College, had collaborated with Bateson on several family studies of human characters. Pearson heard that Mudge was also collecting data on families with albinism. He told Nettleship that Mudge was "no good" (Pearson, K., 1907). Usher had presented microscopic sections of albino eyes to a meeting of the Ophthalmological Society in 1906. Mudge asked to review this material three years later. When Pearson heard about this act, he was incensed that Usher should share clinical material with the other camp in the hereditary debate (Usher, 1909c). He thought that Usher did not realize "the effect of this courtesy to Mudge." He believed that Mudge was doing all he could "to discredit [our] paper before its appearance..." Pearson was convinced, "It is impossible that any work with which I am connected shall not be dealt with in an improper manner by Bateson and his pupils" (Pearson, K., 1909b).

The albinism project did clarify why Pearson and Bateson had developed such enmity. Pearson nicely summarized the state of affairs in a 1908 letter to Nettleship.

> You are quite right about Bateson. I shall not find it possible to take his aid in any way, or to make use of any results reached by him. I trust therefore until we complete this memoir, we may not bring him into the sphere of albinism in any way. My feeling in this matter is a personal one and I cannot give you the reasons for it, but I think we know enough of each other for you to believe that I have reasons for it, or at any rate if you consider me unreasonable that you will respect even the prejudice of a friend (Pearson, K., 1908c).

So there was the nub of the issue. The controversy was not based solely on the merits of one theory over another. It had become a clash of personae.

In contrast to these contentious interactions, Bateson's friendly interactions with British physicians in the same era would help elucidate the working of heredity in the human species, clarifying the usefulness of the competing theories and ultimately resolve this conflict.

BATESON AND THE DOCTORS I

The application of theories of heredity to human families was not always easy. As Ormerod had pointed out earlier, "It might be necessary to refer it for its interpretation to someone who knows the business well" (Ormerod, 1908a, b). The same issue encouraged Nettleship to consult Pearson for his help in interpreting the data on familial eye diseases. Another medical colleague, Wilmot Herringham, a specialist in renal disease at St. Bart's Hospital, suggested to Nettleship, "You had better meet Mr. Bateson of Cambridge, who knows more about heredity than anyone" (Herringham, W.P., 1904).

Bateson already had many friends in the medical profession. His wife Beatrice was the daughter of Arthur Durham, senior surgeon at Guy's Hospital in London. Personal introductions allowed him to access medical opinions on variation which he then used in his 1894 *Materials* book. For many years he had been friendly with Archibald Garrod, physician at St. Bart's Hospital. Garrod had been studying variations in human blood and urine chemistry, and Bateson later noted its relevance to his own work on heredity in the new century (Cock and Forsdyke, 2008c). For several years, the Evolution Committee of the Royal Society had provided Bateson with an annual grant for his studies on heredity. In his December 1901 report to that body, he appended a footnote that marked the beginning of modern medical genetics: the application of heredity to human disease. Bateson had used his breeding data from plants to illustrate how a parent might carry a hidden trait that would then reappear in the offspring. He observed:

> In illustration of such a phenomenon, we may perhaps venture to refer to the extraordinarily interesting evidence collected by Garrod regarding the rare condition known as 'Alkaptonuria.' In such persons the substance, alkapton, forms a regular constituent of the urine, giving it a deep brown colour which becomes black on exposure.
>
> The condition is extremely rare, and, though met with in several members of the same families, has only once been known to be directly transmitted from parent to offspring. Recently, however, Garrod has noticed that no fewer than five families containing alkaptonuric members, more than a quarter of the recorded cases, are the offspring of unions of first cousins. In only two other families is the parentage known, one of these being the case in which the father was alkaptonuric. In the other case the parents were not related. Now there may be other accounts possible, but we note that the mating of first cousins gives exactly the conditions most likely to enable a rare and usually recessive character to show itself. If the bearer of such a gamete mate with individuals not bearing it, the character would hardly ever be seen; but first cousins will frequently be bearers of similar gametes, which may in such union meet each other, and thus lead to the manifestation of the peculiar recessive characters in the zygote [fertilized ovum] (Bateson, W., 1902f).

Here was a mechanism to explain why in-breeding [consanguinity] seemed to increase the frequency of certain hereditary conditions in humans.

After recognizing Garrod's work on alkaptonuria in the 1901 Evolution Committee Report, Bateson and his friend collaborated on a more detailed study of the heredity of this chemical variation. Garrod noted early in 1902, "The subject interests me greatly in its bearing upon chemical as distinguished from structural variations, and it seems to me that alkaptonuria, cystinuria and perhaps albinism also are chemical analogues of malformations." He was also very interested in the inheritance of such chemical variants. Garrod wondered what offspring might result from the "union of two potentially alkaptonuric strains." He was "afraid...that a marriage of alkaptonurics is very unlikely to occur, nor do I see any way of introducing any marriageable alkaptonurics to each other with a view of matrimony!" (Garrod, 1902b). But in more whimsical moments, he may have hoped for just such an event to occur. One of his medical colleagues remembered that Garrod had several young alkaptonuric patients in the London area. He would often admit them to hospital at the same time for demonstration to medical students, in the hope that they might one day find each other attractive and marry. Such a guided experiment of nature might have produced some interesting results (Bearn, 1993b).

Garrod continued his quest for affected families over many more years. By March 1902, he had data from seven families, and in five cases the parents were first cousins (Garrod, 1902d). Such intermarriage, he thought, resulted in "intensification of the family tendencies" (Garrod, 1902c). Garrod also observed the frequent occurrence of cousin marriages in families with albino children (Garrod, 1902e). He sent Bateson another pedigree of a family with first cousin parents and two children born with polydactyly. He suspected recessive inheritance of this character as well and asked for Bateson's opinion (Garrod, 1903a).

Forty cases of alkaptonuria were eventually analyzed late in 1902 when Garrod presented his paper on "Chemical Individuality" in the *Lancet.* He noted that 60% of affected families had first-cousin parents, when the general population at that time had 2-3% such parentage. He observed that the familial pattern for both albinism and alkaptonuria was identical. The trait could remain latent for several generations, but then reappear in the "offspring of the union of two members of the family in which it is transmitted." This peculiar form of indirect heredity "had long been a puzzle," as a trait could appear in "several collateral members of a family...when it had not been manifested at least in recent preceding generations." Garrod observed that Mendel's laws of heredity appeared to offer a "reasonable account of such phenomena." But he also cautioned:

> Whether the Mendelian explanation be the true one or no, there appears to be little reason to doubt that the peculiarity of the incidence of alkaptonuria...[is] best explained by supposing a peculiarity of the gametes of both [parents] is necessary for its production (Garrod, 1902a, 1903b).

This article marked the first description of Mendelism in the British medical literature.

Garrod continued his studies on chemical variation and heredity in man for the next few years. He presented the Croonian Lecture at the Royal College of Physicians in June 1908. His title, "Inborn Errors of Metabolism," summarized his connection of heredity, biochemistry and medicine to elucidate the mechanism of disease resulting from inherited, altered body chemistry. He repeatedly used Mendel's theory of heredity to illustrate the inheritance of altered metabolism in families with alkaptonuria, cystinuria, albinism and pentosuria (Garrod, 1908).

Bateson too delved further into the relationship between Mendelism and the inheritance of human characters, but became dismayed at the difficulties he encountered.

His relationships with the ophthalmologist Nettleship would prove mutually beneficial to both men, as the doctor learned something about heredity, and the biologist learned something about working with humans as experimental subjects (Rushton, 2000).

Nettleship first contacted Bateson in late 1904. He was not sure whether Bateson would be interested in his own work on hereditary eye diseases. "I doubt whether anything I have will be of interest to the workers of experimental transmission, such as yourself, but on the other hand if you can suggest any lines to me I shall be very grateful." He mentioned his work on albinism with Pearson, but found

> the difficulties in getting anything like complete pedigrees of several generations of a human family when one is enquiring about a heritable disease or defect are very considerable for a number of reasons. The facts in regard to a set of siblings are sometimes tolerably complete and sometimes in regard to parents and grandparents, but the collaterals and earlier generations can only be unearthed in very rare instances.

He asked Bateson for suggestions on drawing accurate pedigrees. He noted, "...I expect for a long time to come we (doctors) may have much more to learn from the biometricians (if that is the word) than the latter from us. But I shall be very glad to profit by anything you are kind enough to tell me or suggest" (Nettleship, 1904c).

Bateson responded warmly and invited Nettleship to come out to Cambridge to see the breeding plots of sweet peas "which would give you a clearer idea of what the rules [of heredity] mean than anything else" (Bateson, W., 1905b). The two men thus began a long collaboration on human disorders utilizing pedigree data collected by Nettleship and submitted to Bateson for hereditary analysis. But the pedigrees were often incomplete. Miscarriages and stillbirths frequently went unrecorded. The doctor noted, "In human clinical work one has to take what one can get and hitherto it has been rather seldom that one finds a full record of the unaffected or of sexes or of order of birth or of consanguinity." Nettleship began by collecting pedigrees of albinism, retinitis pigmentosa, color blindness and hemophilia. He was not at all sure of a theory that might explain the observed heredity. He wrote, "I'm sorry that I do not fully understand Mendelianism; I wish it could be put into a formula." He did note that certain diseases were found frequently with consanguinity of the parents. He proposed, "I suppose the latter intensifies, i.e., doubles the influence?" (Nettleship, 1905e).

In collaboration with Nettleship, Bateson began to focus more of his attention on human pedigrees. He reported to the ophthalmologist early in 1907, "I have been spending a good deal of time collecting medical pedigrees lately" (Bateson, W., 1907b). He was concentrating on human neurologic diseases, but the work was frustrating. "The more cases I go through the more I doubt whether they are truly hereditary at all..." (Bateson, W., 1906c). He analyzed some pedigrees of deaf mutism and concluded, "They are not analyzable." Other data from the Royal College of Surgeons on Huntington's chorea showed transmission only through affected individuals, but the ratios of normal and affected were "hopelessly wild." The dentist J.G. Turner sent him a family in which dental enamel hypoplasia appeared to be directly transmitted from parent to child over five successive generations. There were 11 normal and 21 affected offspring. Turner thought this might represent a Mendelian dominant character, but Bateson again could not see how Mendelism might explain the over abundance of affected offspring (Turner, W., no date; Turner, J.G., 1906). Among Leber's amaurosis [blindness] families, he also found too many affected, though the male predominance appeared true in many families. And peroneal atrophy was also transmitted like color blindness with males almost exclusively being affected (Bateson, W., 1906d). The degenerative muscle diseases were inherited irregularly and fit no particular pattern of heredity, except that pseudohypertrophic muscular paralysis also occurred mostly in male children (Bateson, W., 1907b).

Bateson was very puzzled by these findings and had to ask himself whether human disease was hereditary at all, at least in the Mendelian sense. He lamented:

> I am more and more inclined to think that the transmission in some of these at least depends on processes quite distinct from what we ordinarily find in the heredity of variations. With the rarest exceptions all the characters experimentally investigated can fairly easily be shown to follow Mendelian rules, but after making widest allowances for error and misstatements of all sorts, it seems to me most unlikely that the several diseases can be fitted...[to the Mendelian model] (Bateson, W., 1906e).

He wondered whether disease was familial because "a pathogenic organism" was passed from parent to child and then caused maladies in subsequent generations (Bateson, W., 1906d). Nettleship promptly responded to that suggestion. He might know little about heredity, but he had learned a great deal about infections in his clinical years. He told Bateson, "I am very diffident of being ever able to master the theories of heredity..." (Nettleship, 1906g), but about "germs as a cause of hereditary [disease]...I suppose one must not say more than that according to our present knowledge the idea is almost inconceivable." Specific diseases recurred in subsequent generations and were transmitted with exactly the same characters and localizations. He did not think, "it would be fair to the poor over burdened microorganism to run him in for such as that. You must kindly find some other explanation" (Nettleship, 1906e).

They next investigated a large family from France with night blindness. Local physicians and priests were recruited to investigate the details of the family history in different locales. At least nine affected generations were known, probably the most extensive data on any human condition at that time (Nettleship, 1906h). Nettleship presented his findings at a meeting of the Ophthalmological Society in 1907. He thanked Bateson for his interest in the investigation. The complete family tree comprised 2121 individuals over ten generations. Healthy parents never produced affected offspring. The disorder was always directly transmitted from parent to child. The final count in affected branches showed 135 with the disorder of 255 total offspring. There was one case of both parents being affected. They produced two affected daughters. There were eight consanguineous marriages. Affected children only resulted when one parent was already affected. Bateson accompanied his friend to the meeting and was not hesitant to proclaim, "No doubt the paper must prove [to be] a classic." He proposed that the data was consistent with a "simple Mendelian dominant" trait (Nettleship, 1907).

The two men later collaborated on a study of colorblind families. Nettleship had collected many pedigrees over the years with typical male predominant pattern of heredity in which unaffected daughters of affected fathers transmitted the character to their sons. This was the same pattern of inheritance observed in hemophilia and pseudohypertrophic muscular paralysis. There were, however, rare families with colorblind females, whose symptoms were often milder than those in affected males (Nettleship, 1906a). Bateson was particularly interested in this material because it provided a possible example of sexual dimorphism in humans. Bateson wondered whether it was generally the case that color blindness in females was less pronounced than males. Nettleship provided several more pedigrees in which females were only slightly affected (Nettleship, 1908b), but in another family an affected mother was "quite as bad as her sons" who also had the disorder (Nettleship, 1908a). He also found an example of female twins, one colorblind and the other normal (Nettleship, 1912a). Nettleship proposed that there was something in the females' "femaleness that inhibits the action of the colorblind factor when there is only one dose of it...When however there are two doses, the color blindness shows" (Bateson, W., 1908b).

In 1909 Nettleship was asked to present the annual Bowman Lecture at the Ophthalmological Society. His topic was "On some Hereditary Diseases of the Eye." His collaboration with Bateson had convinced him that there were many pedigrees of ocular disorders, that in broad context, "were consistent with the Mendelian theory." Cataract appeared to be a dominant, as was glaucoma. Retinitis pigmentosa, of which he had collected more than 1000 pedigrees, appeared to be of two types. Certain families demonstrated a dominant pattern, while others were more consistent with a recessive type. Stationary night blindness was dominant in some families and sex-limited in others. He thought that continued work in medical genetics would prove enlightening for both the clinician and the biologist. He observed, "Whether the Mendelian theory, or any one of the current doctrines of heredity, contains the whole truth, is perhaps doubtful, but one may rest assured that sooner or later, a ground will be discovered upon which the advocates of the various theories can meet in common" (Nettleship, 1909).

Archibald Garrod thought Mendelian theory might also help elucidate some of the myriad rare neurologic diseases that also recurred in successive generations of certain families. He urged Bateson to accept an invitation to speak before the Neurological Society in February 1906 (Bearn, 1993a). In some respects Bateson appeared to be an unlikely lecturer before such a clinical body. He told the audience that he wondered "whether anything I can say would have a sufficiently direct bearing on the subject in which you are interested." He titled his paper "Mendelian Heredity and its Application to Man," realizing that such application was "rather for the future than for the present." Utilizing results from his breeding studies in plants and animals, he illustrated the features of Mendelian heredity: unit characters, segregation in the gametes, homozygote and heterozygote types, dominant and recessive characters.

He noted that the "application of Mendelian rules to mankind had not made the progress that was to have been expected." But he was able to show pedigrees of several families with dominant traits (brachydactyly and cataract), recessive traits (alkaptonuria and perhaps albinism) and sex-limited characters (color blindness and hemophilia). He expressed his gratitude to Garrod and Nettleship for assisting with such human material. Bateson requested that the medical men in the group join in the search to better understand human heredity. Although few human characters had been well studied, he was certain that if "members of your profession were to take the matter up and study the phenomena of inheritance...the list will be very soon increased." He advised physicians to record both normal and abnormal family members. He hoped that "when complete information had been obtained, it is to be expected the definite rules of transmission" would become evident (Bateson, W., 1906a, b).

Nettleship was also present at the meeting. He wrote to Bateson the following week that the "nerve men" had received a "not un-needed fillip," a little push to study human heredity and disease in their own patients (Nettleship, 1906f). The neurologist Frederick Batten of the National Hospital for the Paralysed and Epileptic in London then contacted Bateson about several families with varied neurologic disorders. Direct parent to child transmission was evident, but far too many affected offspring were counted, again raising the question for Bateson whether Mendel's laws generally could be applied to humans (Batten, 1908).

A young London physician, Alfred Gossage, began to correspond with Bateson in 1907. The two men attempted to analyze pedigrees of the bleeding disorder hemophilia. Typically unaffected females transmitted the disease from their own fathers to half of their sons; and half of their daughters were also expected to be carriers, according to the Mendelian theory. One family demonstrated such a pattern for heredity through seven successive generations. But anomalous pedigrees did appear with too many affected males, again challenging the notion of sex-limited Mendelian inheritance (Gossage, 1907a, b, 1908c, d, e). Gossage also collected pedigrees showing the inheritance of several other conditions: tylosis palmaris et plantaris [dry palms and soles], curly hair and the eye abnormality heterochomia irides [different iris color]. Through multiple generations, the characters were transmitted directly from one parent to about half the children. Gossage acknowledged that Bateson had given him "constant help and criticism," and was able to designate these as dominant characters (Gossage, 1908b).

The inheritance of exostoses [extra knots of cartilage on bones] was the next object of their study. One family had 13 of 15 children affected in a single generation (Gossage, 1909). But typical families showed direct heredity for at least three successive generations (Gossage, 1910c). Gossage eventually collected 67 such families. The character was passed from parent to child, affecting about half the offspring. Males and females were equally involved. When he presented this material to the Westminster Medical Society he could confidently label exostosis as a dominant trait (Gossage and Carling, 1910; Gossage, 1910c).

The two workers continued to collaborate on other human disorders. A disease of muscle spasms, myotonia congenita, was inherited in the same fashion and was a "clear dominant" (Gossage, 1910a). Malformation of the skull and the clavicle [cleidocranial dysostosis] also showed direct heredity in 17 pedigrees collected by Gossage. He suggested dominant inheritance as the most likely mechanism for its heredity (Gossage, 1910b).

George Mudge was a physician on the faculty at the London Hospital Medical School who also recognized the importance of applying heredity to the understanding of human disease causality. Although G. Archdall Reid had complained earlier that no medical school in the world provided systematic instruction in the area of heredity (Reid, 1902), Mudge sent Bateson a circular in January 1908 announcing a lecture series "On Inheritance" to be held at the medical college (Mudge, 1908b). To further publicize the importance of this work, Mudge collaborated with Bateson and Hurst at Cambridge to establish the *Mendel Journal* which first appeared in October 1908 (Kim, 1994g; Cock and Forsdyke, 2008d). His own article in the first issue summarized the evidence that several human characters did segregate in accordance with Mendelian laws: albinism, brachydactyly, night blindness and asthma (Mudge, 1909b). The *Mendel Journal* only published three volumes and then continued thereafter as the *Journal of Genetics*.

The Scottish physician Harry Drinkwater was another young pedigree collector. He contacted Bateson in May 1907 after finding a "somewhat remarkable family" in Staffordshire with an inherited deformity of the hands and feet. Shortened digits [brachydactyly] occurred in about half the children of the family, affecting the sexes equally. Drinkwater thought Bateson was "a careful student of heredity" and asked for suggestions to investigate the family history (Drinkwater, 1907a). A more complete pedigree eventually showed five and later seven affected generations (Drinkwater,

1907b). Drinkwater presented his findings to the Royal Society of Edinburgh. The paper was "very well received" and generated discussion on the connection between such clinical findings and the Mendelian theory of heredity (Drinkwater, 1907c).

Bateson then sent Drinkwater a copy of a 1905 paper by W.C. Farabee from Harvard University in America. A family with similar hand and feet abnormalities had been noted and also exhibited a dominant pattern for inheritance (Farabee, 1905). Drinkwater already knew that one affected individual had emigrated from England to America (Drinkwater, 1907d). He wondered whether the two families could be related. He wrote to Farabee and learned that the two families had similar last names. Farabee also reported that his family claimed to have heard of affected individuals back in England (Drinkwater, 1907c, 1914). Drinkwater presented this data at the Liverpool Medico-Chirurgical Society in 1908 and designated the character brachydactyly as a dominant trait (Drinkwater, 1908a). Bateson also presented their work on brachydactyly at the newly formed Section of Cytology and Genetics at the International Zoological Congress in 1907 (Bateson, W., 1907a).

Further studies on asthma continued the collaboration. Drinkwater sent Bateson a three-generation pedigree to review. Affected children were born only from an affected parent. About half the offspring had asthma (Drinkwater, 1908b). The final pedigree revealed 10 normal and 10 affected offspring. Drinkwater labeled affected individuals as heterozygotes. The expected ratio of normal to affected children was "in accord with Mendel's theoretical 50%" (Drinkwater, 1909). He presented this and other examples of Mendelian heredity in human disease when he spoke before the Denbigh and Flint Division of the British Medical Association in 1908 (Drinkwater, 1908c).

The public forum "Science Lectures for the People" had been a regular fixture of intellectual life in Manchester since the 1870s. Many well-known scientists of the day had presented their findings to a layperson audience as a means of explaining the importance of science for the English public. Drinkwater presented "A Lecture on Mendelism" there early in 1910. He described how the mechanisms for heredity applied to various plants and animals. As a physician he was particularly interested to show that the same principles governed human heredity as well. Examples of brachydactyly, night blindness and hemophilia were utilized to support his claim that Mendel's work was indeed relevant for people (Drinkwater, 1910).

Another physician with an early interest in heredity was Redcliffe N. Salaman, general practitioner in Barley, about 10 miles south of Cambridge. Since early in 1906, he had been studying the segregation of traits in potatoes grown in his own garden. Bateson had suggested this as a means to learn about heredity, and Salaman was able to describe his results in Mendelian terms (Salaman, 1910a). Coming from a Jewish background, Salaman also noted that specific hereditary conditions appeared almost exclusively within Hebrew populations. The absence of alcoholism and the neurologic disorder amaurotic family idiocy [Tay-Sachs disease] were examples of such characters that resulted from inbreeding among the Jews for more than 2000 years. A "certain stable or homozygous combination of factors" would have resulted from such consanguinity. The recessive inheritance of these traits then followed "in accordance with the laws of Mendel..." (Salaman, 1910b).

The first decade of the new century concluded with the publication of the first British M.D. thesis based on the Mendelian theory of heredity. Edward Stainer (b 1869) had graduated from the St. Thomas's Hospital Medical School in 1897. He then specialized in skin diseases and was appointed head of that department at his hospital in

1902. He had become interested in heredity of human disease, and had collected pedigrees for many conditions over the years. He collaborated with both Pearson and Bateson in supplying family data to them for genetic analysis. He decided to prepare a dissertation for the Oxford M.D. degree that was accepted in 1910. His work presented more than 80 pedigrees of diverse human anomalies. He could demonstrate direct heredity for coloboma irides and ectrodactyly, and the sex-limited pattern so characteristic for the inheritance of hemophilia, color blindness, ichthyosis and retinitis pigmentosa. He carefully explained the hereditary patterns in each family in light of the Mendelian theory (Stainer, 1910; Munk, 1955).

William Bateson's opinion on the relevance of Mendelism to human disease underwent a complex metamorphosis in the early part of the twentieth century. His initial hint that the theory might explain the incidence of rare diseases in consanguineous families was eroded by the complexity of pedigrees for other more common disorders. By 1906, he was ready to admit defeat in trying to analyze human conditions. It had all seemed so simple and straightforward in his plant and animal studies. But, the careful pedigree collection by his physician colleagues eventually convinced Bateson that Mendel's laws did indeed apply to humans as well as other living creatures. His personal relationships with many physicians allowed him to analyze human pedigree data and then to show the physicians themselves how Mendel's theory explained the segregation of diverse human traits. Bateson, his Cambridge colleague Reginald Punnett, and the physicians who understood the relevance of Mendel's work to the daily practice of medicine appeared before numerous medical society meetings before 1910. A summary of these venues, as well as the professional journals that carried articles they wrote about the new theory of human heredity, is summarized in Table 12.2.

The 1908 Royal Society of Medicine Meetings

Toward the end of the first decade of the new century, Bateson and his medical colleagues were prepared to explain the issues of human heredity to a wider professional audience. Reginald Punnett had been appointed Bateson's research assistant in 1904. He worked extensively on the heredity of plants, rabbits and poultry. On 28 February 1908, Punnett presented a lecture on "Mendelism and Disease" before the Epidemiology Section of the Royal Society of Medicine in London. This event marked the first major conference to consider this topic in England. He explained that each human egg or sperm carried only one hereditary character for each trait. A pair of such characters was required for the expression of the trait, and this state resulted from the fusion of the egg and sperm to produce the zygote, the fertilized ovum. Subsequent cell division went on to produce a new offspring. He used plant and animal examples to illustrate concepts of dominant and recessive inheritance.

Then he discussed the human characters that also seemed to conform to Mendelian expectations. Brachydactyly, ectopia lentis and hereditary chorea acted as dominants. Alkaptonuria was a recessive trait. He also suggested that such a hereditary trait could result in the "failure of metabolism...the absence of a specific intra-cellular ferment." This was an early hint that an altered genetic element could result in an altered enzyme required for normal cellular metabolism. Colorblindness and hemophilia then rounded out the human cases as examples of sex-linked disorders (Punnett, 1907-1908).

The medical men in the audience found the lecture interesting, but questioned whether it was relevant to daily medical practice. The Oxford physician Horace Vernon complained that the Mendelians largely ignored the "vast amount of work done by Galton and Pearson" on the blended heredity of more common disorders such as insanity and gout. In his opinion, "For the average medical man a knowledge of the laws of ancestral hereditary...appeared more important than a knowledge of the segregated transmission of a few very rare diseases, interesting as such cases were" (Vernon, 1908). Major Greenwood of the London Hospital Medical College complained that Punnnett thought Mendelism to be "the theory instead of a theory of heredity..." (Greenwood, 1908).

Punnett countered that, in fact, the Mendelian theory was useful to physicians because of its predictive value in individual families segregating hereditary diseases.

> There is little doubt that a knowledge of Mendel's principles must be of value in the study of disease, for once Mendelian analysis has established the operation of the law, and the nature of the characters concerned, we are in a position to predict, always the probable, sometimes the inevitable result of the given mating (Punnett, 1907-1908).

He summarized his thoughts as follows, hoping to encourage the physicians in the audience to consider heredity in their daily practices.

> Mendelian inheritance has been demonstrated for numbers of most diverse characters in plants and animals. It is also been shown to hold for a few simple cases in man where the evidence has been collected carefully and critically. How far it applies must be a matter of opinion until much more in the way of accurately recorded pedigrees is forthcoming. Facts alone can decide this matter, and if this paper did a little to stimulate the collection of such facts it would be amply repaid whatever pains went to the making of it (Punnett, 1908).

The general response from the medical community to Mendelism was quite positive. An expanded conference titled "Heredity and Disease" was sponsored by the Royal Society of Medicine over four days beginning in November 1908. There were 18 speakers representing diverse interests and opinions on the relevance of heredity to the understanding of human disorders (Church, 1909). The ophthalmologist N. Bishop Harman commented, "...the medical profession is profoundly interested in the question of the applicability of the laws of heredity as propounded by Mendel" (Harman, 1908). One observer noted, "The place was filled" (Mudge, 1908c).

Initial comments by William Gowers, prominent neurologist from the National Hospital, urged caution. He thought, "We are only in the stage of random observations [regarding heredity and man]. The scientific study of heredity...cannot be fully applied to the diseases of man. The human race is not open to Mendel's essential methods, and its mere complexity of development involves numerous differences from lower forms of life, the effects of which may be greater than we...can realize" (Gowers, 1908a). He claimed there was too little data regarding human heredity. "Potential fallacies surround almost every inference that can be drawn" (Gowers, 1908a). But he did recognize that heredity played an important role in neurologic diseases such as Friedreich's ataxia, muscular dystrophy, Huntington's chorea and myotonia. At this point in time, he thought, "It is useless even to apply the hereditarian terminology to facts..." (Gowers, 1908c). Gowers did present several intriguing pedigrees in his talk. He noted epilepsy in four successive generations of one family. In another example, he observed Dejerine facial muscle atrophy in five successive generations, observing that the character was "almost Mendelian" in its pattern of inheritance (Gowers, 1908b).

` Table 12.2
Bateson and the Doctors
1900-1910
Impact on the British Medical Community

Person	Public Forum	Publications
Bateson	Neurological Society Ophthalmological Society Royal Society of Medicine	*Nature, British Medical Journal, Transactions of the Ophthalmological Society of the United Kingdom, Brain, Proceedings of the Royal Society of Medicine*
Punnett	Royal Society of Medicine	*Proceedings of the Royal Society of Medicine*
Garrod	Royal College of Physicians Royal Society of Medicine	*Lancet* *Proceedings of the Royal Society of Medicine*
Turner	Odontological Society	*Transactions of the Odontological Society*
Nettleship	Ophthalmological Society	*Transactions of the Ophthalmological Society of the United Kingdom, Royal London Ophthalmic Hospital Reports*
Gossage	Royal Society of Medicine	*Quarterly Journal of Medicine, Proceedings of the Royal Society of Medicine*
Mudge	Royal Society of Medicine	*Mendel Journal, Nature, Lancet, British Medical Journal, Proceedings of the Royal Society of Medicine*
Drinkwater	Royal Society of Edinburgh British Medical Association Science for the Public Lecture Liverpool Medico-Chirurgical Society	*Proceedings of the Royal Society of Edinburgh* *British Medical Journal, Liverpool Medico-Chirurgical Journal*
Salaman		*Journal of Genetics*

Bateson was a keynote speaker at the conference and claimed that it could now be convincingly demonstrated that Mendelism did indeed apply to humans. He stated, "I think I shall have no difficulty in showing you that the conclusions to which Mendel came are applicable in many cases with considerable precision to the descent of diseases or congenital defect in man" (Bateson, W., 1908a). He acknowledged the assistance provided by his medical colleagues in collecting well-researched pedigrees illustrating the segregation of human diseases. The list of human characters that followed Mendelian patterns continued to grow. Chorea, ectopia lentis, distichiasis, ptosis and brachydactyly acted as dominant traits. Albinism and alkaptonuria were common in consanguineous families as expected of recessive disorders. Hemophilia, muscular dystrophy and color blindness followed the unusual pattern of affected males with unaffected female carriers that fit the pattern for sex-limited segregation (Bateson, W., 1908a).

Other physicians presented families with different traits that also appeared to follow the Mendelian model. George Mudge recorded families with hair color, eye color and asthma acting as dominants, whereas in other cases, albinism segregated as a recessive character (Mudge, 1908a). He also clarified the distinction between the competing schools of heredity. The biometric theory collected masses of pedigree data for statistical analysis, while the Mendelian approach focused on detailed study of individual pedigrees. The former would advise society on improving its future heredity; the latter sought to counsel individuals regarding their personal genetic future. Mudge thought Mendelism more accurately reflected the needs of medical practitioners (Mudge, 1908a).

Gossage discussed his pedigrees for two skin disorders. Epidermolysis bullosa and tylosis palmaris et plantaris families had equal numbers of affected and normal individuals. This is exactly what was predicted under the Mendelian segregation of a dominant trait. He concluded:

> In order to explain these facts [of heredity], one necessarily required a theory, and the only theory which offered an explanation was that of Mendel...Importantly that theory did not merely depend on human observations, but had in fact been validated by breeding studies on plants and animals where experimental investigations in the laboratory could be conducted (Gossage, 1908a).

Henry Robinson, surgeon at St. Thomas's Hospital, presented a family with ectrodactyly in four successive generations. Gossage interpreted the data to show that about half of the offspring in affected lines inherited the character. This was most consistent with a Mendelian dominant trait (Robinson and Bowen, 1908).

Karl Pearson, the statistician from the Galton Eugenics Laboratory at University College London, challenged the medical audience to carefully consider these claims that Mendelism could explain human heredity. In his opinion, "...There is no definite proof of Mendelism applying to any living form at present" (Pearson, K., 1908a). Hence, it was too early to even consider using a theory to explain complex human heredity, let alone that in less complex lower forms of life. His comments on the work presented at the conference pointed out that Mendelism required the presence or absence of the character under consideration. In his own observations on albinism and brachydactyly, there was in fact a continuum from normal to very abnormal, not the simple plus or minus required by Mendelian theory. He urged physicians to assist in the collection of more family pedigrees because, "When we have more data, then we shall be able to draw theoretical conclusions." He was being "very dogmatic" at the meeting, purposely, to incite a wave of inquiry as to family histories "collected by the medical profession." He did agree with Bateson on one point.

> If only one medical man in ten would once in his life construct two such pedigrees we should have in the course of a generation all the material needed to answer these questions on the inheritance of deformities and the constitutional tendency to special diseases (Pearson, K., 1908a).

One of the pedigrees of albinism used by Pearson demonstrated a woman bearing albino children by two successive husbands. He thought the likelihood of two men from the population carrying such a rare condition was exceedingly unlikely on a statistical basis. This was a somewhat surprising statement, considering all the albinism data collected from hundreds of families by his laboratory and showing numerous examples of the effects of inbreeding. Mudge learned that the family in question was, in fact, from Scotland where albinism was rather frequent. Inbreeding in the villages around Glasgow and Edinburgh was also quite common; he added, "They are all cousins in those communities." In such consanguineous marriages, the likelihood that parents carried rare traits was not at all unexpected. The result of such unions producing albino children was just what one would expect in the inheritance of a Mendelian recessive character. Mudge reported that the audience had a "good laugh against Pearson" (Mudge, 1908c). Mudge also noted, "...Professor Pearson's very comprehensive statement that there is no evidence for Mendelism becomes as incomprehensible as it is unjustified" (Mudge, 1908a).

The perception of Pearson and Bateson by the broader medical community was profoundly affected by their performances at the 1908 Royal Society of Medicine meetings. The acceptance or rejection of the competing theories clearly hinged on the clinical usefulness of each approach as physicians attempted to interpret family data on heredity and disease.

Bateson and the Doctors II

Bateson benefited immensely from his collaboration with British medical men. In 1906 he was almost ready to forget the notion that Mendelian heredity applied to man. But by 1909 extensive work with physicians had convinced him that, in fact, many human characters followed the patterns of inheritance predicted by that theory. The positive reception of these ideas on heredity by the physicians at the Royal Society of Medicine conferences also encouraged him to continue research in this area. When he prepared the book titled *Mendel's Principles of Heredity* in 1909, he acknowledged his debt to the many physicians who had worked with him over the years. The dominant, recessive and sex-limited characters that he identified as Mendelian at this time are listed in Table 12.3 (Bateson, W., 1909a).

The author thanked Nettleship for helping him organize his thinking on the possible connection of color blindness and sexual dimorphism in man. Bateson believed that there was evidence of such dimorphism "among spermatazoa" from color blind men. Those "destined to take part in the production of females bear the color blindness

Table 12.3
Mendelian Heredity and Human Characters 1909

DOMINANT

Short, woolly hair
White forelock
Brachydactyly
Ectrodactyly
Pre-senile cataract
Tylosis palmaris et plantaris
Xanthoma
Multiple telangiectasis
Monilithrix
Porokeratosis
Diabetes insipidus
Stationary night blindness
Distichiasis
Ptosis
Hereditary chorea
Coloboma irides
Ectopia lentis
Glaucoma

RECESSIVE

Alkaptonuria
Albinism
Retinitis pigmentosa

SEX-LIMITED

Hemophilia
Colorblindness
Pseudohypertrophic muscular paralysis

Reference: Bateson, W., 1909a

factor, while those destined to fertilize the male ovum are free from this factor." This would explain the observed fact that daughters of affected man could transmit the trait to half of their sons, while sons of the same fathers were unaffected and could not transmit it (Bateson, W., 1909b). The greater medical community also came to recognize the importance of this work. One reviewer in the neurology journal *Brain* noted that Bateson had reduced the complexities of hereditary theory to the simplest possible form ("Review," 1909).

Over the next few years, Bateson continued his work with physicians who sought to understand hereditary aspects of human disease. The aural surgeon P. Macleod Yearsley was investigating heredity and deafness. He noted consanguinity in 7% of 309 families with congenital deafness, but in 592 families with acquired deafness, only 0.3% of parents were related. Deafness, therefore, acted like a recessive trait, being much more common in inbred families (Yearsley, 1914). Yearsley consulted with Bateson to be "sure of his facts" because the relationship between heredity and deafness was a complicated business. The surgeon assured Bateson that he had carefully studied this material and "didn't want you to think that I am an ignorant ass..." (Yearsley, 1913a, b).

While Nettleship and Bateson continued their work on the heredity of eye diseases, other ophthalmologists also took note of their efforts. The president of the Ophthalmologic Section at the Royal Society of Medicine commented that when he was a young physician, the doctrine of heredity was "rampant," and all sorts of diseases were attributed to it. Then the pendulum swung in the opposite direction, and "one was told that heredity was nonsense." The fact of the matter was that all physicians had seen instances of hereditary disease affecting several generations of particular families (Nettleship and Thompson, 1912), and therefore an understanding of heredity in human disease was vital for the modern practicing physician.

Bateson and Nettleship also spoke at another meeting of the Ophthalmological Society in 1911. Nettleship presented pedigrees segregating nystagmus through five generations. In most examples, only males were affected while the trait was transmitted through unaffected females. Bateson explained to the doctors the Mendelian mechanism that could account for this type of sex-limited inheritance (Nettleship, 1911; Bateson, W., 1911a).

Bateson then heard about a case of night blindness from a Cambridge physician and asked Nettleship to investigate the family history. This appeared to be a different form of night blindness than he had previously encountered. Seven generations were affected; unaffected females appeared to transmit the disease only to their sons. Unlike the dominant form of night blindness, the sex-linked Cambridge variant also was associated with myopia (Nettleship, 1912b).

The inheritance of other sex-limited characters such as colorblindness also provided a fertile field for collaboration. Bateson heard about several unusual color-blind families and asked Nettleship to investigate them. Two pedigrees showed apparently identical female twins, one color-blind and one normal sighted. Another family demonstrated several color-blind sisters whose sons were affected and daughters normal (Nettleship, 1912c). Clearly, there was much more to be learned. The details of sex-linked heredity would not be fully understood for several more decades.

Medical men who collaborated with Bateson were now recognized before a wider audience. Salaman and Drinkwater attended the Fourth International Congress of Genetics that was held in Paris during 1913. Salaman discussed the details of his Mendelian breeding studies in potatoes (Salaman, 1913). Drinkwater presented a five-generation pedigree that showed direct heredity of brachydactyly. There were 26 normal and 21 affected individuals in the family. He characterized the trait as a Mendelian dominant (Drinkwater, 1913b). The hand abnormality appeared in 44.6% of offspring in affected branches of the family, as expected for a dominant character (Drinkwater, 1912).

Despite the demands of a busy general medical practice and the care of the wounded generated by the World War, Drinkwater continued his studies on heredity and anomalies of the hands and feet. Different types of brachydactyly were discovered, but each bred true in specific families (Drinkwater, 1913a, 1916a). He expanded the Farabee Anglo-American pedigree to include six generations and found 51.02% abnormals in the affected branches (Drinkwater, 1914). It was clear that in all cases, different forms of brachydactyly acted as dominant disorders.

Drinkwater examined another hand and foot anomaly involving absent distal phalanges with bifid thumbs and great toes. This character was transmitted through five successive generations and affected the sexes equally. It also demonstrated the dominant pattern for inheritance (Cragg and Drinkwater, 1916). Perhaps the most striking example of Mendelian heredity at this time involved ankylosis [fusion of the joints] involving the proximal and middle phalanges 3, 4 and 5 of the hands. Affected family members were direct descendants of John Talbot, first Earl of Shrewsbury, who was killed in battle near Bordeaux in 1453. His body was buried at Whitchurch beneath a stone effigy showing the digital anomaly in question. Family tradition stated that the Earl broke his femur in the battle and died after sustaining an ax blow to the head. Restoration of the church in 1874 caused the tomb to be opened. Photographs of the skeleton showed fractures of the femur and the skull. The fingers demonstrated the same ankylosed condition noted in members of the current generation. The pedigree was believed to demonstrate direct transmission of a Mendelian dominant trait through 14 successive generations (Drinkwater, 1917b; Clippingdale, 1918).

The careful pedigree analysis performed by Drinkwater convinced him that the Mendelian laws of heredity applied to man, as well as to plants and animals. He thought that his fellow physicians were in an ideal position to record and then to study examples of heredity and disease encountered in their daily clinical work (Drinkwater, 1917a). He commented to Bateson that he wished to encourage "medical man to work out pedigrees of cases they come across..." (Drinkwater, 1916b).

Before the War, Bateson continued his round of lectures on heredity and human disease to medical society meetings throughout England. In June 1911, he spoke before doctors at Westminster Hospital and outlined Mendel's inheritance patterns. He showed pedigrees for cataract, diabetes insipidus, Huntington's chorea and colorblindness (Bateson, W., 1911b). He also appeared at the 1913 International Congress of Medicine in London and hoped that his discussion would influence "the development of genetic study in the medical world." The basic outline of Mendelian inheritance was once again presented with examples of 24 dominant, five recessive, and five sex-linked human disorders that segregated in families according to the Mendelian model (Bateson, W., 1913).

Bateson was appointed Fullerian Professor at the Royal Institution in London for a three-year term, beginning in 1912. Three public lectures were to be given each year (Bateson, B., 1928b). The lectures attracted medical practitioners as well as the general public who became increasingly aware of Bateson's interest in human heredity. A local ophthalmologist, Ernest Clarke, attended one such lecture and then sent Bateson a copy of an article he had published in 1903 reporting a family with hereditary nystagmus in five generations. Only males were affected, and females appeared to transmit the character in successive generations (Clarke, 1903). Clarke thought Bateson might be interested in the family and told him to "use it as he saw fit" (Clarke, 1910). Bateson recognized the sex-limited pattern of heredity and included it in his 1913 list of human hereditary characters presented at the International Congress of Medicine (Bateson, W., 1913).

One of Bateson's most ambitious interactions with the medical profession involved his presidency of the British Association for the Advancement of Science in 1914 which resulted in a trip to Australia for the annual meeting of the organization. Local medical men and scientists in general suffered from a commonly held "tyranny of distance" from the European centers of learning. Those at the periphery of the Commonwealth felt isolated from advances in the professions. At the time, London and the two major universities at Oxford and Cambridge were viewed as <u>the</u> centers for learning. Practitioners in the English provinces, and especially those at more distant sites around the globe, were viewed with contempt and characterized as rustic folk by those back home. Keeping abreast of developments in one's specialized field was not easy when the mail boat took six weeks to carry the latest issue of professional journals from England to Australia (Knight, 1991; Chambers, 1991).

The impact of the B.A.A.S. meeting in 1914 cannot be overestimated. The organization had held foreign meetings in prior years—Toronto in 1897 and even South Africa in 1905. But the planning for this event literally on the other side of the world began as early as 1909. The Australian government and the universities there collaborated on plans for the sessions to be held in several cities throughout the country from late July until late August. Conference participants left England in mid-June as the trip out was 12,740 miles and took at least five weeks. The clouds of an impending European war did not prevent the local people from vigorously supporting the conference meetings. More than 5000 Australians joined the organization during the event, far in excess of those who paid for membership at prior events elsewhere in the world (Bateson, W., 1915a). Australian newspapers reported every detail of the conference sessions. There was great public interest in the proceedings as senior English scientists gained some sense of Australian work in the various disciplines. The event seemed to mark the "scientific coming-of-age of Australia" (MacLeod, 1988).

Bateson gave his Presidential Address on "Heredity" in two sessions: one in Melbourne, and the second a week later in Sydney. He proclaimed, "The outstanding feature of the meeting must be that we are here—in Australia." He then outlined recent experimental work in plants and animals on the details of hereditary mechanisms. One area of controversy related to whether chromosomes had anything important to do with heredity. He observed that the chromosomes of closely related creatures could be quite different in terms of number and size. He also was not certain whether the hereditary factors in the egg and sperm were "in a literal sense material particles." He thought it more likely that their hereditary properties depended on "some phenomenon of arrangement" (Bateson, W., 1915c).

Bateson also noted the accumulating data on dominant, recessive and sex-linked human diseases. He particularly mentioned advances in the understanding of hereditary eye diseases due to the labor of his recently departed colleague Nettleship. The ophthalmologist routinely examined all accessible family members, and the resulting carefully constructed pedigrees were "models of orderly observation and recording." He hoped Nettleship's work would inspire the younger physicians to collect family hereditary data as well (Bateson, W., 1914a, b, 1915b).

Even before Bateson's speeches, Australian physicians had become aware of new developments relating heredity and human diseases. The speaker at a 1913 meeting of the Western Australian branch of the British Medical Association recognized, "It is unpleasant to have to alter our theories and to view things in a new perspective, but science fortunately has no frontiers, and her kingdom is extended with each acquisition of discovered fact." Mendel's work on breeding was reviewed to introduce the concepts of genetic segregation, and dominant and recessive characters. It was expected that this new theory would have implications for human society as well (Shaw, 1913).

E. Pockley attended the B.A.A.S. meeting in Sydney and found Bateson's presentation fascinating. " It was very interesting to see the mathematical accuracy with which the dominants and recessives showed up in definite proportion as a result of certain crosses [in experimental plants and animals]...Possibly transmission of characteristics follows just as immutable laws in man..." Pockley then presented a family segregating Leber's disease [hereditary optic atrophy]. His pedigree showed that the disorder acted like color blindness with unaffected females transmitting the trait only to males (Pockley, 1915). Using Mendelian principles, the psychiatrist John Catarinich from Victoria's Beckworth Mental Hospital analyzed the inheritance of the degenerative neurologic disease Huntington's chorea. His pedigrees showed transmission from parent to child through two and three generations. He thought this represented the Mendelian dominant pattern of inheritance (Catarinich, 1914).

After returning to Europe following the 1914 B.A.A.S. meeting, Bateson did not appear before many other audiences of scientists or physicians specifically interested in human heredity.[9] During the World War, he continued his interactions with British physicians and even received questions from the battlefield. George Gask was a military surgeon with the British Expeditionary Force in France. He had been interested in tissue grafts, both endogenous and heterogeneous, such as skin, bone and tendon. Dissimilarity of donor tissue and recipient usually meant that "a distinct toxic effect" occurred, and the graft failed. He had been wondering whether heredity played some role in graft acceptance. With the advent of the War, Gask had developed great experience with blood transfusions. Many lives had been saved by the technique. But in a small percentage of cases, the recipient became ill very quickly. The transfusion produced a toxic effect with hemolysis of the red blood cells. Agglutination tests had recently become available that defined "blood groups," and allowed compatible blood to be transfused. He thought that blood groups were hereditary and followed the Mendelian law. In this sense, transfused blood acted like a tissue graft. Gask wondered if tissues had "type" as blood did. Perhaps that factor explained the successes and failures of tissue grafting. He asked Bateson if a genetic study of tissue type was possible in experimental animals and perhaps man himself (Gask, 1918).

Bateson had by now worked for more than ten years with Garrod, Nettleship, Gossage, Drinkwater and the many other physicians who applied Mendelism to the questions of human hereditary disease. He felt they were prepared to continue their own investigations on heredity and clinical disease.

Pearson and the Doctors II

While Bateson and his ideas on Mendelian heredity were received in a positive sense by the physicians at the 1908 Royal Society of Medicine meetings, Pearson's appearance must have caused great personal distress to himself. Physician observers noted his somewhat illogical statements, while Pearson complained that the reporting of the conference in the *Lancet* was "mangled" in his opinion (Pearson, K., 1908b). And the fact that the physician audience actually laughed at him must have been a profound blow to his ego (Mudge, 1908c).

Over the previous few years, Pearson had become weary of the constant bickering with the Mendelians. His own thinking about the antagonistic theories had, in fact, begun to shift. As early as 1904, he declared, "...We have no fundamental antagonism between the Mendelian and biometric standpoint" (Pearson, K., 1904e). One year after the Royal Society of Medicine conference, he published a paper titled "On the ancestral gametic correlations of a Mendelian population mating at random" in the *Proceedings of the Royal Society*. He concluded that the two approaches to heredity were, in fact, complementary.

> The striking point, however of the present investigation, is that the values now shown theoretically to exist for the ancestral gametic correlations in a simple Mendelian mixture are very close to those determined for somatic characters in biometric investigations (Pearson, K., 1909c).

Therefore, he had to conclude,

> ...There remains not the least antimony between the Mendelian theory and the law of ancestral heredity, if we confine our attention to gametic constitution. The Mendelian ancestry is connected with the offspring in a series of descending or geometrical progressions, and the regression is linear (Pearson, K., 1909c).

Two years later the Scottish statistician John Brownlee, from the London School of Tropical Medicine and Hygiene, also published mathematical formulae based on Mendelian postulates to analyze the inheritance of more complex human traits such as stature. He likewise concluded that everything in the coefficients of inheritance expected on the biometric model could be explained on the basis of Mendelian inheritance as well (Brownlee, 1910).

Pearson found himself in a difficult position. He and Weldon had argued for years that Mendelian inheritance would only be applicable to particulate inheritance involving very specific characters. But, his more recent work had demonstrated that the theory could also be applied successfully to traits inherited in a population continuum. And, their claim that the Mendelian theory had not been demonstrated to successfully explain any human character could no longer be maintained, either. Pearson refused to admit that Bateson and his medical colleagues were right, and that he was wrong. Instead he decided to forego any further discussion of inheritance theories and to pursue a different course at the Galton Laboratory.

After Weldon's death, Pearson undoubtedly felt somewhat lost in the world of the biologists. He had noted to Weldon a decade earlier that he could only do this inheritance research with his colleague's assistance on the biology side, because he [Pearson] did not have the "necessary knowledge" of even basic biology (Magnello, 1998). Pearson now concluded, "The mission of science was not to explain [with theories], but to describe..." (Porter, 2004k). So Pearson embarked on a research program in human heredity to describe mathematical correlations in a "theory-free fashion" (Norton, 1975).

Having made this decision, there was no room for argument or discussion. The American biologist C.B. Davenport had been a member of the *Biometrika* editorial board since the journal was founded in 1901. In 1910 he recommended publication of work supporting Mendelian heredity. Pearson was outraged. He wrote, "It is a disadvantage to the journal and the course I have at heart to be told that the sub-editors of the journal are opposed to the principles for which it was founded" (Kevles, 1980). Pearson responded by firing the entire editorial board. Davenport responded to Pearson:

> ...Bateson urged that I should withdraw my name on the ground that *Biometrika* stands not for biometry but for a special set of ideas which all experimentalists have found not in accord with the facts. I demurred at the time that I thought it stood primarily for quantitative work in biology without regard to any speculative ideas, but it appears that he was right and I was wrong, and what he suggested logically follows (Davenport, 1910).

Raymond Pearl, another member of the board, noted to Pearson, "[You want] no one associated with you in the editorship of *Biometrika* who does not think exactly as you do on questions of theoretical biology" (Kevles, 1980). Clearly, Pearson viewed these challenges as an affront to his journal. This latest development also involved a reversal of policy promulgated by Pearson himself when the journal began, i.e., that the publication was to be open to all and "not intend[ed] to be exclusive..." (Provine, 1971e).

Thereafter, Pearson was very consistent in the application of his opinion. The numbers of articles that discussed Mendelism in all the publications from the Galton Laboratory between 1900 and 1930 are presented in Figure 12.1. The black bars signify negative application of the theory, while the white bars represent positive applications. Before 1916, there clearly was evidence for give-and-take between the conflicting theories. After 1910, only negative opinions regarding Mendelism were permitted with two exceptions. Edward Cockayne, a young physician at St. Bart's Hospital, traced the inheritance of piebaldism through six generations of a family from Suffolk. His 1914 report in *Biometrika* explained that the character segregated as a Mendelian dominant trait (Cockayne, 1914). The Laboratory established another journal called *Annals of Eugenics* in the 1920s which published a report from 1928 originating at the Peking Medical College on malformations of the human hand. Two families were described in detail with pedigrees. One exhibited brachydactyly through three generations and showed direct parent to child transmission. No particular comments regarding heredity were noted. The second family demonstrated phalangeal ankylosis [fusion of the joints] through seven generations. Direct parent to child transmission was again evident, and about 50 percent of the offspring were affected. The author, G.A.M. Hall, thought that the character behaved as a simple Mendelian dominant (Hall, 1928). Pearson's sharp eye apparently missed only these two instances in twenty years experience as editor.

Around 1910 Pearson was seeking to involve more physicians in the work of the Galton Laboratory. He planned a memoir series to be called the *Treasury of Human Inheritance.* It was to be a collection of pedigrees of diverse human characters—both normal and abnormal. Importantly, Pearson proposed, "...there will be an entire absence of purely theoretical discussions" (Pearson, K., 1908d). This was to be Pearson's theory-free unbiased collection of human data upon which future research on heredity could be performed (Pearson, E.S., 1938b). He noted, once the project had begun, that,

"...Medical men were coming and giving us splendid material...often confidential and personal histories" (Gillham, 2001b).

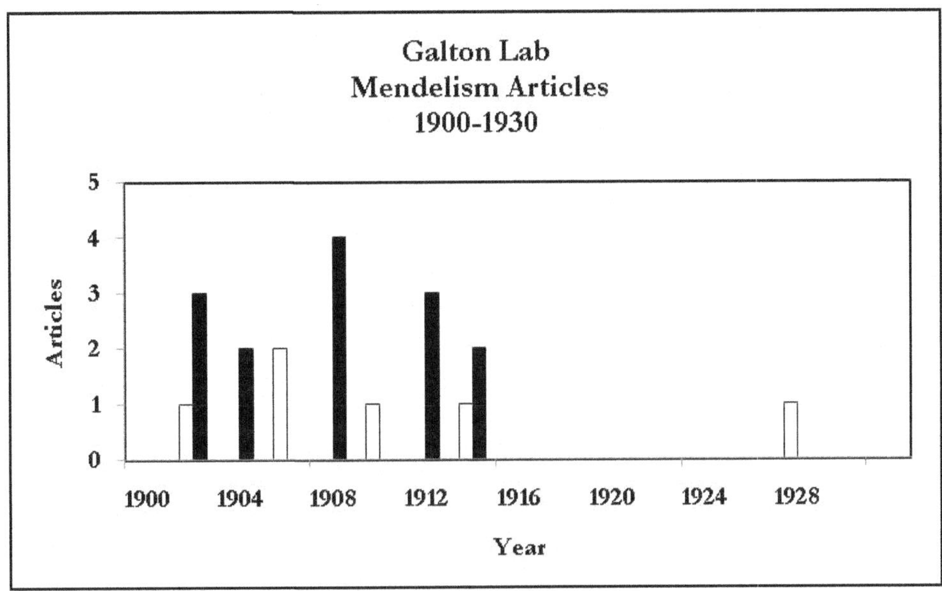

Figure 12.1

The sections of the *Treasury* published from 1909 to 1951 are listed in Table 12.4. The general scheme of the work involved the collection of pedigrees coordinated at the Galton Laboratory and the preparation of each memoir by physicians selected by Pearson as general editor. No theorizing was allowed, but the series remains even today as a monumental work of immense value to human heredity researchers. The *Treasury* recently figured in a suspense novel, *The Blood Doctor.* A British MP investigating whether hemophilia was present in his own family had consulted the Bulloch and Fildes *Treasury* memoir on disorders of the blood (Vine, 2002).

Pearson's non-theoretical approach appeared to influence physicians even when they were not writing for his own organization. Fildes presented a lecture on hemophilia at The London Hospital in 1909. He mentioned the upcoming Galton Laboratory memoir on the disorder. He noted that females typically transmitted the disease, but remained unaffected themselves. Fildes avoided any discussion of how the character was transmitted in such a hereditary pattern (Fildes, 1909). Bulloch sent Pearson numerous pedigrees of both hemophilia and color blindness between 1909 and 1915 (Bulloch, 1909, 1911-1915). When a colleague followed his rules, Pearson could be a true friend. These two men did develop quite a warm friendship. Several years later, Bulloch's father died, and the physician greatly appreciated Pearson's sympathy. "I take your letter as a further sign of the friendship which you have always extended to me and which I greatly appreciate and value" (Bulloch, 1913).

When Pearson planned the *Treasury*, he hoped that physicians of all theoretical stripes would feel free to contribute to the opus. He noted, "Is it too much for our Mendelian friends to give us cooperation in this matter...?" (Pearson, K., 1908d). Several physicians from the Mendelian camp did indeed collaborate with Pearson and the Galton Laboratory project. George McMullan sent a copy of the paper on brachydactyly that he had presented to the Reading Pathological Society in 1910. He concluded that the character over four generations behaved as a dominant trait (McMullan, 1910). Harry Drinkwater also sent Pearson a report on a seven-generation family with brachydactyly. He noted,

> My own observations were undertaken primarily with the object of recording facts and without any bias resulting from the study of Mendel's published works. However, one can hardly fail to recognize the support that these facts give to Mendel's laws of inheritance (Drinkwater, 1907e).

Nonetheless, he thought that the Eugenics Laboratory was the "most suitable repository of this information" (Drinkwater, 1911).

The preparation of the monograph on albinism provided an example of how Pearson's opinions influenced the scientific output of his colleagues. The work comprised four parts. Pearson, Nettleship and Usher completed the last part that included the pedigree charts and the entire bibliography for the work. Their plan in 1913 was to issue this fourth part and then "get on with the third part dealing with albinism in other animals, heredity and statistics" (Pearson, K., 1913). But by an intriguing twist of historical fate, the third part of the monograph was never published. Pearson's biography reported that the advent of war early in 1914, "took Pearson from a subject to which he never found time to return" (Pearson, E.S., 1938a; Williams, 1997).[10] Nettleship had died at the end of 1913, and the statistical skills of the laboratory staff were devoted to the war effort, analyzing economic data, aeronautics and ballistics rather than continuing strictly original research efforts (Farrall, 1985b).

Because Part III of the monograph was never published, the proposed detailed analysis of the hereditary aspects of albinism was not completed. A few brief comments on this topic were included in Part II. The authors attempted to analyze a series of albino dog crosses utilizing Mendelian concepts of dominant and recessive inheritance. They concluded that the numerical results did not support the Mendelian theory (Pearson, K., Nettleship and Usher, 1911). They agreed that albinism was a continuous character with many degrees of affectedness. But, they disagreed on the importance of the different theoretical explanations for its transmission from one generation to the next. Pearson as editor observed, "Mendelism is at present the mode—no other conception of heredity can even obtain a hearing. Yet one of the present writers at least believes that a reaction must shortly set in, and that the views of Galton will again come by their own" (Pearson, K., Nettleship and Usher, 1911). Pearson was thus able to avoid open conflict with his medical colleagues over the relative applicability of Mendelian and biometric theories in explaining this inherited trait.

Pearson had planned the inclusion of a medically qualified staff number at the E.R.O. as early as 1911 to enhance the collection and analysis of human data on both normal and abnormal conditions. However, budgetary constraints prevented the addition of a medical officer to his staff until late in 1922 when Percy Stocks joined the group to assist with "the medically oriented research of the laboratory" (Farrall, 1985d). He immediately set to work examining a four-generation family segregating facial spasm. With one exception, direct parent to child inheritance was noted in the *Biometrika* report

(Stocks, 1922). He also prepared the section of the *Treasury of Human Inheritance* on the bony disorders that appeared in 1925 (Stocks, 1925).

The frequency of tuberculosis was examined next using statistics from Belfast. Parents of affected children had an increased rate of infection among themselves compared to the general population, as did the children of affected parents. More children were diseased if both parents were infected. The report in the *Annals of Eugenics* concluded that this pattern of affectedness was due to a hereditary susceptibility to the infection (Stocks, 1927, 1928). Another study examined the incidence of cancer in families of 255 patients compared to a control group. There was no evidence of increased cancer rates in families of affected persons, suggesting little effect of heredity on the development of human cancers (Stocks and Karn, 1933). The work of Stock was clearly relevant to the practice of medicine in Britain, but his work at the Galton Laboratory was published in memoirs from that organization and not in the general medical journals that would have been read by a broader physician audience.

Other work from the Laboratory did, however, attract a great deal of physician attention and helped to formulate an opinion in the minds of British physicians on the nature and quality of the research work at this institution. Amy Barrington had studied mathematics at Girton College Cambridge, but had left without completing a degree. She worked at the Galton Laboratory and was assigned to study the relationship between defective vision and heredity. Nettleship assisted in the review of the ophthalmological literature on this topic. The general opinion of most physicians, based upon observations of many families, was that heredity did contribute to a certain degree in the development of poor eyesight. The statistical work at the laboratory agreed that heredity provided a "constitutional weakness" in the eyes that became realized "with growth or suitable environment" (Barrington and Pearson, 1909a). The report concluded that environment at school or at home did not alter children's eyesight; most refractive error was due to a hereditary character (Barrington and Pearson, 1909b). The report finally published in 1909 concluded that hereditary visual defect was a potential problem not only for the current generation of children, but for the future visual health of the population as well. The eugenic solution was clearly stated: "The first thing is good stock, and the second thing is good stock, and the third thing is good stock, and when you have paid attention to these things, fit environment will keep your material in good condition" (Barrington and Pearson, 1909c). The call for better breeding then was paramount rather than attempting to merely improve conditions in nutrition, school or housing for the English population.

The response of the medical community to this memoir agreed that heredity certainly played an important role in causing visual defects in children. However, the statement that "good stock" was the only important factor in the development of healthy young eyes appeared to over-reach the available data ("Vision," 1909).

Table 12.4
Treasury of Human Inheritance

Section	Title	Authors
Volume I		
Ia 1909	Diabetes insipidus	W. Bulloch MD
IIa	Split foot	T. Lewis MD
IIIa	Polydactylism	T. Lewis MD
IVa	Brachydactylism	T. Lewis MD
Va	Pulmonary tuberculosis	W. Bulloch MD, W. River MD
VIa	Deaf mutism	J. Horne MD
VIIa	Ability	Laboratory staff
VIIIa	Chronic trophedema	W. Bulloch MD
IXa	Angioneurotic edema	W. Bulloch MD
Xa	Hermaphroditism	W. Bulloch MD
XIa	Insanity	A.R. Urquhart MD
VIb	Deaf mutism	Laboratory staff
VIIb	Ability	Laboratory staff
XIIa	Hare lip/cleft palate	H. Rischbieth MD
VIg	Deaf mutism	Laboratory staff
XIIIa	Cataract	N.B. Harman MD
XIVa	Hemophilia	W. Bulloch MD, P. Fildes MD
XVa	Dwarfism	H. Rischbieth MD
Volume II		
Part I 1922	Retinitis pigmentosa Stationary night blindness Glioma retinae	J. Bell MD
Part II 1926	Color-blindness	J. Bell MD
Volume III		
Part I 1925	Diaphysial aclasis Multiple enchondromata Cleidocranial dystosis	P. Stocks MD

Table 12.4, *Continued*
Treasury of Human Inheritance

Section	Title	Authors
Volume II		
Part III 1928	Blue sclerotics and fragility of bone	J. Bell MD
Part IV 1931	Hereditary optic atrophy	J. Bell MD
Part V 1932	Structural anomalies of the eye Glaucoma	J. Bell MD
Volume IV		
Part I 1934	Huntington's chorea	J. Bell MD
Part II 1935	Peroneal progressive muscular atrophy	J. Bell MD
Part III 1939	Hereditary ataxia and spastic paraplegia	J. Bell MD
Part IV 1943	Pseudohypertrophic muscular dystrophies	J. Bell MD
Part V 1947	Dystrophia myotonica	J. Bell MD
Volume V		
Part I 1951	Brachydactyly and symphalangism	J. Bell MD

A second study on heredity and important human characters appeared in the following year. Ethel Elderton had studied mathematics at Bedford College at the University of London and had learned statistical analysis in her work with Pearson at the Galton Laboratory. Elderton and Pearson attempted to study the effects of alcoholism in mothers and its effects on the children. They did find evidence that childhood mortality was increased in families with alcoholic mothers, but there was no measurable difference in intelligence, physique or specific diseases in surviving children born of alcoholic mothers, compared to children with unaffected parents. The conclusion was that heredity was more important in these areas than intrauterine environment. They felt that heredity was approximately 4 to 10 times more potent than environmental factors in the formation of healthy children (Elderton, 1910). Elderton summarized the importance of the work as follows, "The only way to keep a nation strong mentally and physically is to see to it that each new generation is derived from the fitter members of the generation before" (Elderton, 1909). The eugenic message again was that better breeding was much more important to society then improved sanitation or other public health measures.

The medical community had generally believed that alcoholism was a serious disease and had dire consequences not only for those affected adults, but also for the children born into such families. Most of the physicians of the day generally agreed with temperance organizations that the control of alcohol consumption would certainly enhance the general health of the population. One can easily imagine that the laboratory memoir claiming no effect of maternal alcoholism on childrens' health was viewed as unbelievable and outrageous. One commentator thought the report had achieved an "extraordinary conclusion" (Sturge and Horsley, 1911). How could physicians think this was a truly scientific study if such illogical conclusions had been reached? Some suspected that the laboratory staff was mistaken. Two physicians commented, "They have concealed the truth by a mass of mathematically formulated conclusions, which being calculated on misstated data, are necessarily also erroneous" (Sturge and Horsley, 1911).

Even the medically trained staff of Pearson's own organization was sensitized to the claims emanating from the Laboratory. Major Greenwood was a physician who taught physiology at London Hospital Medical College. He had worked with Pearson to learn the application of statistics to medical science, but left in disgust when Pearson's staff claimed that nutrition had no demonstrable effect on the performance of children in the classroom. While he agreed that heredity was important in providing human potential for learning, he refused to accept that environmental factors such as inadequate protein intake would not affect the intellectual health of children. He called such eugenic notions, "Simply SHIT from beginning to end" (Kevles, 1985c)

After episodes like this, Pearson realized that he had to carefully state his findings on socially relevant issues of heredity in such a way that would not offend British physicians. He wanted and needed the medical community to support the work of his laboratory and did not wish to drive them away as he made eugenic claims which spoke against their generally held opinions based on clinical experience.

Because of his desire not to alienate the British medical community, Pearson was also careful in his dealings with the social eugenics movement that developed before the World War. Middle-class society in England was increasingly concerned about the rise of the pauper class. The underlying cause of such unfortunate families was widely believed to be hereditary defect. With their rapid breeding rate, control of such an underclass was clearly in the best interests of the more sophisticated elements of society. Attempts to control the fecundity of the paupers would certainly enhance the commonweal for the future.

The Eugenics Education Society (E.E.S.) had been formed in 1907 with just such a social purpose in mind. Its members were educated middle-class folk. The historian Lyndsay Farrall has designated them as "middle-class radicals" (Mazumdar, 1992a). The organization began publishing *The Eugenics Review* in 1909 with summaries of articles on the importance of good breeding for the health of the nation. Pearson was concerned that the public would confuse the Eugenics Record Office with the Eugenics Education Society. He noted that if the work of the Record Office had been, "mixed up in any way with the work of Havelock Ellis, Slaughter or Saleeby [from the E.E.S.], we shall kill any chance of founding eugenics as an academic discipline" (Gillham, 2001b). He also feared that the radical eugenics of these men would act as "red rags to the medical bull, and if it were thought that we were linked up with them we should be left seriously alone" (Gillham, 2001b). One physician complained that eugenics meetings brought out all the "Neo-Malthusians, anti-vaccinationists, anti-vivisectionists, Christian scientists, Theosophites, Mullerites, vegetarians and that lot of society" (Kevles, 1985c). Pearson was concerned that the E.E.S. was too much propaganda and too little science (Kevles, 1985d).

The openness of the eugenics community to Mendelism also grated against Pearson's opinions on heredity and true science. Leaders of the E.E.S. accepted both the biometric and Mendelian approaches to human heredity. Pedigrees were collected from socially-misfit families, and direct evidence of transmission of social traits from one generation to the next was interpreted to mean that Mendelian factors were at work. Public education lectures also brought speakers from both camps before the eugenics community. The E.E.S. President, the lawyer Montague Crackantharpe, noted as early as 1910:

> The Mendelian thesis that inherited characters may be 'patent' or 'latent' militates somewhat against Professor Pearson's results, which being based on the statistical line of inquiry are derived from the observation of patent characters only. But I beg you not to infer from this that Mendelism has therefore superseded biometry. It would be a thousand pities if the Mendelians were to say to the biometricians, 'We have no need of you,' or if the biometricians were to say to the Mendelians, 'We have no need of you,' for Eugenics requires the services of both, as a little reflection will show (Mazumdar, 1992b).

The Society's first lecture series in 1911 featured G.P. Mudge speaking on Mendelism, while David Heron discussed the biometric work of the Galton Laboratory. Ethel Elderton examined the issue of first cousin marriages, and A.D. Darbshire presented material on "the inheritance of sex" (Mazumdar, 1992b). In January 1913, the educational series on eugenics was transferred to Imperial College London and presented an even-handed selection of topics from both biometric and Mendelian points of view (Mazumdar, 1992c; Kevles, 1985d).

The E.E.S. also sponsored the First International Congress of Eugenics that met in London in July 1912. Pearson was conspicuous by his absence. He again avoided close association in public with the popular eugenics movement. The President of the Congress was Leonard Darwin, son of the famous naturalist. He argued that man's future clearly rested on inborn qualities. The role of society leaders then was to encourage the reproduction of those desirable qualities in subsequent generations and to prevent the continuation of socially undesirable characters from the pauper class (Gillham, 2001c). The pathologist F.W. Mott from the London County Asylum presented his analysis on heredity and insanity (Mazumdar, 1992d). Inbreeding appeared to enhance the character. Pauperism, idiocy and consumption all appeared in large families to pass directly from affected parents to their children (Gillham, 2001d).

Reginald Punnett, Professor of Genetics at Cambridge, agreed that feeble mindedness appeared to segregate as a simple Mendelian recessive trait (Gillham, 2001e). But he cautioned his audience that research in human heredity was not straightforward.

> ...[Man] must be regarded as unpromising [for genetics study] not only from the small size of his families, the time concerned in their production, and the long period of immaturity, but also because full experimental control is here out of the question. For these reasons, man is of interest to the student of genetics, chiefly insofar as he respects problems of heredity which are rarely to be found in other species and can only be studied in man himself...Though the direct [experimental] method is hardly feasible in man, much may yet be learned by collecting accurate pedigrees and comparing them with the standard ones worked out in other animals. But it must be clearly recognized that the collection of such pedigrees is an arduous undertaking demanding high critical ability and only to be carried out satisfactorily by those who have been trained in and are alive to the trend of genetical research (Punnett, 1912).

The relevance of eugenics ideas for physicians appeared obvious to the Congress participants. One noted:

> Medicine...has confined its activities almost entirely to single individuals of its own generation. This science has hardly concerned itself at all with the well-being of future generations: on the contrary, it is bringing to future generations many evils by its protection of those people who are at present physically or mentally unsound (Bluhm, 1912).

Hence, the physician should not only be a healer of current ills, but a judge of those who deserved to reproduce. H.E. Jordan of the American Association for the Study and Prevention of Infant Mortality also attended the Congress in London. In his opinion, "Modern medicine is becoming more preventive than curative." Doctors therefore should become "guardians of public health," rather than caregivers of individuals with disease (Jordan, 1912). When Jordan spoke of "public health," he clearly meant the genetic health of future generations. Physicians would be expected to counsel young people "to prevent weakness in themselves and in their offspring" (Jordan, 1912).

After his absence at the Congress, Pearson did accept an invitation to present the Cavendish Lecture to the West London Medico-Chirurgical Society in 1912 (Eccles, 1912). He hoped to explore common goals that his organization, the Eugenics Record Office, and practicing physicians had "towards increased social welfare" (Pearson, K., 1912). He noted that the Galton Laboratory had sought the co-operation of physicians in collecting pedigree data from its inception. He acknowledged that practicing physicians were the primary resource of such family data on human disease. Pearson also recognized that the primary goal of the general practitioner was to enhance the welfare of the individual human being and the relief of individual suffering. But he also encouraged the audience to think of the public health as well. In daily practice, physicians had access to large amounts of public health statistics, but they did not have the training or interest in analyzing such data in a scientific manner. The E.R.O. could function to analyze the data and help the doctors understand how eugenic measures could enhance the health of future generations. He argued that deformities and disabilities of all types had a strong hereditary basis. Therefore, only through eugenic policy could one hope to improve the health of society's children. He recommended that his physician audience act as advisers to the families in their practices to effect healthy marriages. In this manner, medicine and eugenics together would enhance the well being of the nation (Pearson, K., 1912).

Having encouraged the physicians to work with him on the eugenic health of society, Pearson then made a disparaging remark that reflected his opinion of how physicians really functioned on a day-to-day basis. He quipped in parting, "It has been the first medical audience he had known in which professional duties had not called at least one or two members" away to care for their ill or injured patients (Pearson, K., 1912). Although Pearson did not retire from active research work until 1933, he would never again appear before another medical audience for the rest of his life.

Pearson clearly did not think much of medical practitioners because they often appeared to be more interested in caring for their patients than in learning about science as he defined it. He thought much of current medicine was "full of humbug," and concluded that physicians needed more scientific, and especially statistical, training (Porter, 2004j). There is no question that he was correct about the mathematical innocence of most physicians. J.S. Manson observed:

> The highly abstract mathematical doctrines of the law of averages, the theory of probability involved in the correlation of coefficients [in biometry], make this method more attractive to the mathematical experts than to the ordinary medical practitioner...As a rule to the ordinary individual its conclusions are vague and unconvincing (Manson, 1928).

The difficulty in applying biometry to specific cases involved the calculation of correlation coefficients to connect one generation to the next. Because these varied in each case, physicians without mathematical expertise were obliged to turn to Pearson's "rival and antagonist" William Bateson (Mercier, 1913).

For the physician of the day, it appeared that the two schools of hereditary thought focused on different issues. The biometric approach analyzed large numbers of individuals in many different families. Mendelism, on the other hand, focused on specific cases involving the offspring of one set of parents. Physicians primarily dealt with individual patients and their families in daily practice. G.P. Mudge commented:

> Someday the mathematicians will succeed in learning that living structures are not dead marbles, and the mathematical conceptions and formulae which may legitimately be applied to the latter have not always a solid application to the former (Mudge, 1909a).

In other words, any theory of heredity which would prove useful to the practicing physician had to address the central aim of medicine which was the care of individual patients, or in mathematical terms, the statistic of one.

The Mendelian approach appealed to physicians because they learned from its daily application that, "by the careful and exact study of a few cases, [we can] materially assist in the advancement of [genetic knowledge]" ("Nature and nurture," 1912). The family data often did, indeed, appear to fit the expectations of the Mendelian model. By the end of the decade, physicians could observe,

> Data obtained from the minute analysis of their compounded factors in carefully studied pedigrees, and their accordance with Mendelian principles, will prove of enormous importance in our studies of their heritage of disease (Bevan-Lewis, 1909).

Because of this type of observation, it could therefore be argued, "It is necessary to insist that the biological method is supremely that which is proper for the physician to study...by it alone can we hope to unravel the problems of genetics" (Bevan-Lewis, 1909).

Pearson and his colleagues were not impressed. He collaborated with David Heron on the 1913 book titled *Mendelism and the Problem of Mental Defect.* Pearson argued,

> New scientific methods, new standards of logic and accuracy [that is to say statistical methods and arithmetical standards] have fought their way to the front and in both pure science and in medicine much of the current [work]...can only be looked upon as dogma or quackery ("A censor," 1915).

From the physicians' point of view in dealing with individuals, Pearson seems to have missed just that key point. One anonymous writer from the *British Medical Journal* observed:

> No one has a keener eye for both the absurdity and the weakness of an opponent's position than Professor Pearson, but surely no one has ever been more blind to the weaknesses of his own [position]. He never realizes that medicine includes the art of treating individual cases, or that in treating individual cases, a knowledge of means and averages is useless...("A censor," 1915).

Until Pearson recognized his bias against a personal analysis of one person and his family, the practicing physicians of the day did not feel that the biometric approach to heredity fit their needs very well.

Thirteen

The Maturation of Mendelism in Medical Practice 1910-1930

The Royal Society of Medicine meetings in 1908 and the publication of Bateson's 1909 book *Mendel's Principles of Heredity* strongly influenced both the scientific and the medical communities of the era. The Mendelian theory for heredity appeared to explain many problems in human heredity better than any competing model. The botanist R.H. Lock summarized the current state of opinion in his *Recent Progress in the Study of Variation, Heredity and Evolution*, where he noted, "A study of numerous pedigrees has enabled Bateson to show that there is great probability that in the case of the human race certain congenital diseases are simply transmitted from parent to offspring in accordance with Mendel's law." The key question, according to Lock, that would be examined by physicians over the next decades was, "How far the influence of the Mendelian principle may extend." He admitted at this time, "[that] we do not know" (Lock, 1909).

The development of ideas on heredity and human disease in articles by Frederick W. Mott, pathologist at Maudsley Hospital and the London Asylum, provided an example of how one physician recognized both the strengths and the limitations of the new theory. He discussed the general issues of heredity and disease before the Manchester Medical Society in October 1911. First, he wished to end the Pearson-Bateson controversy. Although it was often supposed that the two men's theories were contradictory, Mott agreed with Yule that the two, in fact, complemented each other. The biometric theory examined the average of the race, while Mendelism examined individual pedigrees.

There had to be some physical particles that carried the hereditary information in the egg and sperm from one generation to the next. Mott thought it likely that the chromosomes were the vehicles for inheritance. He then presented pedigrees to illustrate the dominant, recessive and sex-limited forms of inheritance for specific human disorders (Mott, 1910, 1911a, 1912).

Over the course of several years, Mott had collected data on both physical and psychological characters from hundreds of London families. In his 1911 presidential address to the Neurology Section of the Royal Society of Medicine, he concluded that temperaments as well as physical characters could be influenced by heredity (Mott, 1911b). Two years later he addressed The Psychology Section of the same organization on the heredity of mental disease. He admitted that:

> How far such [hereditary] analysis could be carried we do not yet know, but we have the certainty that it extends far, and ample indications in supposing that we shall probably be right in assuming that it causes most of the features, whether of the mind or of the body which distinguish the various members of a mixed population like that of which we form a part (Mott, 1913b).

Certainly, not all characters that appeared to be hereditary could easily be explained using the Mendelian theory. Mott studied families with mental disorders for more than a decade. His opinion in 1913 was that Mendelian hereditary had not been shown to have much influence in families with such "complex human traits" (Mott, 1913a). In October 1925, he delivered the Harveian Oration to the Royal College of Physicians. At that time, his analysis of families with insanity, schizophrenia and depression showed cases in several successive generations, but the pattern for heredity did not readily fit any simple Mendelian model he could discern (Mott, 1925).

However, the Mendelian theory did work in many other cases. Fleming M. Sandwirth, Professor of Physic at Gresham College, noted the applicability of Mendel's laws to several human conditions. The old question on the heredity of acquired characters was again raised. He thought the modern data should put such notions to rest forever (Sandwith, 1915). Ernest Reynolds, Professor of Clinical Medicine at Manchester University, spoke on this same topic before the Royal College of Physicians two years later. In his opinion, however, the habits or environment of parents could produce "hereditary disease" in the children. "Whether it was due to an action on the somatic plasm or the germplasm is a matter of more or less indifference to the physician," he thought. He held that heredity combined the effects of infections such as syphilis and tuberculosis or of toxins such as lead and alcohol with nervous instability to produce symptoms of epilepsy (Reynolds, 1917). Clearly, he lacked a precise definition of hereditary disease as opposed to congenital disease, i.e., one present at birth.

The issue of heredity and acquired disease was particularly important during the War when injured servicemen considered having children of their own. The surgeon William Eccles from St. Bart's Hospital reviewed the literature and could find no well-documented cases of injury such as amputation being transmitted to offspring of an affected parent. Hence, it was acceptable for women to marry war veterans without fearing for the physical health of the children that they might bear in the future (Eccles, 1918).

The on-going collection of human family data by British physicians further helped to elucidate the role played by heredity in different human disorders. Standards for pedigree construction using male and female symbols were outlined. Darkening the symbol indicated that an individual was affected by the character in question (Smith, P., 1910b). G. Archdall Reid presented pedigrees of families showing dominant brachydactyly, recessive alkaptonuria and sex-limited hemophilia in the 1910 edition of his book *The Laws of Heredity*. But at that time, he was not convinced "that Mendelian inheritance is the norm for human heredity" (Reid, 1910a).

Although Reid was not completely satisfied with the applicability of Mendelism to human characters, he did outline the scientific approach that could be used to accept or reject the utility of any such theory. He noted:

> If the hypothesis is true, it will generally be possible to infer deductively from it facts which had not been before explained or which had even been unobserved (Reid, 1910b)...If a hypothesis enables us to predict correctly...it is in all probability true, and it is the more certainly true (and useful) in proportion to the numbers of different correct predictions it enables us to make...Such deduction appeals to reality...and enables us to perceive the relations between the several laws so as by linking the laws together to advance toward the harmony of knowledge which is one of the principle aims of science (Reid, 1910c).

The accurate prediction of outcome and the logical union of several related theories were therefore viewed as important tests for the validity of any theory of heredity.

To many physicians of this era, it became evident that the combination of microscopic study of cell division coupled with an understanding of the details of human heredity could have a profound effect on the understanding of many human ills. As James Barr, physician at the Liverpool Infirmary, recommended, "It would be well if the medical profession were obliged to study Mendelian laws" (Barr, 1922).

Was it possible to actually discern the physical representation of hereditary elements in action? To do so could transform mere theory into actual facts of heredity in practice. The botanist and microscopist D.J. Scourfield cited earlier German work demonstrating the connection between the behavior of chromosomes and the segregation of hereditary factors. He argued that chromosomes where the "actual material bearers of the hereditary tendencies." He noted that individual chromosomes retained their identity during cell mitosis. They also existed in pairs—one from each of the parents. Different chromosomes produced different physiological effects. Normal embryonic development required an intact set of all the chromosomes (Scourfield, 1905-1906).

The zoologist Leonard Doncaster from King's College Cambridge reviewed this concept before the Swansea branch of the British Medical Association in 1910. He acccepted as fact that the human chromosomes carried the hereditary units. Egg and sperm cells each appeared to contain 24 chromosomes. Fertilization of the egg restored the chromosome number to the normal 48. Different combinations of chromosomes from each parent thus produced the variation that made each human unique (Doncaster, 1910).

The discovery of how sex was determined also provided evidence that specific chromosomes carried specific hereditary elements. In many species, including man, the development of one particular sex had been associated with the possession of one particular "accessory" chromosome. The segregation of the Mendelian sex-limited characters also provided parallel evidence for hereditary factors on specific chromosomes providing specific human characters (Doncaster, L., 1913). J.A. Jenkins consulted with Bateson in 1912 on the inheritance of sex-linked diseases such as color blindness (Jenkins, 1912a, b). He thought the human female was homozygous and the male heterozygous for the sex factor. Sex-linked diseases segregated with the sex-determining factor. A color blind male only required one abnormal factor to be affected, but the homozygous female only could be color blind if she inherited abnormal factors from both her mother and her father (Jenkins, 1913).

Doncaster noted that if sex was determined by chromosomes, "it is almost impossible to reject the belief in a similar connection with Mendelian factors." He thought that chromosomes each carried more than one hereditary element. Such "coupled characters" were detected in experimental plants and animals. One model proposed that chromosomes were like beads on a long string, each bead representing one hereditary "factor" (Doncaster, L., 1913)

American workers provided much of the basic genetic and cytological research that developed this chromosome theory of heredity. The biologist E.B. Wilson appeared before the Royal Society in 1914 and summarized recent work which showed that the chromosomes were indeed the bearers of the hereditary units (Wilson, E.B., 1914). The major publication that popularized this theory was the 1915 book *Mechanism of Mendelian Heredity* by the Columbia University biologists Morgan, Sturtevant, Muller and Bridges. Their work on *Drosophila*, the common fruit fly, had suggested the following points:

1. The hereditary material is on the chromosomes;

2. The behavior of chromosomes during mitosis and meiosis mimics Mendelian segregation of hereditary factors;

3. Coupled characters or linkage groups are "genes" on a particular chromosome. Each specific gene resides at a particular physical location on a specific chromosome;

4. During meiosis, crossing-over and exchange of corresponding chromosomal segments can occur. The frequency of such crossing-over is proportional to the physical distance two genes are separated on the chromosome.

The utility of the latter two points allowed the construction of physical maps for each chromosome linkage group (Morgan, Sturtevant, Muller et al., 1915; Brush, 2002).

T.H. Morgan subsequently presented the 1922 Croonian Lecture to the Royal Society on "Mechanisms of Heredity." He summarized the experimental data that showed the correlation between the segregation of Mendelian characters and individual chromosomes during both meiosis and mitosis (Morgan, 1922a, b). The Society presented him with the Darwin Medal for his work which had "thrown light on the relation of the factors of heredity to the chromosomes...These researches mark an advance in the science of heredity" (Brush, 2002).

Doncaster appreciated the importance of the chromosome theory of heredity, noting it is "the only one which seems at all nearly to approach the truth" (Doncaster, L., 1920b). He commented elsewhere:

> It is impossible to read the facts presented...without being impressed by the great strength of the evidence for Morgan's theory that Mendelian factors are borne by chromosomes and arranged in definite sequence within them. Difficulties arise, but a theory which enables predictions to be made and verified cannot lightly be disregarded (Doncaster, L., 1920a).

The ability of such a theory of heredity to actually predict results of mating of particular parents was one of the factors suggested by Reid as a measure of robustness of any theory. By the end of the war, British physicians had begun to carefully consider the chromosome theory for heredity, although their mentor Bateson had decided against its usefulness. When Bateson left Cambridge for the John Innes Institute, he did not sponsor any cytological work, focusing strictly on breeding studies of various plants and animals. Around 1916 he concluded that sex linkage of certain characters and the segregation of the sex chromosomes were connected. Not until he visited Morgan in New York in 1921 did he carefully review their findings and finally concede that the chromosome theory was solidly supported by experimental data. He noted in 1924, just two years before his death:

> There are endless reasons why the chromosomes should not do all the things they are supposed to do, but these reasons have somehow to be reconciled with the fact that by representing the chromosomes as doing these things we get a consistent representation, not merely of linkage etc. etc., but a great many unforeseen facts, for example, those associated with the idea of non-disjunction (Cock, 1983, 1989; Brush, 2002).

Bateson's medical colleagues, however, rapidly accepted the chromosome theory and began to apply it to human material as well. In the Croonian Lecture of 1917, J.G. Adami criticized Bateson for refusing to even imagine a physical structure like the chromosome to be the bearer of hereditary units (Adami, 1917). By the 1920s, there was general agreement in the British medical community on the correctness of the modern theory of heredity. Francis A.E. Crew, physician from the Animal Breeding Research

Department, University of Edinburgh, spoke before the British Medical Association at Dundee and outlined the current theory for heredity. The nuclear chromosomes were the bearers of heredity from one generation to the next. Application of the genetic laws was universally applicable to plants, animals and humans. Concordance of the segregation of sex-limited traits and the X-chromosome in humans was used to illustrate the chromosome theory for heredity (Crew, 1925). He proposed, "Knowledge of inheritance in humans is essential for accurate diagnosis and prognosis in medicine" (Crew, 1926).

The model for the chromosome as a string of beads with each bead representing a specific gene that determined the development of a particular character was also presented at a Birmingham Medical Society meeting. The available data indicated that human heredity was governed by the same Mendelian laws as in plants and other animals (Humphreys, 1928). An Edinburgh review pointed to the genes as "packets of chemicals," arranged in definite order along the chromosome. Experimental work in fruit flies had also shown that several different genes could affect one particular organ. The color of the fruit fly's eye was controlled by at least 25 different genes. Complex human traits, such as intelligence, must also be controlled by many different genes (Clarkson, 1927).

Francis Crew presented the first William Wuthering Lecture at the University of Birmingham Faculty of Medicine in 1927. His title, "Organic Inheritance in Man," emphasized the union of cellular mechanisms and heredity. He prepared his material to educate the general practitioner on recent developments in human heredity. First, he emphasized that "many of the physical and physiological characteristics of the human are subject to laws of inheritance revealed through the study of other forms [of life]" (Crew, 1927b). The experimental evidence indicated that the chromosomes were the germplasm, the physical "bearers of hereditary factors." Each factor or "gene" had a characteristic location on one of the chromosomes. Studies were underway to construct chromosome maps for several organisms (Crew, 1927c). He presented pedigrees to illustrate the nature of human heredity. Crew's selection of more than 200 dominant, recessive and sex-linked human traits that appeared to segregate in a Mendelian fashion are included in Table 13.1 (Crew, 1927a).

Education for physicians in this new field of human heredity was clearly necessary if they were to accurately assist the affected families who consulted them in clinical practice. Humphrey Rolleston, Regius Professor of Medicine at Cambridge and Physician to King George VI, commented on the necessity of sound education in the basic sciences. He did not wish to make all physicians into "highly skilled bacteriologists," for example, but he wished them to retain "a working knowledge of these fields for daily diagnosis and treatment of disease" (Rolleston, H., 1927). Crew summarized his opinion: "No medical school can be regarded as completely equipped until it includes a section devoted to the study of human genetics" (Crew, 1928). And yet, no such faculty existed in Britain at the time.

By the 1920s, the question of what constituted one of the genes, the hereditary elements, was being considered because changes in the genes, or mutations, appeared to result in human genetic variation, for good or ill. R.R. Gates elaborated the concept of mutation during observations on plant heredity. In his opinion, new Mendelian characters arose through a physical alteration in one particular region of the chromosome. Such changes could either involve a change in chemistry, or in some cases,

Table 13.1
Mendelian Inheritance in Man 1927

Dominant	
Achondroplasia	Ear, bilobed
Acoustic tumor	Ectopia lentis
Adenoid disposition	Elephantiasis
Adiposity	Epicanthus
Alopecia	Epilepsy
Angioneurotic edema	Exostosis
Aniridia	Eye color, tortoiseshell
Anonychia	Eyelids. Constricted
Arteriosclerosis	Flat foot
Asthenia	Fragilitas ossium
Asthma	Freckles
Atheroma	Gall stones
Atrophy of auditory nerve	Glaucoma
	Glomerulonephritis
Baldness (early male)	Glycosuria, mild
Brachydactyly	Goitre
Bimanual synergia	Gout
Camptodactyly	Hemorrhagic telangiectasis
Carcinoma	Hallux valgus
Carpal displacement	Hare lip
Cataract	Hay fever
Cerebellar ataxia	Hemeralopia
Chondrodystrophy	Hereditary epistaxis
Chorea	Hereditary tremor
Cleft palate	High blood pressure
Clinodactyly	Hyperextension, joints
Clubbed fingers	Hyperidrosis
Coloboma irides	Hypermetropia
Compulsive insanity	Hyperphalangia pollicis
Colon hypertrophy	Hypertrichosis
Corneal opacity	Hypospadius, male
Corpulence	Hypotrichosis
Cystinuria	Hysteria
Dermatosis Darier	Ichthyosis vulgaris
Diabetes insipidus	Infundibular thorax
Dysostosis, cleidocranial	Inguinal hernia
Dysostosis cranio-facialis	Insanity, manic
Ear, absence	Jaundice, hereditary

Table 13.1, *Continued*
Mendelian Inheritance in Man 1927

Dominant	
Keratosis follicularis	Pterygium
Keratosis palmaris et plantaris	Ptosis
Lagaopthalmus	Rachitis
Leuconychia	Radioulnar olisthy
Luxatio coxa	Radiolulnar synostosis
Migraine	Relaxation, eyelids
Monoletrichosis	Retinitis pigmentosa
Myopia	Rounded back
Myotonia atrophica	Sclerosis
Myotonia congenita	Scoliosis
Neurasthenia	Sickle cell anemia
Neurofibromatosis	Spastic paraplegia
Nystagmus	Spastic spinal paralysis
Oedema of legs	Splenomegaly
Osteopsathyrosis	Split foot
Otosclerosis	Stammering
Oxycephaly	Stenosis, mitral valve
Paroxysmal myoplegia	Strabismus+hypermetropia
Patella, absent	Struma sporadica idiotypica
Pernicious anemia	Suicide
Polycystic kidneys	Syndactyly
Polycythemia	Urticaria
Polydactyly	White forelock of hair
Prognathism	Xanthomatosis
	Zygodactyly

Table 13.1, *Continued*
Mendelian Inheritance in Man 1927

Recessive	
Albinism	Hydrophthalmia
Alkaptonuria	Hypoplasia
Amaurotic family idiocy	Hypotrichosis
Anencephaly	Ichthyosis congenita
Anophthalmia	Infantalism
Anophthalmia	Keratoconus
Astigmatism	Keratosis universalis
Ateliosis	Microbrachycephaly
Club foot	Microcephaly
Calvaria absence	Micromelia, infantile
Cretinism	Microphthalmia
Crypophthalmus	Muscular dystrophy
Cyclopia	Myoclonus epilepsy
Dementia praecox	Myopia
Deaf mutism	Nyctalopia
Dementia amauroticans	Paralysis agitans
Diabetes mellitus	Pemphigus connatus
Distichiasis	Pseudohermaphroditism
Dupuytren contracture	Retinitis pigmentosa
Embryotoxon	Scarlatinal nephritis
Enuresis nocturnal	Schizophrenia
Epidermolysis bullosa	Spasmodic torticollis
Epilepsy, muscle clonus	Split hand
Epispadius	Steatorrhea, congenital
Friedreich's ataxia	Strabismus
Glioma	Teeth, absent canine
Glycosuria, severe	Teeth, absent molar
Hereditary spinal ataxia	Torsion neurosis
Heterochromia iridis	Trophoneurosis
Hydro-aestivale	Xeroderma pigmentosum

Table 13.1, *Continued*
Mendelian Inheritance in Man 1927

Sex-linked
Anhidrosis
Anodontia
Ectopia pupillae
Epilepsy
Gower's disease
Hemophilia
Megalocornea
Myopia, hemeralopia
Neuritis optici
Nomadism
Optic atrophy
Pityriasis versicolor
Progressive muscular atrophy
Red-green colorblindness
Retinitis pigmentosa

Reference: Crew, 1927a.

alteration in three-dimensional space, a stereo-chemical modification in a chromosome (Gates, 1915, 1925, 1926a).

J.S. Manson had been studying heredity of eye and neurologic diseases in his practice and had consulted Bateson in 1911 to ask basic questions about Mendelism (Manson, 1911). He recognized his mentor's "powerful advocacy of the Mendelian conceptions" of genetics as one of the foremost scientific advances of the day. But he went beyond Bateson and argued that the chromosomal work had provided a clear material basis for the Mendelian genetics factors. Manson noted that both protein and nucleic acids were present within the cell nucleus. Some studies appeared to indicate that 40% of the chromosomes were comprised of nucleic acids. He wondered whether, "The influence of the nucleic acids [could] rival those of the amino acids in proteins in their vital importance" (Manson, 1928). Were genes made from nucleic acids, just as proteins were made from amino acids?

Sudden changes in human genes, mutations, were certainly rare in humans. But Archibald Garrod, named Regius Professor of Medicine at Oxford, thought much could be learned from such alterations of nature. In a lecture titled "The Lessons of Rare Maladies," he echoed the suggestion of William Harvey almost 300 years earlier that physicians should pay particular attention to the rare changes from the "normal" that are encountered in clinical practice. Garrod argued that mutations could be dominant or recessive, and certainly could be transmitted to the next generation. Such genetic behavior might cast a "light upon problems of heredity and the development of our bodies and of living processes of which they are the seats, and on the liabilities of individuals to specific forms of disease." Mutations then could shed light upon both normal and pathologic anatomy and physiology (Garrod, 1928).

Clinical Applications of Mendelian Heredity

By 1910, the British medical community at large began to recognize the applicability of the new theory to the daily clinical practice of medicine. A reviewer of Bateson's 1909 book noted that he had reduced the complexities of the theory to their simplest forms. This approach did appear useful in predicting for families the segregation of specific characters ("Review," 1909). The application of Mendel's laws to humans appealed to British physicians because it was a logical extension of the rule of thumb observations they had used every day in understanding heredity and disease. For a generation, they had been using the pedigree format to summarize inheritance of human conditions (Leslie, 1881). The French psychologist Theodore Ribot published his observations on patterns of disease and heredity in English translation in 1875. He recognized three distinct patterns of human inheritance that were also widely used in the British medical literature.

1. Direct: successive parent to child transmission of the trait;
2. Indirect: traits which ran in the family, often occurring in several siblings of one generation, often recurring in collateral relatives such as aunts, uncles and cousins;
3. Sex-limited: a characteristic indirect pattern of affected males, and unaffected females transmitting the character to their sons (Ribot, 1875).

Clinical examples of such characters were well recognized by 1900. These patterns of heredity and several clinical examples of each are illustrated in Figure 13.1. The advent of Mendelism helped explain how segregation of hereditary elements in egg and sperm could produce such recognizable patterns for the inheritance of specific human characters. The direct pattern was Mendelian dominant. The indirect pattern was Mendelian recessive. The sex-limited pattern was characteristic of the Mendelian sex-linked form of heredity.

By 1910, Bateson and his medical colleagues had successfully communicated in understandable terms the potential and important role for Mendelian heredity in providing workable solutions to the day-to-day problems of human inheritance. The translation of theory into practice over the next few decades was certainly not automatic. It was fraught with missteps, misinterpretations, and frank mistakes in the application of theory to the imperfect human pedigrees collected by the medical practitioners. Examples in the next section will illustrate the remarkable shift in understanding of the heredity of many human disorders. Physicians were able to not merely describe pedigrees of disease, but also to utilize Mendelian mechanisms to explain the inheritance pattern they observed.

Blood and Blood Vessel Disorders

Hereditary hemorrhagic telangiectasia [Osler-Weber-Rendu disease] had long been regarded as a form of hemophilia. But analysis of the pedigrees of affected families showed a different pattern for the inheritance of this character, not the sex-limited pattern for hemophilia. William Osler, Regius Professor of Medicine at Oxford, found a family with 31 affected individuals in four successive generations. It was not a particularly pleasant disorder. One of his patients reported with "quiet humour" that he had been in the "habit of bleeding to death" (Osler, 1908). The same direct pattern for heredity was noted in families with two (Ballantyne, 1908; Kelly, 1907), three (Kelly, 1906; Phillips, 1907; Langmead, 1909; East, 1926; Mekie, 1927), four (Weber, F.P., 1907; Mackay and McKenty, 1927), and even five successive generations affected (Paul, 1918). Bateson noted this as most consistent with a dominant character in 1913 (Bateson, 1913). Later, a second five-generation family also demonstrated a pattern of inheritance consistent with the segregation of a dominant trait (Foggie, 1928).

An unusual form of periodic anemia termed acholuric jaundice also appeared to be hereditary; both sexes were affected (Hawkins and Dudgeon, 1908). In one family, the four affected persons had enlarged spleens as well (Hutchinson, 1910). Detailed study showed that the red blood cells of affected persons were unusually fragile. Periodic hemolysis produced jaundice and anemia. About half of the offspring appeared to inherit the character directly from an affected parent. One family demonstrated five affected generations, both sexes were equally affected, and affected children were only born of affected parents. This was recognized as an example of a "dominant Mendelian character" (Campbell and Ware, 1926; Cowen, 1922; Rolleston, H., 1928). A similar pattern of direct heredity was also recognized in families with pernicious anemia, but no specific comments were made regarding a mechanism for inheritance (Hurst, A.F., 1925).

By 1920, the inheritance of the major human ABO blood group was recognized to follow a dominant Mendelian pattern as well (Dyke and Budge, 1922; "Human blood relationships," 1922; Waugh, 1928). In one family, a child possessed a blood group which could not be explained by inheritance of the characters from his parents. It was then believed to represent a case of false paternity which, as one physician commented,

Mendel and Ribot—Patterns of Inheritance

Pedigree Charts	Ribot's Class	Clinical Examples	Mendel's Class
	Direct heredity	Ectopia lentis Huntington's chorea	Dominant
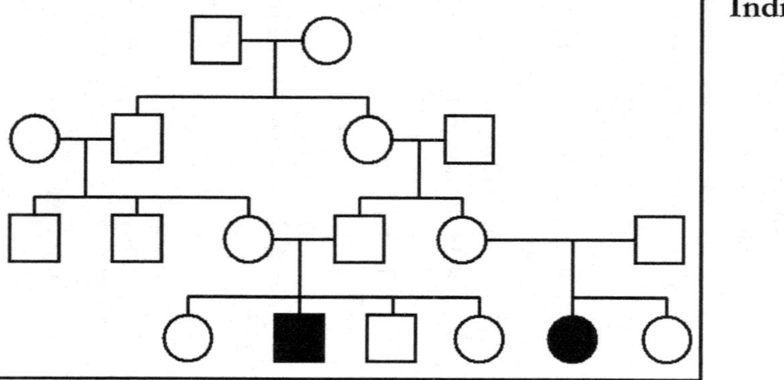	Indirect heredity	Optic atrophy Friedreich's ataxia	Recessive

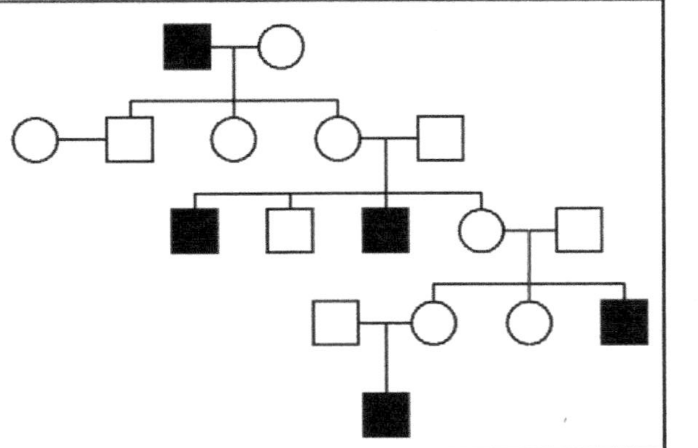

Sex-limited heredity	Colorblindness Muscular dystrophy	Sex-linked

Figure 13.1

"may afford a valuable medico-legal test" (Learmonth, 1920) for forensic purposes in the future.

Hereditary lymphedema [Milroy's disease] appeared in two (Rolleston, H.D., 1902; Sutherland, A.G., 1908), three (Rolleston, J.D., 1917), and even five (Hope and French, 1908a, b) successive generations. William Bulloch of the London Hospital prepared a review of affected families for the *Treasury of Human Inheritance* (Bulloch, 1909b), but did not discuss the heredity of the disorder. Bateson identified lymphedema as a dominant trait in 1913 (Bateson, 1913).

Angioneurotic edema produced life-threatening swelling in the throat and obstruction of the airway. It was a frightening hereditary trait in susceptible families and was commonly observed in two or three successive generations (Griffith, T., 1902; Prior, 1905; Savill, 1909; Cameron, 1920; Bulmer, 1929). Byram Bramwell from the Edinburgh Royal Infirmary reported a family in which an affected woman had married twice and produced affected children in both families (Bramwell, 1907a). Another family demonstrated direct transmission through six successive generations. It was clear that those who escaped were less liable themselves to transmit the condition to their offspring than those who were affected. Bulloch reviewed affected pedigrees for the *Treasury of Human Inheritance* (Bulloch, 1909a), but again without any hereditary analysis. Bateson was later able to characterize this as a dominant character (Bateson, 1913).

Hemophilia had traditionally been known as "one of the most marked hereditary diseases" (Wilson, J.J., 1905). Numerous families had produced affected sons born of unaffected mothers, whose fathers also had the bleeding tendency. Women clearly transmitted the trait, as one mother had affected sons by two different husbands (Finlay and Drennan, 1916). The disorder was observed worldwide. A four-generation family was reported from India (Macnicol, 1910). J. Muir from South Africa spent decades examining wills and church registrars to prepare a 12-generation pedigree encompassing over 600 people with 46 males affected by hemophilia (Muir, 1906, 1928). In rare instances, female bleeders certainly did occur (Bramwell, 1907c; "A case of hemophilia," 1909). In some of these families, the affected women merely had a tendency to bruise easily (Wilson, M.G., 1920). In other cases, the severity of hemorrhage from minor lacerations, nosebleeds and bleeding into the joints was just as severe in the sisters as in the affected brothers (Swanton, 1907; Osler, 1910). One affected woman lost consciousness due to hemorrhage after a dental extraction, and later bled for weeks after a cut on her hand (Warde, 1923). The monumental work by Bulloch and Fildes on hemophilia in the *Treasury of Human Inheritance* series recorded hundreds of pedigrees from affected families (Bulloch and Fildes, 1911). Bateson identified the consistent pattern as sex-linked inheritance in all affected families (Bateson, 1909, 1913).

Bone and Muscle Disease

Various forms of brachydactyly [shortening of the digits in the hands and feet] were common anomalies that often recurred in at least five or six generations of affected families (Marshall, L., 1902; Mathew, 1908; Webb, 1901). Henry Drinkwater reported his large pedigree of a family with brachydactyly in Edinburgh and Liverpool as early as 1907 (Drinkwater, 1907, 1908). Seven generations were affected; about half of children born of affected parents inherited the character. Sexes were equally affected. He was able to designate brachydactyly as a dominant character (Drinkwater, 1908). The same consistent dominant pattern of inheritance was noted in subsequent families reported over the next two decades (Drinkwater, 1912, 1913b, a, 1914, 1916; Lipscomb, 1915; Gilmore, 1927; Marshall, R., 1929).

Drinkwater also examined another family comprising five successive generations with a different hand anomaly. The thumbs and great toes were bifid, while the distal phalanges were absent. Both sexes again were affected. The abnormal children always were born of affected parents. The inheritance pattern generally followed the Mendelian dominant, though in this case, there was an excess of affected persons (Cragg and Drinkwater, 1916).

Ankylosis [the fusion of digital joints] also followed a characteristic hereditary pattern. One family of three generations exhibited affected members with tightness of all the hand digits (Sawyer, J.E.H., 1907). Drinkwater reported another family with strict ankylosis of digits four and five. This family was descended from the first Earl of Shrewsbury who also appeared to have had the characteristic hand abnormality. This dominant Mendelian character apparently had descended unchanged for 14 successive generations (Drinkwater, 1917).

At times, the pattern for heredity of a trait was not so characteristic. J.L. Bunch from the Queen's Hospital for Children in London noted a family segregating Dupuytren's contracture involving the tendons of the hands. The digits involved were the same in all the family members he could examine. The family history indicated that the character had been present for more than 300 years. Only males were affected, transmitting the trait directly to their sons. This pattern of inheritance differed from sex-limited traits such as hemophilia, and did not match either simple recessive or dominant characters (Bunch, 1913). Other unidentified factors may have been involved to produce the abnormality in only one sex.

Lobster-claw deformity of the hands and feet [ectrodactyly] resulted from the absence of several middle digits and the development of a long thumb with three phalanges. H.B. Robinson presented a family to the Royal Society of Medicine that he believed was related to another family reported in 1887 (Parker and Robinson, 1887). Four generations were affected involving both sexes. There was some degree of variable expression of the character in individual persons, but all those affected still could transmit the character. Gossage interpreted the pedigree as most consistent with a Mendelian dominant pattern (Robinson and Bowen, 1908). Bateson also agreed in 1913 (Bateson, 1913). Lewis and Embleton from University Hospital in London updated several families with ectrodactyly that had been presented in the previous generation (Anderson, 1886; Tubby, 1894). In these families as well, the character was transmitted from affected parent to child with some variation in different generations. In this example, there were 44 affected and 32 normal, an excess of the "dominant" type. These reports were published in *Biometrika*, and the authors were not so sure about the hereditary mechanisms involved.

> It may be the case that Mendelism applies to certain human deformities, but the conclusions which are being drawn, or implied...are at present ahead of the facts at our disposal...[The]...evidence has not yet been produced which warrants the statement that any human sport is transmitted along the lines of Mendelism (Lewis and Embleton, 1908).

The *Treasury of Human Inheritance* series included a further report by the same authors (Lewis, 1909a). An excess of affected individuals was also observed in another family reported after the War (Rutherfurd, 1919).

Polydactyly [extra digits on hands and feet] was another disorder frequently seen in three to five successive generations (Mott, 1910; Greene, 1907; Hunter, O.G., 1909; Crivelli, 1920). Lewis prepared a monograph on this disorder for the *Treasury of Human Inheritance* series, but did not make any particular comments regarding its heredity (Lewis, 1909b). Syndactyly [webbing] of the fingers also ran in certain families. Typically, several fingers and toes were involved. A father and three children were affected in one family (Clark, 1916). The combination of syndactyly and polydactyly was also observed in a five-generation Welsh family. About 50% of the offspring were affected, and the character acted like a Mendelian dominant trait (Manson, 1915). But in another family with polydactyly alone, four generations were affected. Of 48 total members, 26 were affected: 17 males and 9 females. However, the author could find "no marked Mendelian feature..." (Atkinson, 1921) to explain the hereditary pattern.

Webbing of the toes alone appeared to be a distinct hereditary trait. Bramwell reported a family with direct transmission of the character through three successive generations. He noted that Mr. Gunn, the medical student involved with the family at the Edinburgh Royal Infirmary, had taken the time to carefully investigate the matter because he was interested in the hereditary aspect of the disorder (Bramwell, 1907d). Another three-generation family demonstrated segregation of the character from parent to child, again consistent with a Mendelian dominant course (Newsholme, 1910).

Other more generalized forms of skeletal malformation also appeared to run in families. The dwarfing condition achondroplasia was sometimes reported in three successive generations with direct parent to child transmission (Keyser, 1906; Porter, 1907; Hunter, D., 1928; Ord, 1925). As early as 1910, D.B. Hart had questioned whether a hereditary growth factor could be involved in the production of this disorder. He noted that Mendel had studied a hereditary factor in peas which affected their ultimate size. He then suggested that a mutation, resulting in the loss of a human growth factor, and inherited in a Mendelian pattern, could explain the development of the abnormality in affected families (Hart, D.B., 1913). Several years later, a large family was reported with irregular inheritance of achondroplasia in three generations, and direct transmission in the two most recent generations. Bangson suggested that the character acted like a recessive in the earlier generations, and as a dominant trait in the latest two generations (Bangson, 1926). Rischbieth reviewed the literature on achondroplasia for the *Treasury of Human Inheritance* (Rischbieth and Barrington, 1910).

The surgeon Duncan C.L. Fitzwilliams of St. Mary's Hospital in London examined the heredity of cleidocranial dysostosis [abnormal formation of skull and collarbone] and ultimately collected 60 cases. Direct parent to child heredity was repeatedly observed. In one family an affected woman produced affected children through marriages to two unaffected men (Fitzwilliams, 1910). Gossage and Bateson had also investigated this disorder and classified it as a dominant (Bateson, 1913).

Multiple exostoses [abnormal growth of cartilaginous knots on bones] were commonly observed in several family members, demonstrating its "well-marked hereditary history" (Francis, 1902). In 1915, a family from the Federated Malay States was reported in which an affected man had affected children by two unaffected women (Cox, 1915). Gossage collected pedigrees from 67 families and found typically about half the offspring were affected, males and females equally. Very occasionally the character was transmitted via an unaffected female. He thought the trait acted most likely as a dominant trait in the males and occasionally as an incomplete dominant in the females (Gossage and Carling, 1910).

Osteogenesis imperfecta is a disorder of bone and connective tissue that results in frequent fractures due to softened bones, premature deafness due to abnormality of the ear ossicles and blue sclerae [the outer surface of the eyeball]. It appeared to be hereditary, but the pattern for inheritance varied in different families. In some, affected children were born of normal parents (Heaton, 1903; Haward, 1902), sometimes with affected more distant relatives (Rolleston, J.D., 1911), suggesting a recessive inheritance pattern. Variable expression of the character was also a frequent occurrence. Not all those with blue sclerae had fragile bones. Generally, the character was noted in successive generations, passing directly from parent to child for two, or even five generations (Whitchurch Howell, 1924; Cockayne, E.A., 1926; Stobie, 1924; Kidd, 1910; Wise, 1920; Buchanan, 1923; Alexander, 1922; Adair-Dighton, 1912; Cockayne, E.A., 1913, 1914; Burrows, 1911). One affected woman had affected children in each of two marriages (Stewart, H., 1922). The ophthalmologist Sidney Stephenson of Queen's Hospital for Children in London thought the trait followed the "knight's move"[11] of sex-limited disorders, but his own investigation noted four generations with direct heredity involving 21 affected individuals (Stephenson, 1915a, b). E. Bronson of Edinburgh reported two other families with three and four generations involved. Direct transmission from parent to child was again evident; no affected children were born of unaffected parents. He also thought the disorder followed the "knight's move" as seen with hemophilia or color blindness (Bronson, 1917, 1918). An editorial in the *Edinburgh Medical Journal* reviewed this report and noted Bronson's error. In fact, the disorder appeared to be inherited as a simple Mendelian dominant ("Fragilitis ossium," 1917). Blegvad from Norway agreed that the disorder generally fit the Mendelian dominant mode for heredity (Blegvad and Haxthausen, 1921).

Various types of muscle disease were also noted to be hereditary in specific families. Myotonia congenita [Thomsen's disease] was often transmitted directly from parent to children (Dreschfeld, 1905). A. Birt from the Medical College at Dalhousie University in Nova Scotia suffered from this disorder and investigated his own family history. He noted the disorder in his own siblings, but not in his parents. Affected cousins on his mother's side were also known (Birt, 1908). Another Canadian family had a similar pattern for heredity (Rudolph, 1910). Direct heredity through three generations was observed in a third family. The investigation noted this pattern was not "sex-linked," but no further comments about the pattern of heredity could be made (Rosett, 1922).

Peroneal muscle atrophy [Charcot-Marie-Tooth disease] was another muscle disorder that ran in families. Different patterns for inheritance were again observed in different families. In some instances, affected children were born of asymptomatic parents. One such family had eight affected children (Collier, J., 1903). In other cases, the affected children were noted to have normal parents, but affected collateral relatives such as cousins (Bryant, 1905b) or, in another instance, a great uncle (Bryant, 1905a), suggesting a recessive form of inheritance. Direct transmission from an affected parent was more commonly observed in two (Warrington, 1901; Collier, A.J., 1908; Guthrie, 1910), three (Symonds and Shaw, 1926; Spillane, 1940; Hamilton, 1911), or four (Halliday and Whiting, 1909) successive generations. J. Raffan from the Aberdeen Royal Infirmary reported an anomalous family. A six-generation pedigree was presented with overwhelming male predominance of affected individuals (ten male and three females). In one branch of the family the character was transmitted via two unaffected women (Raffan, 1907). This report suggested to Bateson that peroneal muscle atrophy could sometimes be a sex-linked human character (Bateson, 1913).

Pseudohypertrophic muscular paralysis [Gower's or Duchenne's disease] was characteristically evident in boys born of unaffected mothers (Ness, 1908). Such mothers of affected sons often had two or three affected brothers among their own siblings (Hunter, W.K., 1900; Parkinson, 1912). One woman had a sister who also produced an affected son (Rankin, 1900). Bateson noted this pattern of the "knight's move" that was, in fact, characteristic of the sex-linked Mendelian pattern (Bateson, 1909, 1913).

The indirect hereditary pattern for another muscle disorder was evident in a family with spastic paraplegia noted at the London School of Clinical Medicine. Unaffected parents without consanguinity produced eight affected sons, including one set of twins (Jones, E., 1907).

CANCER

The belief that cancer had an important hereditary component reached a low-ebb early in the 1900s. Hillier of Middlesex Hospital in London reviewed 3000 cases in 1902. Of 2368 females, 14.6% had a positive family history, and among males only 7.8% had other family members affected as well (Hillier and Tritsch, 1904). Pearson then correlated these results with data from patients of the general hospital wards and found no difference in family history of the disease (Pearson, 1904), arguing against the general notion that cancers were hereditary.

Specific cases of familial cancer continued to raise the question of whether heredity was one of several important etiologies in this type of disorder. Hodgkin disease appeared in male twins (Peacocke, 1905). Osteosarcoma in a father reappeared in both of his sons (Battle and Shattock, 1907). Another type of bone tumor, osteochondroma, was directly transmitted through three generations (Houghton, 1925). Neurofibroma of the acoustic nerve also appeared to be directly transmitted from parent to children in three generations (Felling and Ward, 1920).

Cancer of the bowel recurred frequently in successive generations. A father and three of five children were affected (Watkins, 1904). By the 1920s, systematic investigation of such cancer families had begun in London hospitals. John Lockhart-Mummery of St. Mary's Hospital reported several affected families with direct transmission through three generations (Lockhart-Mummery, 1925; Dukes, 1926).

Glioma of the retina appeared to be a cancer with several different hereditary patterns. It could appear in only one generation, affecting two or three siblings (Snell, 1904, 1905; Ridley, 1902). But in one large family of 16 children, two died at a young age, four were healthy and 10 had gliomas (Newton, 1902). Parents in such families could be unaffected themselves, but have affected collateral relatives such as uncles or cousins (Owens, 1905; Berrisford, 1916). Direct heredity was also evident in many other families. An affected parent might produce two or three afflicted children (Griffith, A.H., 1917b, c; Traquair, 1919; Letchworth, 1928; Sym, 1928), while instances of four (Griffith, A.H., 1917a, b), and even five of seven children were reported (Griffith, A.H., 1917c; Bride, 1923). A similar tumor, sarcoma of the choroid membrane of the eye, was also found to be directly transmitted from parent to children through four successive generations of another family (Davenport, 1927).

Many reports appeared in the medical literature of this era claiming to have definitive evidence for a microbe that caused cancer in experimental animals and man (Goring, 1909; Young, 1925; Loudon, 1925; Loudon and McCormack, 1925). However, the majority of practitioners in medicine were unconvinced by these claims (McDonagh,

1926). Lockhart-Mummery noted, "The relationship between heredity and disease is one of the most interesting and at the same time one of the most difficult problems of modern medicine." He believed that hereditary predisposition was certainly one important factor in the etiology of cancer (Lockhart-Mummery, 1925). The dermatologist Edward A. Cockayne reviewed the data on both the rare and the more common forms of familial cancers. He concluded that several did, in fact, segregate in familial patterns consistent with Mendelian dominant hereditary, namely multiple exostoses, neurofibromas, retinal glioma, as well as colon and breast cancers (Cockayne, E.A., 1927).

Diseases of Metabolism

The "inborn errors of metabolism" as defined by Garrod continued to attract the attention of physicians at this time. A.R. Gunn from the University of Edinburgh noted that one abnormality, albinism, as a hereditary condition could lend itself to the application of Mendelian methods of investigation. He urged medical men to refer such patients to him as early as 1907, and he would then investigate the history of their families (Gunn, 1907). Aaron Levy of the Royal London Ophthalmic Hospital reviewed the pedigree of an inbred albino family at a meeting of the Ophthalmological Society. The presence of albinism in collateral branches of the family seemed to him to "illustrate Mendel's theory of the intensification of qualities through inbreeding" (Levy, 1907). Affected children born to cousin parents were quite common (Butler, 1908; Paton, 1907). J.E. Adler and J. McIntosh from the Bacteriological Laboratory of London Hospital reported a similar family in *Biometrika.* They observed, "From a Mendelian view, both parents might be considered as carrying recessive albinism" (Adler and McIntosh, 1909). Bateson also thought the hereditary pattern for albinism was quite consistent with a Mendelian recessive trait (Bateson, 1909).

Although the detailed statistical analysis of albinism, which had been planned in Part III of Pearson's monograph, was never published (Pearson, Nettleship and Usher, 1911a), he nonetheless had claimed that human albinism did not fit the expected inheritance pattern for a recessive Mendelian character. The French pediatrician, Eugene Apert from the Hotel Dieu in Paris, examined the 691 pedigrees on albinism which had been reported in the monograph. He calculated the theoretical proportion of affected individuals born if both parents were unaffected heterozygotes. He concluded, contrary to Pearson's opinion, that the results fit the Mendelian predictions very closely (Apert, 1914).

Garrod continued his own studies on other inborn errors of metabolism. Familial steatorrhea, in which the stools were full of greasy fat, appeared in several children born of unaffected parents. He noted again that the parents were frequently consanguineous. He thought that steatorrhea was "an inborn error...on a par with such anomalies as alkaptonuria and cystinuria" and, from a hereditary point of view, it was a "Mendelian recessive character" (Garrod and Hurtley, 1912). Another case from Paddington Green Children's Hospital was noted in a family with unrelated parents. If present, consanguinity would "undoubtedly have the effect of emphasizing and unmasking a family tendency" (Miller and Perkins, 1920). Garrod subsequently helped analyze another case of alkaptonuria in a child born of first cousin parents, again consistent with a "recessive character" (Cuthbert, 1923).

Walter Brain, a neurologist from London Hospital, reported a family with goiter in which direct transmission from parent to child was observed through four generations. It was well-known that lack of iodine was a common cause of goiter, but he proposed the existence of a Mendelian dominant trait that produced a defect in the metabolism of iodine and predisposed affected persons to develop the disease more frequently than their neighbors (Brain, 1927). He also noted another form of goiter associated with deaf mutism in which affected children were born of unaffected parents. He noted 12 affected children in five different families. This pattern of inheritance was most consistent with a recessive trait. In 1927, he also wondered if the hereditary association of goiter and deafness could represent an example of human genetic linkage (Brain, 1927).

Richard T. Williamson of the Manchester Royal Infirmary recognized the recent interest in the heredity of human disease as evidenced by the 1908 Royal Society of Medicine conferences. That same year he had reported cases of diabetes mellitus in several branches of his own family: two brothers and a sister, three other sisters, a father, his son and their paternal aunt (Williamson, 1908). William Bosanquet of Charing Cross Hospital presented another family with an affected father, sons and paternal cousin. He also noted the "hereditary influence of diabetes in this case" (Bosanquet, 1908). Bramwell reported another family with two affected children, paternal uncle and maternal aunt (Bramwell, 1907b). Percy J. Cammidge reviewed 800 of his own diabetic cases and found 28% had a positive family history. Pedigrees showed affected children as well as affected collateral relatives, acting like a typical recessive trait. He also noted a few families in which the character acted like a dominant trait. He knew little of distant relatives in such families and thought these cases might, in fact, represent marriages of carriers. Cammidge studied the segregation of blood sugar levels (glycemia) in experimental mice as well. He reported that hypoglycemia was recessive to euglycemia in three generation breeding crosses with the expected Mendelian proportions (Cammidge, 1928).

The disorder of water metabolism diabetes insipidus had been noted to recur in several successive generations. Bateson labeled it as a dominant character as early as 1909 (Bateson, 1909). Lillian Chase of Saskatchewan reported the disorder segregating through five generations in one family. The character was directly transmitted from parent to child, affecting at least 20 members of the family. She also concluded that the character acted like a dominant trait (Chase, 1927).

Eye and Ear Disorders

All ophthalmologists were familiar with hereditary eye diseases. Early in the new century, Nettleship had capitalized on his broad interest in this field by noting in a 1906 post-graduate lecture at Oxford University:

> The chief interest in heredity of eye disease lies, like that of all heredity, in the light that a study of the subject may throw upon the laws of inheritance; and we, the medical profession, can often contribute to the elucidation of the problem, even though our researches are hedged in by many limitations from which the experimental biologist is free...The eye is, in many respects, particularly suitable for the clinical study of the inheritance of peculiarities, deformities and disease (Nettleship, 1906b).

One of the first extensive hereditary studies carried out by Nettleship himself involved the investigation of a large family in France segregating stationary night blindness. Previous families in the nineteenth century had been reported showing direct heredity through two and five generations (Hudson, 1903; Sinclair, 1905). Nettleship traveled to the continent and collaborated with local physicians and priests to gather information on ten generations in this particular family. The completed pedigree encompassed 2121 individuals. In the affected branches, 53% of the offspring were affected: 72 males and 63 females. Healthy parents never produced affected children; direct transmission was the rule. Bateson participated in the analysis of the case and labeled night blindness as a Mendelian dominant character (Nettleship, 1907a, b).

Several years later Nettleship investigated another family with night blindness coupled with myopia. The pattern of heredity in this case was quite different. In a seven-generation family, unaffected females appeared to transmit the disorder only to their sons. A different hereditary mechanism was clearly involved in this particular example (Nettleship, 1912a, 1911a), most consistent with a sex-limited pattern for heredity (Nettleship, 1909).

Color blindness had been known to affect males in certain families for several hundred years. The pattern for heredity typically showed unaffected daughters of affected fathers who then transmitted the character to their own sons. The same mode for heredity was observed in families with hemophilia and pseudohypertrophic muscular paralysis. But rare cases of colorblind females did occur; their degree of disability was often milder than their affected brothers. Nettleship began to collect pedigrees from such families with colorblind females. He discussed his findings with Bateson, attempting to understand the hereditary mechanisms which could explain these results. In each family, the expected pattern for inheritance to males was observed with an occasional affected female also born of a mother who could also be affected or be a normal-sighted carrier for the trait (Nettleship, 1906a, 1908a, 1912c, 1914). Bateson concluded that color blindness was most consistent with a sex-limited pattern for heredity (Bateson, 1909, 1913). Detailed evaluations over the next few years also indicated that in all cases of female color blindness, the anomaly followed a typical sex-linked pattern in which other unaffected females in the family had colorblind fathers and produced colorblind sons in the next generation (Schiotz, 1920).

Nettleship additionally presented reports on two different five-generation families segregating hereditary nystagmus. Only males were affected; transmission occurred through normal females. Bateson was also present at the meeting of the Ophthalmological Society when Nettleship reviewed his findings. Bateson concluded that the disorder segregated as a sex-limited character. He urged the medical men in attendance to collect information from other families with apparent sex-limited disorders, because the data would help elucidate the whole concept of the heredity of male- and female-ness in humans (Nettleship, 1911b; Bateson, 1911). Another large six-generation family was reported several years later. In this example, both sexes were affected by nystagmus, and direct transmission through at least four generations was evident. The pattern for inheritance in this family did not match the sex-limited type proposed by Nettleship, but the author was unable to analyze the situation any further to suggest an alternative mechanism for the heredity of this character (Nicol, 1915).

Many different types of cataract appeared to have a hereditary basis as well. Senile cataracts were the most common, developing in the elderly. Nettleship reported four- and six-generation families in which the character appeared to be directly transmitted

(Nettleship, 1905). He also studied an unusual family where both parents had senile cataracts. They produced ten children: three were normal and seven were affected. Nettleship proposed that the parents were "impure dominants," each carrying the "normal character obscured or hidden but not destroyed by the cataractous character..." According to Mendelian expectations the ratio of affected to normal in such a case would be 3:1, approximating the results obtained in reality (Nettleship, 1908c).

Congenital or pre-senile cataracts were present at birth or developed during young childhood. Many multi-generation families were noted to have typical direct inheritance (Nettleship, 1905; Nettleship and Ogilvie, 1906; Harman, N.B., 1910). Nettleship studied the heredity of this type of cataract through seven generations in one family. Affected children were only born of affected parents (Nettleship and Ogilvie, 1906). Bateson thought this was quite consistent with a Mendelian dominant pattern (Bateson, 1909). N. Bishop Harman, ophthalmologist at London Hospital, noted a four-generation family also with direct transmission of the trait from parent to child. He was not able to examine all family members, but found 19 of 57 affected. The Mendelian prediction for offspring in such cases would have been 50% affected (Harman, N.B., 1909a). The Professor of Ophthalmology at the University of Birmingham, Priestley Smith, discussed his observation of several other families segregating congenital cataract at a meeting of the Midland Medical Society. In four generations, direct transmission was apparent. Affected children were only born of affected parents. About 50% of the offspring in affected lines inherited the cataracts themselves. The disorder clearly represented a dominant trait. The Cambridge zoologist Leonard Doncaster was present and outlined other examples of human traits that were inherited in recessive and sex-limited Mendelian patterns (Smith, P., 1910a).

Smith later reported a seven-generation family with a third form of cataract—Doyne's discoid type. He used parish church records in Leicesterhire to trace the family lines. Affected children were only born of affected parents. In the affected branches of the family, 26 of 51 were affected; 15 males and 11 females. He thought the pattern of inheritance best fit the Mendelian dominant mode (Smith, P., 1910c). A similar pattern for inheritance was observed in families with posterior polar cataracts (Harman, N.B., 1909b; Nettleship, 1912b; Harman, N.B., 1914b).

Several large families with lamellar cataracts were reported at this time. Nettleship found evidence of direct transmission through three and six generations of two families (Nettleship, 1905, 1908b). Harman observed the same disorder in two-, three-, four- and five- generation examples (Harman, N.B., 1909b, 1910a, 1914b). Another family with direct transmission prompted a more detailed genetic analysis. Ali Khan mistakenly noted that such a pedigree did not fit the expected Mendelian results for recessive or dominant characters, although it did illustrate "quite well the influence of heredity in lamellar cataract" (Ali Khan, 1926).

Direct heredity of coraliform cataract was observed in two and three successive generations of affected families as well (Fisher, 1905; Harman, N.B., 1910). Stellate cataracts were noted to be transmitted directly from parent to child through five generations of another family (Adams, 1909). Harman reviewed the hereditary aspects of cataracts in a monograph for the *Treasury of Human Inheritance* (Harman, B., 1910b), and thanked Nettleship for his work on the classification of the many different types of lens disease. Nettleship concluded that most types of cataract did follow the dominant pattern for inheritance (Nettleship, 1909).

Abnormalities of the muscles around the eyes also appeared to have a hereditary basis. Ptosis [drooping of the eyelids] had been known to pass directly from parent to child (Lane, J.K., 1901). Bateson called this a dominant character (Bateson, 1909). The inability to move the eyeball in the orbit [ophthalmoplegia externa] likewise appeared to run in families. A four-generation example with direct parent to child transmission was reported in 1900 before the Ophthalmological Society. The president, G.A. Critchett, commented that, "Modern medicine [tended to] discredit the part played by heredity, but undoubtedly [this paper] throws a considerable weight of evidence to the opposite side" (Beaumont, 1900). Other families with four and five generations affected were later reported. Bradburne noted direct transmission. He observed the character was "congenital, not sex-limited, of continuous descent, and non-progressive." However, the exact hereditary mechanism eluded him (Cooper, 1910; Bradburne, 1912).

Different forms of corneal opacities appeared in successive generations. Robert Doyne, Reader in Ophthalmology at Oxford, reported a three-generation family showing direct transmission from parent to children (Doyne and Stephenson, 1905). Similar patterns of disease transmission were noted in other families (Hancock, 1905; Clegg, 1915). When another family was presented to the Ophthalmological Society in 1909, the President G.A. Berry observed that, "The question of heredity had been carefully considered in recent years in cases before the Society" (Folker, 1909). Clearly, heredity had something to do with the etiology of this disorder. But other cases of corneal opacity appeared in several children born of unaffected parents (Collins, 1905; Dawnay, 1905; Macnab, 1907). F. Moxon from the Royal London Ophthalmic Hospital noted one family in which the unaffected parents were first cousins, and a second family where the parents were second cousins (Moxon, 1913, 1914). The discovery of consanguinity raised questions about other possible hereditary mechanisms that might be involved.

Malformations of the iris which appeared in successive generations were examined as well. The iris could be absent [aniridia] or partially intact [coloboma irides]. Defects were noted in families of two to five generations. Direct parent to child transmission was the rule; both sexes were equally affected (Juler, 1902; Cunningham, 1909; Snell, 1908). Bateson concluded this was consistent with a dominant character (Bateson, 1909). Certain individuals had an iris with one color in one eye and another color in the opposite eye. Gossage noted a five-generation family segregating this disorder termed heterochomia irides. Direct transmission was evident (Gossage, 1908). Charles J. Bond, surgeon to the Leicester Royal Infirmary, described four other affected families in 1912 (Bond, 1912). The character clearly behaved as a Mendelian dominant.

Dislocation of the lens [ectopia lentis] was also observed in successive family generations. An affected mother produced seven of nine affected children in one example (Adams, 1909). A.R. Gunn reported direct transmission through four generations in another family. He found an excess of affected individuals and thought the trait did not act like a recessive character (Gunn, 1912). Bateson, on the other hand, thought it was quite consistent with a dominant trait (Bateson, 1909). C.H. Usher, too, reported direct heredity in a three-generation family in *Biometrika*, but made no further comments regarding hereditary mechanisms (Usher, 1924).

Myopia[12] was found commonly in many related people. Typically, it was passed directly from an affected parent to children. Harman reported one such pattern for heredity over four generations (Harman, N.B., 1914a). But another ophthalmologist reviewed 654 of his own cases and found that only 56% gave a positive family history for myopia. One example of a four-generation family was noted in which males were affected, having inherited the disorder through unaffected females (Worth, 1906). J.A. Wilson from the Ophthalmic Institution in Glasgow compiled a more detailed analysis of myopic heredity in 1914. He collected the family histories from 1500 patients; about 58% had evidence of myopia in relatives. He observed direct heredity in most cases. Eight families provided examples in which both parents were myopic. About 70% of their children were also affected. In 105 families with one myopic parent, about 40% of the offspring were affected. His data indicated that not all offspring of the doubly affected parents were affected, suggesting to him that the disorder did not fit either the Mendelian recessive or dominant pattern for heredity. He felt it was most compatible with the biometric theory for inheritance (Wilson, J.A., 1914). If affected parents were generally heterozygotes, the union of two of them would result in offspring affected in a 3:1 ratio (75 percent). When only one parent was affected, offspring would be affected in a ratio of 1:1 (50 percent). In fact, Wilson's results of 70 and 40% were approximately what would have been expected on a Mendelian model for heredity.

Glaucoma [increased pressure inside the eye] generally was typically transmitted directly from parent to child. Nettleship assisted Lawford in the collection of five pedigrees which documented this pattern over two and three generations (Lawford, 1908, 1914). Bateson concluded that glaucoma also acted as a dominant trait (Bateson, 1909). Subsequent studies of other families showed the same pattern for heredity (Holland, 1924; James, 1927).

Retinitis pigmentosa is a degenerative disorder of the retina, producing defective eyesight over time. Simeon Snell, Professor of Ophthalmology at the University of Sheffield, collected several extensive pedigrees showing the direct transmission of retinitis pigmentosa in successive generations. Both sexes were equally affected (Snell, 1903, 1907a, b). Nettleship's monumental study collected more than 1000 families. He could document direct heredity in 230 families. One family had five generations involved; another had seven successive generations affected. About half of children were affected when one parent was also affected. This was most consistent with a dominant Mendelian character (Nettleship, 1907c, 1909).

But, in a small percentage of families, another pattern for heredity appeared to be at work. Consanguinity was often present among these parents, and other relatives in collateral lines of the families were affected. Direct heredity was not the rule here. One woman with normal eyesight had two successive husbands also with normal eyesight. Both marriages produced children affected with retinitis pigmentosa. Bateson and Nettleship concluded that two different types of disease must therefore exist in the population. The second form would be most consistent with a recessive form of heredity (Bateson, 1909; Nettleship, 1909). Similar patterns for inheritance were noted in subsequent families, but no further genetic analysis was reported (Usher, 1914; Hine, 1928; Oliver, G.H., 1913; Bradburne, 1916).

Leber's disease [hereditary optic atrophy] exhibited a different form of heredity. Large families typically showed only males to be affected, while normal females appeared to transmit the character to their sons (Hawkes, 1900; Bickerton, 1904; Batten, R., 1909; Bramwell, 1904). William Hancock, ophthalmologist at the Royal London Ophthalmic Hospital, noted affected males in five successive generations of one family (Hancock, 1908). Nettleship did find rare affected females in families with the typical male-predominant pattern for heredity (Nettleship and Thompson, 1912). Albert Worton, ophthalmic surgeon to the Princess Beatrice Hospital, concluded in 1913 that Leber's disease was most likely a sex-limited disorder (Worton, 1913). It acted like color blindness in producing affected males born from unaffected transmitting females (Worton, 1913; Taylor and Holmes, 1913a, b; Pockley, 1915). Consistent with this mechanism for heredity, in one family an unaffected mother produced affected sons with two different husbands (Taylor and Holmes, 1913a).

The incidence of hereditary optic atrophy appeared to be particularly elevated in parts of Australia. Large affected family pedigrees were collected on that continent and from Tasmania that showed the consistent pattern of females transmitting the disorder only to males through four or five generations (Pockley, 1915; Moriet, 1921; Hogg, G.H., 1928). This pattern for heredity was similar to that of hemophilia, following the Mendelian sex-linked pattern (Burroughs, 1924).

British ophthalmologists had been challenged by Nettleship's leadership in carefully examining family histories and then reporting cases of hereditary eye diseases to medical societies. One speaker in 1928 commented that he had presented a case of retinitis pigmentosa because Charles Usher, president of the Ophthalmological Society at the time, "has made the investigation of familial eye diseases his hobby" (Hine, 1928).

As early as 1907, Charles Hurst, biologist from Cambridge, had examined the eye color in children born of 139 pairs of parents from one village in Leicestershire. He defined human eye color in two simple patterns—light or dark. Light-eyed parents always produced light-eyed children. Dark-eyed parents produced two patterns of offspring. Some families had all dark-eyed children; a second had predominance of dark-eyed to light-eyed in a ratio of about 3:1. Dark-eyed parents crossed with light-eyed parents also produced two classes of offspring. In some families only dark-eyed children were present; and in others both types appeared in approximately equal numbers. Bateson assisted Hurst in the analysis of the data and concluded that human eye color followed a Mendelian pattern with dark being dominant to light. The two different patterns of offspring from dark-eyed parents were consistent with parents being either heterozygous or homozygous for the dark allelomorph (Hurst, C.C., 1907).

James Galloway, ophthalmologist at the Eye Institution in Aberdeen, subsequently worked with Pearson to counter the Mendelian interpretation of Hurst's data. Nettleship and Pearson had earlier realized the difficulty in classifying human eye color as they studied albinism together. Galloway believed that it was not possible to accurately grade eye pigment as merely light or dark. Using his own scale for eye color, he found families in which the children's eye colors did not show Mendelian proportions for the inheritance of the character (Galloway, 1912).

Another indefatigable worker in the field of ophthalmic genetics was Madge T. Macklin from the Medical School at the University of Western Ontario. Macklin had graduated from Johns Hopkins Medical School in 1919 and was appointed part-time instructor at the medical school in Canada two years later. She was passionate about the importance of teaching medical students about human genetics, but was never able to organize a formal course for the students at her own medical school (Mehler, 2000). She re-addressed the issue of eye color in Canadian children and found it reasonably possible to grade individual eye color that she categorized as blue or brown. Her segregation analysis showed brown dominant to blue, consistent with the segregation of a Mendelian character (Macklin, 1926). In 1927 she published a series of articles in the *Canadian Medical Association Journal* that essentially constituted a monograph on the Mendelian heredity of different disorders of the eye (Macklin, 1927a, b, c, d, e, f, g, h). She was convinced that a thorough knowledge of genetics would aid physicians in diagnosing much human disease and in guiding their patients' reproductive choices for future generations (Mehler, 2000).

The hereditary nature of deafness was another matter examined at this time. In one family normal parents produced three affected children among six total offspring. The author of the report could not classify this case "on the Mendelian basis." Pearson's hypothesis would predict normal parents producing only normal children. Hence, neither competing theory of heredity appeared sufficient to explain such a pattern of inheritance (Bowen, 1908). P. Macleod Yearsley, aural surgeon from the Royal Ear Hospital, examined hundreds of families for instances of consanguinity. In 309 families with congenital deafness, first cousin marriages were evident in 7% of cases. But in 592 families with acquired deafness, only 0.3% of parents were consanguineous. He concluded that deafness was a recessive Mendelian trait, and that inbreeding intensified such characters and made them more likely to appear in offspring (Yearsley, 1914). James Love, another aural surgeon from the Glasgow Royal Infirmary, agreed that deafness was often due to the inheritance of a recessive trait (Love, 1920, 1921). Both experts also agreed that persons affected with hereditary deafness should not marry, because of the high likelihood of them having affected children.

Hair and Skin Diseases

Variations in the form and color of hair often passed through several generations of affected families and were another area of interest to physicians. Gossage observed a four-generation family in England with wooly hair. Although commonly seen in African families, no ancestors of that ethnic background could be determined. Direct transmission from parent to child was evident; more females than males were affected. Gossage labeled wooly hair as a Mendelian dominant trait (Gossage, 1908).

Other families demonstrated normal hair texture, but had white tufts of hair. Usher reported a five-generation family segregating this "piebald" trait (Usher, 1906). The ophthalmologist N. Bishop Harman noted a six-generation family in 1908. The first affected woman had been born in 1730. Direct transmission from parent to child was evident. One affected man had affected offspring by both of his unaffected wives. Harman interpreted the pattern for inheritance as consistent with a dominant trait (Harman, N.B., 1908, 1909c, 1914b). Bateson concurred that this represented a dominant trait (Bateson, 1909), as did M.H. Lane who reported a four-generation affected family (Lane, M.H., 1912). Edward Cockayne observed a family from Suffolk in which the piebald character had been present for seven generations. Both sexes were affected; affected children were only born of affected parents. He collaborated with Pearson and presented the work in *Biometrika*, attempting to classify family members as homozygous or heterozygous for a Mendelian dominant character. But he was unable to successfully use that theory to explain the segregation pattern in this particular family (Cockayne, E.A., 1914).

Abnormal development of skin structures also was known to be transmitted from parent to child in rare families. Ectodermal dysplasia is a syndrome of hypoplastic nails, minimal body hair, dental anomalies and often absence of the sweat glands. Two Canadian family pedigrees demonstrated the important role heredity played in the etiology of this disorder. One five-generation family demonstrated direct parent to child transmission; both sexes were affected (MacKay and Davidson, 1929). Another family had 119 members in five generations. The sexes were again equally affected, and direct transmission suggested ectodermal dysplasia was consistent with a dominant character (Clouston, 1929).

Another rare skin condition involved very dry skin on the palms and soles. Bramwell observed the trait in four successive generations (Bramwell, 1903). The disorder was termed "keratosis palmaris et plantaris." Direct transmission through three generations of a Scottish family was evident (Halley, 1903), while five generations of another family were affected (Jacob and Fulton, 1905). Gossage collected 40 families and noted direct transmission as the rule. Males and females were equally affected. About 50% of the offspring of affected parents inherited the character as well. No affected children were born of normal parents. This pattern was again consistent with a Mendelian dominant trait (Gossage, 1908).

A chronic blistering skin condition called epidermolysis bullosa also was evident in several generations. Individual case reports documented families affected in three (Pernet, 1904; Castle, 1922) or four (Cane, 1909; Castle, 1924) successive generations. Direct transmission was present; the sexes were equally affected. Bateson reported this as a dominant character in 1913 (Bateson, 1913). E.B. Morley then observed the disorder in five generations. Direct transmission was also evident, suggesting also to him that epidermolysis bullosa was a Mendelian dominant trait (Morley, 1914).

A rare disorder involving multiple malignant skin lesions, xeroderma pigmentosa, was widely known as a familial disease, often affecting several children in one generation who were born of normal parents. In one family from India, for example, two daughters and one son were affected. The parents and eight other children were healthy (Drury, 1910). Cockayne later reviewed the hereditary nature of several human tumors and labeled xeroderma pigmentosa as a recessive Mendelian character (Cockayne, E.A., 1927).

Nervous Diseases

The role for heredity as an etiologic factor in neurologic diseases remained controversial. It was clear that many such disorders appeared in several members of certain family, but did that necessarily imply that heredity had actually caused the symptoms of disease in question? Epilepsy was often present in several members of a family. J. Ferguson of the Toronto Western Hospital was convinced that heredity did play an important role in predisposing individuals to develop seizures (Ferguson, 1903). Another Canadian report demonstrated epilepsy in a mother and her son, uncle and three cousins of one family (Peters, 1905). In a family from St. Vincent in the West Indies, eight epileptics were observed among the 38 children born of six brothers (Branch, 1905). William Gowers, physician at The National Hospital for the Paralysed and Epileptic in London, reviewed more than 2400 of his own patients and found a positive family history for epilepsy in 40%. He attended the 1908 conference at the Royal Society of Medicine and presented pedigrees from families with direct transmission of epilepsy in three and four generations. He did not believe that the theory of Mendel could explain much about human heredity, but he did admit that such cases made epilepsy seem "almost Mendelian in its pattern of inheritance" (Gowers, 1908a, b). Walter Brain, neurologist at London Hospital, later recorded his own analysis of family history and epilepsy. He found examples of two and three generations affected. Nonetheless, he concluded, "Our present knowledge is not sufficient to render practicable the application of Mendelian principles to the inheritance of epilepsy" (Brain, 1926).

Henry Head, another neurologist from London Hospital, reviewed the heredity of spastic paralysis. A woman and four of her six children were affected (Head and Gardner, 1904). He commented in 1908 that such diseases "did not accord with the Mendelian law," although they clearly were hereditary (Ogilvie, 1907). However, Bateson was convinced that the pattern of inheritance was consistent with a dominant character (Bateson, 1913).

Hereditary tremor was also evident in successive generations of affected families. Three generations of affected people were not uncommon (Harris, 1904; Hertz, 1912). Bateson likewise labeled this as a dominant character (Bateson, 1913).

Cerebellar ataxia was frequently directly inherited from parent to child (Morris, 1908), but the many different clinical types of the ataxias made study of their pathology and heredity problematic (Holmes, 1907). Brain discussed the hereditary ataxias and noted both recessive and dominant forms. He proposed a dominant heredity factor that was required to produce the disease, and possibly another recessive modifying factor which segregated independently in affected families. His analysis of inheritance patterns in a very large family appeared consistent with the segregation of two Mendelian characters ultimately causing the ataxia (Brain, 1925). This 1925 proposal was one of the earliest to suggest that interaction between several Mendelian genes could result in human pathology.

Direct transmission was likewise evident in families with neurofibromatosis [Von Recklinghausen's disease]. Recurrence in two and three generations was well described (Parsons, 1906; Telling and Scott, 1905; Sutherland, G.A., 1906; Rolleston, J.D., 1910; Adie, 1925b), but discussions of hereditary mechanisms were lacking at this time.

Hereditary chorea [Huntington's disease] was reported from numerous families in the medical literature of this era. The striking progression of chorea and mental instability when affected individuals passed through middle age was a frightening specter as the illness segregated from one generation to the next. It was a "hereditary severe degeneration" and affected successive generations in almost all cases (Jollye, 1902). A selection of choreic pedigrees is listed in Table 13.2. Direct heredity was the inevitable pattern. Because the disease typically had its onset in the fourth or fifth decade of life, women who had the trait may have died in childbirth before being diagnosed with clinical disease. This may explain the slight male predominance in number of affected individuals. When Bateson began his own investigation on chorea, he was worried about the excess number of affected offspring in the families he studied. More complete pedigree analysis convinced him by 1909 that Huntington's chorea was a dominant trait (Bateson, 1909). Frederick Mott then discussed heredity and chorea at a meeting of the Manchester Medical Society in 1911. He reported a family affected in four successive generations and also labeled the disorder as a dominant character (Mott, 1911a, 1912). G.A. Shannon from Canada also described two affected families and agreed, "The Mendelian law of dominant inheritance was followed by nine patients, each of these having a choreic father or mother" (Shannon, 1913). The Australian psychiatrist John Catarinich reviewed the histories of families with three affected generations. He too agreed that the chorea acted as a Mendelian dominant (Catarinich, 1914). But fifteen years later, the London neurologist Charles Worster-Drought was still not convinced.

Table 13.2
Huntington's Chorea
1900-1930

Generations Affected	Males Affected	Females Affected	References
2	2	2	Jollye, 1902
4	6	2	Hogg, C.A., 1902
2	1	1	Jones, R., 1905
3	1	3	Deachell, 1905
2	1	1	Mill, 1906
1	2	2	Buzzard, E.F.,1907
2	3	1	McIntosh, 1907
3	2	1	Evans, 1908
4	1	3	Eager, 1910
3	2	6	Sawyer, E.H., 1910
4	3	5	Mott, 1911b
3	3	0	Buzzard, A., 1916
4	14	7	Jones, H., 1917
3	6	1	Back, 1926
2	1	2	Yealland, 1926
4	4	5	Oliver, J., 1912
4	4	4	Mott, 1912
4	3	4	Mott, 1911a
3	3	4	Worster-Drought, 1929
Total	62	53	

He observed a family affected in three successive generations and then stated that he could not analyze the available data to explain the "method of inheritance with the known laws of heredity" (Worster-Drought and Allen, 1929).

Another neurodegenerative disorder with a distinctive pattern for inheritance was amaurotic family idiocy [Tay-Sachs disease]. Mental deterioration, seizures and then blindness typically developed before age two years. Several affected children in families were described, often of Jewish origin. A selection of reports from the literature before 1930 is presented in Table 13.3. The pedigrees generally were incomplete, emphasizing the number of affected children rather than the total children in each generation. Relatedness or consanguinity was often assumed in families of Jewish ethnicity, but first cousin marriages were also commonly seen in non-Jewish families as well (Cockayne, E.A. and Attlee, 1914; Levy, 1922; Mandel, 1922; Ledbetter, 1925; Hart, B., 1910). Frederick Poynton examined many families with this disorder at the Hospital for Sick Children in Great Ormond Street London. His pathological examination of the brains of the children who had died indicated, "The disease is due to some inherent biochemical property of the protoplasm of the cells which results in degeneration of the neurons" (Poynton, 1906).

Because physicians lacked an understanding of the hereditary nature of this disorder, there could be tragic consequences for the families involved. One mother who had borne two affected children asked a physician whether it would be wise to have any more children. She was told, "There was no reason to believe the next child would be afflicted" (Carlyll and Mott, 1910).

A juvenile form of the same disease also was recognized in other families. The symptoms began later in childhood and then progressed more slowly. But the pathology in the eyes and brain was very similar to that found in the classical infantile disease (Batten, F.E., 1903, 1914; Batten, F.E. and Jukes, 1914). The pattern for heredity of this variant was similar, as indicated by the reports listed in Table 13.3. More complete pedigrees showed predominance of normal versus affected children in these families. The juvenile form also appeared frequently in non-Jewish families; consanguinity, however, was a common feature. The neurologist W.J. Adie noted that both forms of the disease had an abnormal accumulation of lipoid pigment in the ganglion cells of the nervous system (Adie, 1925a).

The hereditary mechanism for classical Tay-Sachs disease was finally understood by 1929. The segregation pattern was most consistent with a Mendelian recessive character. As was seen in albinism and alkaptonuria, consanguineous parents were heterozygous for the disease, and could produce homozygous recessive, and therefore, affected offspring (Stewart, D.S., 1929; Platt, 1929).

The same pattern for familial recurrence among siblings was also noted in cases of Friedreich's ataxia. In 1917, Litchfield presented a family in which three of nine children were affected. It was obvious that the disorder ran in families, but it could not be labeled "hereditary," because it rarely was passed from parent to child (Litchfield, 1917). Consanguinity was a common feature in these families as well (Rankin, 1902; Batten, F.E., 1902a; Palmer, 1906; Moody, 1910). When Frederick Mott discussed Friedreich's disease at the Pathology Section of the British Medical Association in 1905 he noted, "Convergent heredity may have been the cause for focusing a disease strain of remote ancestral origin." This suggested to him that the Mendelian "doctrine" for heredity might be applied to such cases (Mott, 1905).

Table 13.3
Amaurotic Family Idiocy
Tay-Sachs Disease
1900-1930

Affected Children	Normal Children	Consanguinity	References
CLASSIC FORM			
1	3	+	Poynton and Parsons, 1905
1	5	+	Poynton, 1906
1	4	+	Poynton, 1906
1	4	+	Poynton, 1906
2	0	+	Poynton, 1908
2	3	+	Carlyll and Mott, 1910
1	2	+	Smith, E.B., 1910
3	3	+	Weber, F.P., 1910
2 twins	1	+	Baildon, 1912
3	2	+	Hume, 1914
2	6	+	Battenand Mayou, 1914
1	0	+	Cockayne and Attlee, 1914
8	2		Paterson, 1921
4	2		Torrance, 1922
1	1	+	Levy, 1922
1	1	+	Mandel, 1922
1	1	+	Ledbetter, 1925
1	0	+	MacGregor, 1926
6	6	+	Steward, 1929
42	42	Totals	
JUVENILE FORM			
2	6		Batten, F.E., 1903
3	3	+	Mayou, 1904
1	11		Turner, 1912
2	4		Batten, F.E., 1914
3	2		Batten, F.E., 1914
3	2		Batten and Jukes, 1914
1	0	+	Weber, F.B., 1916
2	4		Greenfield, 1925
1	2	+	Riddoch, 1922
2	4		Hine, 1923
4	2		Adie, 1925a
3	4		Hay and Naish, 1923
2	4		Holmes and Paton, 1925
31	48	Totals	

Several other degenerative neurologic disorders presented the same familial pattern with frequent consanguinity. Samuel A.K. Wilson was born in the United States and emigrated to Edinburgh to study medicine. He received further training in neurology at the National Hospital in London (Critchley, 1940). In 1912, he reported a disorder involving degeneration of the brain and the liver called hepatolenticular degeneration that affected several children in one family. (Wilson, S.A., 1912a). He thought initially that, "No specific heredity appears to be involved" (Wilson, S.A.K., 1912b). Other families with several affected children in a single generation were noted subsequently (Sawyer, J., 1912; Hadfield, 1923; Greenfield, Poynton and Walshe, 1923; Barnes, 1924; Barnes and Hurst, 1925). One family produced ten affected and only two normal children (Paterson and Carmichael, 1924). The disease appeared to involve the storage or accumulation of excess protein or fat in the brain and liver that eventually altered the function of these organs and resulted in clinical disease. Similar recurrence patterns were observed in families with other degenerative disorders: Krabbe's (Krabbe, 1916), Hunter's (Hunter, C., 1916; Hunter, D. and Evans, 1929), and Gaucher's (Graham and Blacklock, 1927) diseases. Consanguinity was evident in one family (Hunter, C., 1916). Future investigation would attempt to assess whether heredity played any role in the etiology of these diseases.

Frederick Batten of the National Hospital reported several families segregating Werdnig-Hoffman disease [spinal motor atrophy]. The function of the spinal nerves deteriorated shortly after birth, producing muscle weakness and eventually asphyxiation. The disorder recurred in children born to unaffected parents. Several families he discovered had up to four affected children (Batten, F.E., 1902b, 1910, 1911; Batten, F.E. and Holmes, 1912). Krabbe investigated another family with first cousin parents and affected second cousins (Krabbe, 1920), again emphasizing the possible hereditary role of consanguinity.

Familial microcephaly [small head circumference] exhibited the same pattern for its heredity. A meeting at the Royal Society of Medicine in 1926 prompted Cockayne to mention that such a pattern for heredity might be compatible with a Mendelian recessive trait (Paterson, 1926). This suggestion would be investigated in more detail during the next decade.

Miscellaneous Disorders

Many other anomalies appeared repeatedly in both parents and children of affected families. One family with hereditary hematuria [blood in the urine] was studied by an entire generation of physicians in several London hospitals. L.G. Guthrie of Paddington Green Children's Hospital first recorded the character in several branches of a family in 1902. Archibald Garrod then analyzed the urine of the children but found only the presence of red blood cells (Guthrie, 1902). Similar problems were noted through four generations of other families (Aitkin, 1909; Kendall and Hertz, 1912). By 1923, the original family had expanded to encompass a third affected generation (Hurst, A., 1923). In 1927, A.G. Alport of St. Mary's Hospital in Paddington re-examined the family and discovered the association of deafness with the hemorrhagic nephritis (Alport, 1927). Direct inheritance from parent to child was evident, but no specific genetic mechanism was described.

Polycystic kidney disease was also noted in successive generations. One family had four affected generations. Both sexes were affected, and affected children were only born of affected parents (Fuller, 1928). A second family demonstrated a similar pattern for inheritance through three generations. However, as late as 1925, Hugh Cairns, physician at the Radcliffe Infirmary, explained, "The available data are insufficient to admit of analysis on Mendelian lines" (Cairns, 1925).

Allergic problems, such as hay fever, were seen through three successive generations (Freeman, 1920). Drinkwater was able to analyze another family segregating asthma via direct inheritance over three generations. Affected children were only born of affected parents. In affected lines of the family, there were ten normal and ten asthmatic offspring. He concluded that this was "in accord with Mendel's theoretical 50 percent" (Drinkwater, 1909) for a dominant character.

Over time, a hereditary trait that at first appeared unanalyzable could be better understood as experience in human heredity developed. In 1906, the dentist J.G. Turner had asked Bateson to review pedigrees segregating dental enamel hypoplasia. The character appeared to be directly transmitted from parent to children over five successive generations. There were 12 affected males and 9 affected females. Overall there were 21 abnormal compared to only 11 normal offspring. Turner thought the transmission was characteristic of a dominant feature. Bateson and Nettleship had noted an excess of affected persons at that time in pedigrees segregating many different human characters. Bateson wondered if Mendelian segregation actually occurred in humans at all, as it clearly did in his experimental plants and animals. He indicated to Turner that, in fact, the dental hypoplasia in the family did not segregate like a Mendelian character (Turner, 1906). After several more years of experience in studying human traits and their patterns of segregation, Bateson changed his opinion. By 1913, he was confident in stating that dental hypoplasia was also a Mendelian dominant trait (Bateson, 1913).

Conclusion

The continued work of pedigree collection and genetic analysis of dozens of human characters had convinced many British physicians of the relevance of Mendelian genetics to clinical practice. A detailed compilation of human genetic characters—both normal and abnormal—appeared at the end of the decade. The book, titled *Heredity in Man,* was published in 1929 and represented the work of Reginald Ruggles Gates, Professor of Botany at King's College London. Born in Canada, he had studied chromosomes and plant evolution in the United States before settling in England after the War. He never limited himself to studying plant genetics, but developed a broad anthropological approach to human heredity as well. Gates was one of the first to apply blood group analysis to different human populations. He recognized Mendelian segregation of physical traits characteristic of specific human ethnic groups when inter-"racial" marriages occurred. By 1929, Gates had developed an international reputation in the field of human genetics (Gates, 1929b; Gates, 1929a, 1926b, 1927; Roberts, 1964; Rushton, 2004).

By 1930, the mechanisms for Mendelian heredity—recessive, dominant and sex-linked—had been successfully applied to explain the familial segregation of diverse human characters. As early as 1908, Pearson had claimed that Mendelism could not explain the inheritance of any single human condition (Pearson, 1909b). The following year he complained, "There is hopeless confusion in such a method of treating Mendelism" when applied to specific cases of disease (Pearson, 1909a). But several years later, his own biometric theory for heredity appeared to have become less appealing to biologists and physicians alike, and he lamented, "No other conception of heredity can even obtain a hearing..." (Pearson, Nettleship and Usher, 1911b).

An analysis of medical articles discussing heredity and disease from 1900 until 1929 reveals that, in fact, Pearson's worst fears were realized. The number of H.D.D. citations for the biometric theory of heredity during this time are shown in Figure 13.2. The black bars indicate favorable references, while the white bars represent negative comments. Medical men generally had a positive attitude toward the biometric approach before the World War. Interest in the theory declined rapidly thereafter, and almost nothing was mentioned about it for more than a decade. The single 1916 reference was a historical review in an article written by a medical student and published in the *University of Durham Medical College Gazette* (Shaw, 1916). The final comment in 1928 was decidedly negative. The biometric scheme for human heredity had become passé.

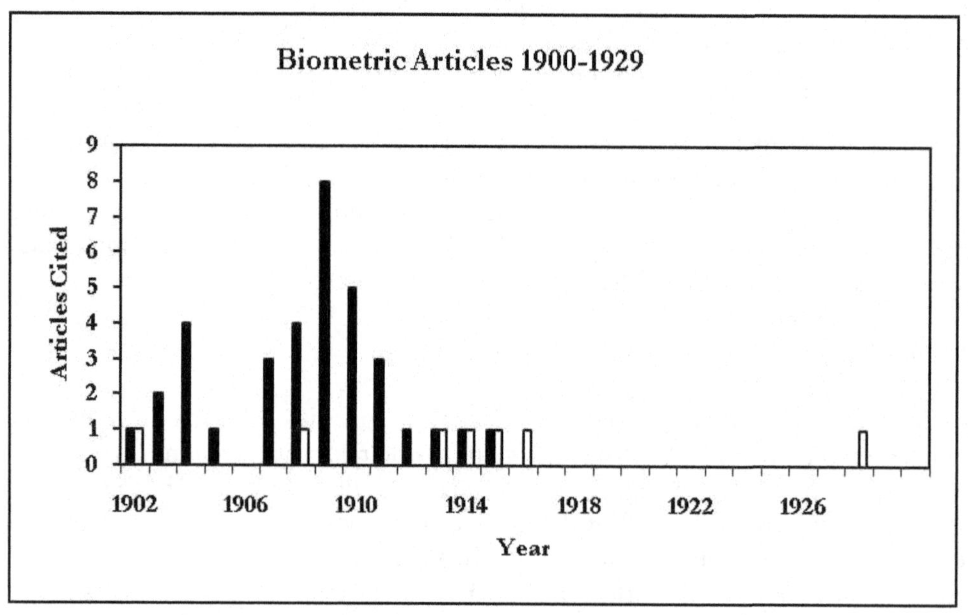

Figure 13.2

The next graph (Figure 13.3) represents the number of H.D.D. articles discussing Mendelism which appeared from 1900 until 1929. Again the black bars represent favorable and the white bars indicate unfavorable citations. Positive interest in Mendelism and human heredity swelled around the time of the 1908 Royal Society of Medicine conferences, lagged during the War and rose again later in the 1920s. The negative opinions changed radically over these years. The far-reaching comments from the biometricians before 1910 claimed that Mendelian heredity had not been shown to be of any usefulness in understanding human inheritance. Thereafter, the negative comments typically involved unsuccessful attempts to explain the hereditary pattern of a condition in Mendelian terms. During the first 30 years of the twentieth century, clinical experience had convinced many British physicians that Mendelism could explain the hereditary aspects of many of the diseases they encountered in their daily medical work.

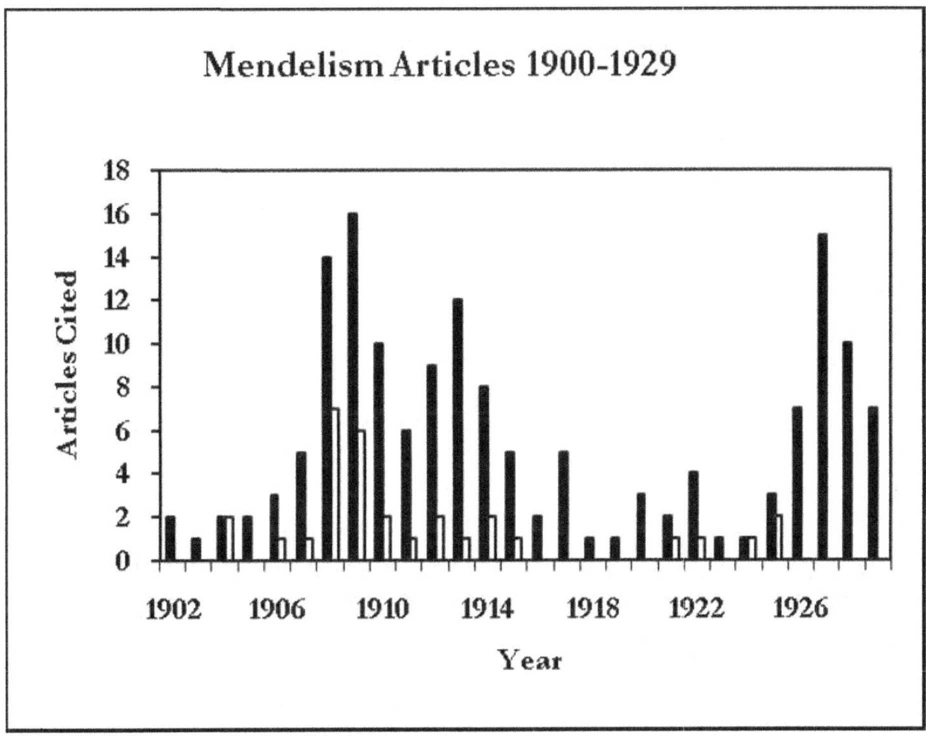

Figure 13.3

Fourteen

The Early Modern Era of Medical Genetics 1930-1940

By 1930, the senior leaders in the British schools of heredity were approaching the end of their professional careers. Bateson had died in 1926. His associate R.C. Punnett was named Professor of Genetics at Cambridge in 1911, where plant and animal breeding was the primary research focus. Pearson retired from the Galton Laboratory in 1933. His leadership roles were divided amongst two younger men. Ronald Fisher succeeded him as Galton Professor of Eugenics, and J.B.S. Haldane was appointed Professor of Genetics at University College London (Jones, J.S., 1993). Fisher had been seeking a unified theory of heredity for many years. Even as an undergraduate at Cambridge in 1911, he stated that he was trying to bridge the gap between the two competing schools of genetic thought (Fisher, 1911). After the War, he did prepare a general statistical theory that unified the biometric and Mendelian approaches (Fisher, 1918). But Bateson, Punnett and Pearson failed to understand, or simply ignored, the younger man's opinions.

The Development of Medical Genetics

In 1933, when Fisher assumed the editorship of the *Annals of Eugenics*, published by the Galton Laboratory of University College London, he sought the collaboration of all workers in genetics and statistics. He pledged to "prevent the perpetuation of the one-sided 'biometrical' and 'genetical' standpoints on human problems" (Fisher, 1934b).

And yet, the manifesto for human genetics in the 1930s came from a most unlikely source—the London School Economics—where Lancelot T. Hogben had just been appointed the first Professor of Social Biology. He had received the Natural Science Tripos from Trinity College Cambridge. After the War, he studied insect chromosomes at the Imperial College of Science and Technology and later collaborated with F.A.E. Crew on amphibian embryology at Edinburgh. Brief faculty appointments in Canada and South Africa prepared him for the London post in 1930 (Wells, 1978; Bud, 2004).

The publication of his book, titled *Genetic Principles in Medicine and Social Science,* in 1931, produced many innovative ideas that resounded throughout the British biological and medical communities. In his opinion:

> At present misguided beliefs about heredity are still widely prevalent in the medical profession owing to the fact that the rapid advances in genetic knowledge in the present generation have not yet had sufficient time to infiltrate the curriculum of medical studies..." (Hogben, L. 1932a).

Difficulties inherent in the study of human heredity were well known:

1. Matings were not controlled;
2. Family size was small;
3. Sexual maturity developed slowly;
4. Family environment was transmitted as well as genetic endowment;
5. Man was not outbred (Hogben, L., 1932b).

The combination of long generation times, small numbers of children and some degree of inbreeding all required a more organized and innovative approach to the study of human genetics. Hogben proposed that specialized research centers be established with professionals from the different disciplines to study in detail what role was played by heredity in the production of human diseases.

Hogben also suggested a research plan to better understand the old question of inherited conditions versus environmental effects on human beings (nature vs. nurture). Careful assessment of relatededness [consanguinity] among parents would signal the possibility of rare autosomal recessive traits that were common in inbred families. The role of the intrauterine environment could be answered by studying the association of birth order and maternal age, and physical disease. Twin studies could also be used to assess the roles of heredity in identical or fraternal types. The importance of the family environment could be assessed by examining differences between adopted children and their naturally born siblings in the same family (Hogben, L., 1932c).

Hogben also proposed the use of human blood groups as genetic markers for linkage studies. If several blood groups could be identified, such as the ABO and MN types, and all were located on different chromosomes, "human genetics would be equipped with the means of mapping the chromosomes of Man" (Hogben, L., 1932d). He reported preliminary studies attempting to detect linkage between the ABO type and several different human traits: diphtheria susceptibility, goiter, hemophilia, allergies, migraine, eye color, polydactyly, feeble mindedness and the direction of the occipital hair whorl. Results to date were all negative (Hogben, L., 1932e). Nonetheless, Hogben was convinced that such linkage studies would transform the field. Thus, "human genetics may be made an exact science, and an object lesson to those who are disposed to construct pretentious hypotheses on the basis of isolated pedigrees" (Hogben, L., 1932f). The mere collection of family histories could no longer be the sole aim of human hereditary studies.

The team approach to the collection and analysis of family data was certainly indicated. An ideal working environment would involve:

> ...genetical investigators working in association with the medical registrars...appointed in hospitals to take charge of the collection of information relating to the families of the patients and given facilities for following up cases suggestive of further inquiry...Little further advance will be made through the work of isolated investigators...Advances in the future will only be made if it is recognized that the further development of the subject presupposes the cooperation of large numbers of workers with facilities for obtaining all the requisite data...
> (Hogben, L., 1932g).

Pearson had requested that physicians send family data to the Galton Laboratory for analysis before the War, but the collaborative efforts faded after 1918. Hogben was convinced,

> Today the prospects of advancing human genetics as an exact science are much higher than they appeared to be twenty years ago. New methods of mathematical

> analysis for testing the applicability of experimentally established hypotheses to human data have been elaborated...It is now legitimate to entertain the possibility that the human chromosomes can be mapped (Hogben, L., 1932h).

He concluded that the laws for heredity applied to all organisms. Genetic linkage studies involving peas, corn and *Drosophila* had been successful. Now the human organism was to be studied in the same way.

The British medical community responded enthusiastically to Hogben's innovative approach to the analysis of human genetic conditions. The *Lancet* noted, "The study of human genetics should be removed from the atmosphere of the drawing room to that of the laboratory" (Mazumdar, 1992a). The *British Medical Journal* observed "a new spirit of hopefulness" that had developed in human genetics with the application of statistical methods to the family data. This approach could mark "the beginning of a new phase in human genetics" ("Genetics and Medicine," 1932; Mazumdar, 1992b).

Application of Genetic Studies to Humans

Hogben did not deny the importance of accurate pedigree collection by his medical colleagues. That was the source of the data, but not the end of study in itself. He thought, "The value of pedigrees lies in the fact, that they can be used to decide whether the frequencies of observed traits conform to the quantitative requirements of the principle of segregation" (Mazumdar, 1992b). The quantitative analysis of large collections of pedigrees with albinism, retinitis pigmentosa, hemophilia, color blindness, Tay-Sachs disease and Leber's optic atrophy all were consistent with the expected Mendelian frequencies in affected families (Hogben, L.T., 1931). The classic inborn error of metabolism, alkaptonuria, was subjected to the same test with data from families with 43 percent of the parents being consanguineous. The pattern for inheritance was consistent with an autosomal recessive trait (Hogben, L., Worras and Zieve, 1932).

Large-scale studies were then begun to discover genetic linkage relationships between many different human traits. An American study had recently shown that the ability to taste the chemical phenylthiocarbamide (PTC) was a Mendelian trait, nontasters being homozygous recessives (Blakeslee, 1932). Hogben combined that marker with the ABO blood groups to seek linkage in a series of families with brachydactyly or Friedreich's ataxia. Many London physicians had agreed to allow their patients with these conditions to participate in the study. Unfortunately, no positive correlations were obtained (Hogben, L.T. and Pollack, 1935). Human eye color, tendency to develop allergies and the blood groups ABO and MN were next studied in another group of families. Again no evidence of linkage was evident (Wiener, Zieve and Fries, 1936; Zieve, Wiener and Fries, 1936). These results were certainly disappointing but not really unexpected. Human cells possessed a large number of chromosomes, perhaps 48. Each one carried many different genes. Hogben concluded that the likelihood of finding linkage was slight: "The yield of relevant information obtained in linkage studies confined to a few genes is very small" (Hogben, L.T. and Pollack, 1935).

Changes were also evident across town at the Galton Laboratory. R.A. Fisher had earlier declined a position to work with Pearson in 1919. Instead, he chose to develop his own research agenda on the genetics of plants and animals in his role as statistician at Rotham Experimental Station. In 1930, he published *The Genetical Theory of Natural Selection* which examined the relationship between natural evolution and the Mendelian theory of heredity (Yates, 1970; Spencer, 2004). When he arrived at University College in 1933, he took advantage of the opportunities for the study of human genetics that had been developed there over the prior two decades. Like Hogben, he was anxious to study human heredity with linkage to genetic markers. The Rockefeller Foundation provided funds to begin studying the correlation between blood groups and different forms of mental and neurologic diseases. Fisher thought that correlation of human hair and eye color, form of the ear lobe, and the blood groups could define such linkages, and then hopefully diagnose predisposition to such disorders before affected persons had any symptoms of disease. Reproductive counseling could then be offered to affected adults in order to decrease transmission of the abnormal genetic conditions to the offspring (Mazumdar, 1992c).

The Galton Laboratory Blood Group Team was founded in 1935 with two physicians (G.L. Taylor and R.R. Race), Fisher as a geneticist and other statistical colleagues. At the same time, Fisher showed mathematically the efficacy of correlating the segregation of a rare autosomal trait such as alkaptonuria with a dominant disorder such as PTC tasting ability (Fisher, 1934b). The first large project at the Galton Laboratory attempted to investigate markers in families with dominant Huntington's chorea. Data on blood groups, PTC tasting, hair and eye color, ear lobe shape and handedness were carefully collected, but no linkage associations were found (Mazumdar, 1992d). A second study examined any relationships between blood groups, attached ear lobes, hyper-extensible joints and the presence of the hemolytic anemia termed acholuric jaundice. The unfortunate negative results were only published years later (Race, 1942).

But, there was one potential success in this early gene-hunting scheme. Fisher reanalyzed the data on the blood groups and Friedreich's ataxia studies previously reported by Hogben (Hogben, L.T. and Pollack, 1935). One of the twelve reported families did appear to show a positive result of co-segregation (Fisher, 1936).

J.B.S. Haldane joined Fisher at University College in 1933. He had spent the decade after the War collaborating with F. Gowland Hopkins, the prominent biochemist at Cambridge, in examining the roles of physiology, chemistry and genetics in Darwinian evolution. When he arrived to accept his new London post, the University charged him with a great responsibility. He was to apply

> ...his great knowledge of biochemistry [which] will enable him to introduce into genetics, which has heretofore been purely morphological in stature, those physiological conceptions which alone can lead to an understanding of the mode of action of the gene on which the hereditary transmission of structure rests...
> (Clark, 1968; "John B. Sanderson Haldane," 1970).

Haldane subsequently developed statistical tools to measure the proportions of homozygous and heterozygous individuals in families segregating hemophilia. His analysis supported the Mendelian expectation that half of the sisters of hemophiliac males were heterozygotes, and these then produced equal numbers of affected and normal male children (Haldane and Philip, 1939). Such pedigree data allowed him to estimate the mutation rate that produced the abnormal hemophilia gene as approximately 1 in 50,000 lives (Haldane, 1935b).

He then analyzed the existence of lethal human genes potentially linked to recessive characters such as albinism. The results showed, in fact, an increase in the frequency of diseased offspring when the parents' degree of consanguinity increased. The fact that the offspring survived argued against any lethal genes being closely linked to recessive disease genes segregating in those families (Bedichek and Haldane, 1937).

Haldane also attempted to correlate structural changes in human chromosomes with some anomalous pedigree data. For example, blood group analysis occasionally produced unexpected results. In one case, an AB mother and O father might produce a child with O blood group. False paternity could have been involved, or one of the blood group genes in the egg or sperm could have mutated. A third possibility would be that the mother was trisomic, in other words carrying three copies of the chromosome involved with the genes for the ABO blood group (Haldane, 1935a). Another unexpected finding was the rare situation in which a woman in a family segregating sex-linked disorders such as hemophilia or color blindness produced daughters all affected and no affected sons. A cytological explanation could involve an attached X chromosome, as documented in *Drosophila* (X^X). In this hypothetical example, a woman would transmit the mutant gene on the double X-chromosome to all her daughters, and to none of her sons (Haldane, 1932).

The ability to analyze human chromosome structure in greater detail would certainly help resolve such confusing situations. Research in Russia at this time showed the feasibility of growing human white blood cells (lymphocytes) in culture (Chrustschoff, 1935). Such a readily available tissue source could then be studied microscopically to examine the human chromosomes for unusual size, shape or number (Haldane, 1932, 1935a). Techniques in use in Britain at this time involved sectioning of tissues into thin strips and then attempting to use the microscope to count the clumped chromosomes. The results were often ambiguous as it was impossible to distinguish individual chromosome size and shape.

The opening of the Galton Laboratory to new ideas on human genetics changed the way the existing staff did their work. Julia Bell (b 1879) had worked with Pearson on human heredity and statistics since 1907. Her interest in medical topics suggested to her that she attend medical school, but Pearson was not enthusiastic. He wondered whether the time required for such study would really enhance her ability to collect and analyze medical statistics. He noted that Major Greenwood was medically trained and had spent time at the laboratory studying statistics. But Greenwood seemed to have had little success combining the two disciplines (Pearson, 1916). Instead, Pearson wanted her to stay at the laboratory and continue to work with him. He knew of her "desire...to get forward with the medical work," but he thought she should put it off for a while (Pearson, 1915).

But she did not follow Pearson's recommendation, and Dr. Bell graduated from the Royal Free Hospital Medical School in 1920. She fully intended to return to the Laboratory and resume her hereditary work there, and asked Pearson for one day each week in which she could develop a small medical practice. Pearson was surprised that she could consider such "divided affection" for the Galton Laboratory. With his typical one-sided thinking, he was astounded at her independent wish, as if "our work would not and could not again supply all your needs" (Pearson, 1919a). But Pearson decided that Dr. Bell was a valued asset and subsequently offered her the next available position at the Laboratory (Pearson, 1919b).

Over the next decade, Dr. Bell prepared lectures on medical topics such as "Heredity in Eye Anomalies" for Pearson's course in medical statistics (Pearson, 1920). She collected and updated pedigrees on eye disorders such as color blindness (Pearson, 1922). But Pearson kept a close hand on her "medical" genetic visibility. He advised against her publication of an article in *Lancet.* Instead he wished to present the material in one of the Laboratory's publications as an advertisement for future work (Pearson, 1922). As Pearson approached retirement, he still would not allow her the personal freedom to follow her own interests. In 1930 Dr. Bell was considering a research position at the Royal Eastern Counties Institution in Colchester, where L.S. Penrose would soon successfully examine the hereditary aspects of mental defect. Pearson thought the position might be only temporary and could also involve a good deal of administrative work rather than be a "free research post." He did not at all encourage Dr. Bell to apply for the position that would mean her termination at the Galton Laboratory (Pearson, 1930a). So, she remained there and held the title Galton Research Fellow from 1926 to 1944 (Jones, G., 2004; "Obituary of Julia Bell," 1979).

In 1932, Hogben proposed that the Medical Research Council establish a Committee on Human Genetics to coordinate funding in this newly expanding field. Haldane was appointed chairman. Julia Bell, E.A. Cockayne, R.A. Fisher, L.S. Penrose, and J.A. Fraser-Roberts were appointed to the panel (Mazumdar, 1992e). In her work at the Galton Laboratory and with other committee members, Bell was able to completely change her research focus. During the War, Pearson had put her to work measuring bones of hundreds of deceased Englishmen in physical anthropology studies (Pearson and Bell, 1917). She had also completed the laborious pedigree collections that were presented in the *Treasury of Human Inheritance* monographs (Table 12.4). But in these memoirs, she had not been permitted to analyze the data to further a detailed understanding of human heredity, because Pearson had designated the *Treasury of Human Inheritance* to be "theory-free."

Beginning in the 1930s, Bell prepared extensive pedigrees for osteogenesis imperfecta, polydactyly, brachydactyly, syndactyly and migraine headaches. All the families showed direct inheritance of the respective trait for many generations. The sexes were equally affected. She was not, however, allowed to interpret the hereditary mechanisms that appeared to explain such familial disease segregation (Bell, 1930a, b, 1931, 1933). However, the issue of the *Treasury of Human Inheritance* that appeared after Pearson retired from the Galton Laboratory reported similar direct inheritance of the neurodegenerative disorder Huntington's chorea. Bell was now able to classify it as a dominant Mendelian character (Bell, 1934). Subsequent studies revealed her skill at deciphering difficult genetic traits. The next issue of the memoir series examined the heredity of Charcot-Marie-Tooth disease [peroneal muscle atrophy]. There appeared to be three different forms of the disorder. It could segregate in a recessive, dominant or sex-linked fashion. About 69% of families demonstrated a dominant form. She also attempted to correlate linkage of this disease with PTC tasting ability in the affected families (Bell, 1935). The volume on Friedreich's ataxia and spastic paraplegia, in contrast, analyzed pedigrees to demonstrate recessive heredity with a high frequency of parental consanguinity. She again emphasized the potential for genetic linkage studies using PTC tasting and blood groups as genetic markers (Bell, 1939; Harper, 2005).

Bell's pedigree analysis eventually led to the development of the first human chromosome map. She had collected six pedigrees segregating two sex-linked traits: color blindness and hemophilia. William Bulloch had earlier reported to Pearson that one of his hemophiliac patients had mentioned that he was colorblind, and knew of other "bleeders" with the same ocular condition (Bulloch, 1928). Bell thought these two sex-linked characters could be demonstrated to segregate on the same X-chromosome. One apparent crossover was observed in a colorblind hemophiliac who had a colorblind non-hemophiliac brother. This event occurred in about 5% of the matings in that family

(Bell and Haldane, 1936). Haldane thought that it should be possible to use other sex-linked markers to devise a map of the human X-chromosome (Haldane, 1936). Bell and Haldane presented their work before the Royal Society in 1937 and offered the first human chromosome map with five genetic markers (Bell and Haldane, 1937). The relative estimated positions on the X-chromosome for the genes involving color blindness, xeroderma pigmentosum, the Japanese form of congenital blindness [Oguichi disease], one type of epidermolysis bullosa, and a rare form of retinitis pigmentosa are shown in Figure 14.1. A contemporary map of the *Drosophila* X-chromosome is included for comparison. The *Lancet* reported this important development to the medical community at large ("Colour blindness and hemophilia," 1937). Julia Bell continued her studies at the Galton Laboratory until she finally retired in 1965 at age 86 years. She lived to celebrate her centennial birthday and died in 1979 (Jones, G., 2004).

The most prominent physician involved in human hereditary research during the 1930s was Lionel Penrose (b 1898). He completed clinical training in 1928 after several years spent studying psychology in Vienna. He was then appointed research medical officer at the Royal Eastern Counties Institution at Colchester and began a series of studies on heredity and mental illness there (Harris, 1973; Cooke, 2004). He completed a monumental seven-year study of 1280 mentally retarded patients, their parents and 6629 siblings. Penrose personally interviewed family members in order to document accurate histories of these illnesses in as many generations as possible. Karl Pearson noted the intensity of such labor and lamented the fact that another Nettleship, who had so carefully studied families with eye diseases, was not available to do the work in these families with mental diseases (Pearson, 1930b). The Colchester report attempted to use statistical tools to discriminate effects of heredity and environment in causing such disorders. It has been called the "last grand manifestation of eugenist problematic in its most traditional form" (Mazumdar, 1992f). Penrose concluded that there was no single answer as to the origin of these cases. Mental illness and mental retardation had heterogeneous causes. Evidence accumulated that both nature and nurture were involved (Harris, 1973).

A detailed study of one particular form of mental retardation—Down syndrome or mongolism—accentuated the best of current genetic analysis. Many prior workers had noted the increased frequency of babies with mongolism born to older mothers. Identical twins could be affected, suggesting, "The essential cause of mongolism must be in the germplasm and could not be an environmental factor." Others argued that the character behaved like a Mendelian recessive trait (Stewart, 1925). As many different body systems were affected in Down syndrome, Macklin suggested that 5-6 Mendelian characters on separate chromosomes could segregate and produce the disorder (Macklin, 1929). Fraternal twins were typically disparate with regard to mongolism—one was affected and the other was normal. But P.M.G. Russell noted a fraternal twin pair where both were born affected. In this case, he suggested the existence of a maternal factor, rather than strictly a genetic defect which resulted in the disorder (Russell, P.M.G., 1933).

It had been suggested that children with Down syndrome were the result of racial cross breeding involving Mongolian ethnicity. Research work done by Gates and others in the 1920s had showed that different racial groups had different frequencies of human blood groups. Penrose examined the frequency of the ABO antigens in mentally defective, normal and Down syndrome patients from England. He could detect no

X-Chromosome Maps

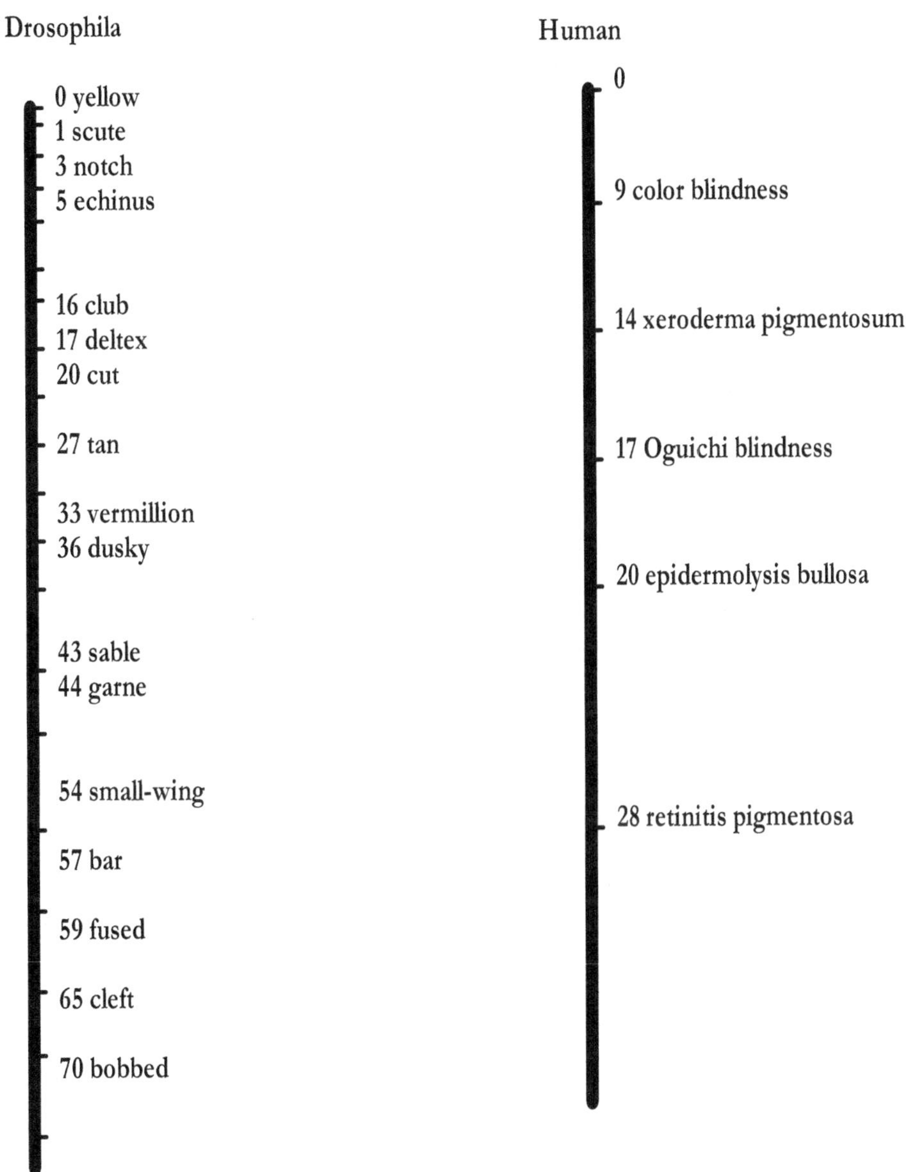

References: Sinnot and Dunn (1932) p. 160 | Bell and Haldane (1936)

Figure 14.1

differences, suggesting that, in fact, all the children derived from the same general ethnic background (Penrose, 1934a).

Maternal effects on reproduction such as age at birth of children with Down syndrome were examined next. Penrose obtained 150 pedigrees with at least one affected child and correlated both maternal and paternal age at the time of birth of such children. Maternal age in the families with Down syndrome was about six years greater than that of a control population (Penrose, 1933, 1934b). About 70% of affected children were born to mothers older than 35 years. The existence of prior children in affected families did not appear to make any difference. Hence, birth rank was of no importance (Penrose, 1934d, e), and the pedigree data did not fit a simple Mendelian recessive pattern for inheritance either (Penrose, 1934c).

Other birth defects showed quite opposite results. Neural tube defects [spina bifida and anencephaly] did not demonstrate any maternal age effect. The order of birth did appear to be important in the development of babies with pyloric stenosis, a narrowing of the muscle at the distal end of the stomach. About 50% of these cases appeared in first-born children (Penrose, 1939).

At this time, theoretical research by Fisher, Haldane, Hogben and Penrose realized the desire of their predecessor, Pearson, for the unification of statistics and human heredity.[13] *The Origin of Theoretical Population Genetics* by William Provine subsequently outlined the historical development of this specialized field of study (Provine, 1971).

Medical Education and Genetics

Human genetics researchers of the day attempted to explain the application of statistics and linkage to medical groups, hoping to elicit the interest of the medical practitioners. Hogben presented the 1933 William Wuthering Memorial lectures at the University of Birmingham titled "The Methods of Medical Genetics." The material was later presented in a book, *Nature and Nurture,* for the general medical and lay public. He reviewed current understanding of recessive, dominant and sex-linked human traits. He also outlined his goal for studying genetic linkage with different blood groups as markers. The role of twin studies to examine the relative importance of heredity and environment also was outlined as a means for understanding how genetics impacted important human conditions (Hogben, L., 1933, 1939). Haldane then lectured on congenital disease at the Royal College of Physicians in 1938. He pointed out that a dominant trait such as brachydactyly often appeared suddenly in a family as the result of a genetic mutation. Penrose had estimated such mutation rates as approximately 1 in 30-40,000 lives (Gunther and Penrose, 1935; Penrose, 1936). Recessive characters such as alkaptonuria or Tay-Sachs disease were typically noted in inbred families. Other specific diseases had different inheritance patterns in different families. Retinitis pigmentosa for example was known to have recessive, dominant and sex-linked variants (Haldane, 1938).

Practicing physicians complained, however, about the lack of opportunity to learn and apply these notions of the new genetics. One reviewer of Hogben's book observed that the application of genetics to medical care had not been too successful, as "genetics has almost no place in the modern curriculum" [of medical education] ("Clinical Genetics," 1934). Madge Macklin from the University of Western Ontario Medical School regularly campaigned for the inclusion of such training in the regular medical course-work. She had already noted in the past,

> Those interested in human heredity have been looked upon as faddists, or as propagandists with interesting material at their command but with nothing of practical value to appeal to the practitioner. [But] heredity as an implement in the armamentarium of the physician is coming into its own (Macklin, 1933a).

She surveyed the medical school curricula in Canada, the United States and the United Kingdom and discussed her findings at the Third International Eugenics Congress held during August of 1932. She found that formal discussions of heredity and disease were typically held during the pre-clinical years. When hereditary diseases were actually encountered in the clinic or hospital ward, physician teachers at that time often failed to explain the role of genetics in actually causing such disease symptoms. Macklin suggested a formal course in medical genetics during the last year of medical school when students had contact with real patients suffering from such conditions. Instruction by a medically trained faculty would serve to emphasize the important role of heredity in human disease (Macklin, 1933c, 1934, 1935a). Hogben summarized the current situation, "Before genetic prognoses can become part of preventive medicine, it will be necessary to introduce the teaching of genetics into the medical curriculum" (Hogben. L, 1932i).

John A. Fraser-Roberts from the Medical Research Department of the Stoke Park Colony in Bristol emphasized the same facts to a medical audience several years later. The General Medical Council in the United Kingdom had recently recognized the importance of teaching genetics as part of the basic pre-clinical biology courses for medical students. However, to be very useful, the material also had to be taught in conjunction with clinical subjects. Utilization of cases from the clinic could certainly illustrate the "technical parts" of human heredity and disease (Fraser-Roberts, 1937). There was a growing feeling that genetics would play an expanding role in all of biology. "Endowment of the subject in our universities" was hoped to educate many on the importance of heredity in modern-day life (Ashby, 1936; Haldane, 1938).

The Application of the New Genetics to Medical Practice

Contemporary medical students and practicing physicians attempted to inform themselves on developments in human heredity by course work, medical society lectures and readings in the medical journals. But some of the senior leaders in the field found it difficult to keep up with new findings. In 1931, Charles Hurst asked Archibald Garrod to attend a meeting to discuss the formation of a British Council for Research in Human Genetics. Garrod answered that he was still interested in the topic, but admitted that he had difficulty following the work of Hogben and the others involved in current genetics (Bearn, 1993). Two years later, he noted to E.A. Cockayne, "I find myself out of my depth in the new Mendelism of Hogben and Haldane..." (Garrod, 1933). The Regius Professor of Physic at Cambridge, Humphrey Rolleston, felt the same way. In his opinion, "The new knowledge of heredity, which like statistics, ha[d] now become too complicated for the plain medical man in the streets" (Rolleston, 1928) to fully comprehend and still required a great deal of explication.

Twins and Genetic Disorders

Work in the new genetics continued to be applied to the human condition. Twin studies were increasingly used to examine the effects of heredity and environment. Macklin studied Canadian population data and concluded that specific cancers were much more common in certain families than chance alone could explain. She found the existence of specific tumors in identical twins to be another powerful argument that heredity played an important role in causing such malignancies (Macklin, 1932). P.A. Gorer from the Lister Institute in London also examined cancer in twins. In cases of both gastrointestinal and female reproductive tract tumors, cancers were found to be much more frequent in identical vs. fraternal twins (Gorer, 1937).

J.A. Wilson from the Ophthalmic Institution in Glasgow examined the effects of hereditary on structures of the eye—the pattern of the iris, the shape of the lens and the pattern of blood vessels on the retina. He found that he could not discriminate monozygotic from dizygotic twins. About 58% of all twins demonstrated identical eye examinations. Brothers and sisters who were not twins had about 30% with identical eye structures (Wilson, J.A., 1932). A second study found 62% of identical twins with identical eye findings, while fraternal twins had 0% with similar eye structures (Law, 1934). Both studies emphasized the relative importance of heredity in producing structures of the eye.

E.M. Watson from the University of Western Ontario Medical School found identical twins that had developed diabetes as young adults (Watson, 1934). Another Canadian study found Dupuytren's contractures in tendons of the hands of identical twins (Couch, 1938). The neurologic disorder tuberous sclerosis was also noted in a set of identical twins (Fabing, 1934). The more frequent occurrence of all these characters in monozygotic twins suggested a hereditary predisposition to the development of such clinical diseases.

In contrast, W. Sheldon at the Hospital for Sick Children on Great Ormond Street in London reviewed 1000 cases of pyloric stenosis. Twenty-three affected twin pairs were recorded; but there was only one case of affected monozygotic twin boys (Sheldon, 1938), arguing against the importance of heredity in this disorder, and suggesting an intrauterine maternal factor producing abnormal development of the muscle in the stomach.

Genetic Linkage and Disease

British physicians also attempted to apply the new genetics in order to determine genetic linkage relationships between human characters, both normal and abnormal. J.C. Thomas completed blood group comparisons between mental illnesses such as manic-depressive disorder and schizophrenia in 526 patients and 374 normal controls. The ABO and MN blood group frequencies were no different in the two populations (Thomas and Hewitt, 1939). When two hereditary diseases segregated within the same family, such co-occurrence did not necessarily imply that the genes for the disorders were linked to the same chromosome. Charles Worster-Drought presented a family to the Royal Society of Medicine Neurology Section in which both myotonic dystrophy and muscular atrophy appeared to be present. The Section President A.S. Barnes offered the suggestion that two unrelated mutant genes happened to the present in the same family (Worster-Drought, C., 1932), because they segregated independently. Another family also demonstrated independent segregation of two dominant traits: periodic paralysis and muscular atrophy (Biemond and Daniels, 1934). The confusing syndrome of blue sclera, frequent fractures and deafness termed osteogenesis imperfecta also could be explained by the segregation of two genetic disorders in one family (Ottley, 1932).

W.J. Rutherfurd of Glasgow shared the hopes of Hogben and the other researchers in human genetics on the practical application of such studies. He described a family with both nail aplasia [atrophic finger and toe nails] and dislocating patella. He observed:

> It is the occurrence of such associations of medical conditions that holds out the possibility of carrying out in some degree for the human species the modern scientific practice of mapping in the chromosomes the exact situation of various characters that has been carried out with such an extraordinary degree of detail in the fruit fly *Drosophila* (Rutherfurd, 1933).

When two apparent genetic defects did segregate together, linkage certainly could be suspected. The ophthalmologist, Arnold Sorsby, presented a family with coloboma irides as well as bifid thumbs and great toes. E.A. Cockayne suggested that these did represent an example of autosomal linkage of defective and adjacent genes. The traits would be inherited together, unless crossing-over during meiosis occurred in subsequent reproduction (Sorsby, 1934, 1935). The Laurence-Moon-Biedl syndrome was another multisystem disorder involving obesity, retinitis pigmentosa, polydactyly and mental retardation. Cockayne noted that consanguinity among parents was common, and about 25% of the children were affected. He described a family with three children with the entire syndrome, six normal children and two others with polydactyly alone. He thought that the digital anomaly was due to one recessive gene and that the other defects resulted from the action of at least one other recessive gene carried on the same chromosome (Cockayne, 1935a). All of the defects generally were inherited together, but crossing-over could result in the inheritance of only one of the genetic traits. Lewis Savin and Sorsby recorded a similar case and reached the same conclusions (Savin, 1935; Sorsby, 1939).

Studies of a family from New Zealand showed myoclonic epilepsy and deafness that appeared to segregate together. The parents were normal but second cousins. This example appeared to represent two separate recessive genetic entities. The fact that they segregated concurrently suggested that they could be linked on the same chromosome (Latham and Munro, 1937). Richard W.B. Ellis from the Hospital for Sick Children reported several cases of chondro-ectodermal dysplasia involving malformations of the skin, nails, teeth and skeleton. Consanguinity in the parents was a common finding. He concluded that this was most likely a recessive disorder. But the multitude of systems involved suggested to him that this condition might result from the linkage of several recessive genes, as suggested in the Laurence-Moon-Biedl syndrome (Ellis, 1940).

Another chromosomal mechanism was postulated to explain unusual segregation patterns of other hereditary diseases. The ophthalmologist M.D. McQuarrie from the University of Liverpool reported two families with a previously undescribed form of blindness. In one family the disorder followed a typical Mendelian dominant pattern through three successive generations. But a second family of four generations presented a segregation pattern more consistent with a sex-linked form of inheritance. E.A. Cockayne suggested that a chromosomal translocation between an autosome and the X-chromsome might explain how the disease appeared to be dominant in one case and sex-linked in another family (McQuarrie, 1935).

Other studies used large samples of patients with various disorders to seek co-segregation and possible genetic linkage. Maddox from Australia examined over 250 families with diabetes. Typically the disorder followed a Mendelian recessive pattern. His patients showed no linkage to cancer, thyroid disease, asthma, hair, or eye color variants. He next planned to test for linkage with the different blood groups (Maddox and Scott, 1935). The ophthalmologist William J. Riddell from Glasgow University investigated linkage of several eye disorders. He noted two families segregating two sex-linked conditions—hemophilia and color blindness. Each trait was inherited independently, implying that the two genetic loci were located on two different X-chromosomes in these families (Riddell, 1937, 1938). He next discovered a family segregating a dominant form of osteogenesis imperfecta and sex-linked color blindness through seven generations. He examined color sense, PTC tasting ability, blood groups and physical evidence of the genetic diseases. He found no evidence of linkage, however (Riddell, 1939, 1940).

The interest of practicing physicians in genetic studies was not purely theoretical. Most clearly stated that the potential for prediction of disease before symptoms began and the possibility of reproductive counseling were the goals of such research. Linkage of a blood group or other common marker to a serious genetic disorder like Huntington's chorea would allow physicians to accurately predict predisposition to disease later in life. Knowing the pattern for inheritance of that particular disorder would then allow prospective parents the opportunity to guide their own reproduction to decrease the risk of transmitting genetic disease to their children (Riddell, 1939).

Application of Human Genetics to the Community at Large

Although there was increasing interest in the study of heredity and health, available data on the genetics of human disease was still inadequate to guide the medical profession in its daily practice. One suggestion proposed that the National Health Service should establish regional genetic offices. Trained research workers could collect pedigrees from many different families. Lectures on the role of heredity and disease could also be sponsored for physicians, medical students, nurses, teachers and social workers. The goal of such a plan was to "complete knowledge of disease, defect and abnormality in the population...in order to obtain data concerning the hereditary factor with the future prevention of morbid inheritance" (Goodall, 1936).

The concept of eugenics that aimed to enhance the reproduction of the fit and decrease the reproduction of the unfit continued to be debated among both the British public at large and the medical profession during the 1930s. A detailed analysis of the role played by British physicians in the Eugenics Education Society and other groups aimed at improving the genetic health of the population is beyond the scope of this monograph. Three authors have carefully detailed the growth of the British eugenics movement prior to the Second World War.[14]

Other less global initiatives were recommended at the same time to enhance the development of human and medical genetics. Lord Harden of St. Bart's Hospital and physician to the Prince of Wales (later Edward VIII) suggested that the Ministry of Health should establish a research unit in human genetics (Harden, 1933). The British National Human Hereditary Committee did, in fact, establish the Bureau of Human Heredity, to act as an international clearinghouse of facts concerning human heredity. A Board of Directors from medical and scientific bodies in the United Kingdom was established. Pedigree and twin studies on all human traits were solicited for consideration. Within the first eighteen months of its operation, more than 600 varieties of human disease were catalogued ("Bureau of Human Heredity," 1936, 1938). Physicians, in particular, were asked to collect careful family histories on their patients and submit them to R. Ruggles Gates at the Bureau office on Gower Street in London (de F. Bauer, 1940).

Local initiative was also evident in the attempts to apply human genetic knowledge to medical practice. Charles J. Bond (b 1856) had retired from the active practice of surgery, but was convinced of the importance of genetics and human disease. He collaborated with the county national health committee in Leicestershire to establish a "Eugenic Consultative Committee" which offered advice to prospective parents about the future genetic prospects of their offspring ("Charles John Bond FRCS-Obituary," 1939a; Kemp, N.D.A., 2004).

Mendelism and Human Disease

Despite the numerous clinical reports on the application of Mendelism to disease, one commentator thought that British physicians still felt that genetics was "an obscure and academic subject, quite unconnected with the wards" [of the hospital] ("Human Genetics," 1939). At the same time, other evidence indicated that physicians of the day had learned a great deal about Mendelism and understood its application to the study of familial disorders. While Mendelism had been discussed at numerous conferences and medical society meetings in earlier decades, this was no longer so commonplace. F.A.E. Crew appeared before the Royal Society of Medicine in 1933 to update the audience on recent understanding of heredity and disease (Crew and Fraser-Roberts, 1933). J.A. Fraser-Roberts spoke before a local medical society in 1937 to review the different types of recessive, dominant and sex-linked human diseases (Fraser-Roberts, 1937). And J.B.S. Haldane spoke to the Royal College of Physicians to remind them of the importance of pedigree analysis in understanding human diseases which could segregate in irregular patterns unique to each family. Retinitis pigmentosa, he noted, was one such disorder that presented recessive, dominant or sex-linked variants (Haldane, 1938). A basic appreciation of Mendelian genetics, albeit imperfect, was expected of practicing physicians. More detailed reports on heredity and human diseases continued to be published during this decade.

Blood and Blood Vessel Diseases

The heredity of various hemorrhagic states was often confusing, but genetic analysis was now used more frequently to differentiate different forms of these diseases. L.J. Witts, Professor of Medicine at the University of London, suggested that physicians should analyze affected family groups rather than attempting to diagnose specific diseases. Patterns of heredity specific for individual families would provide useful diagnostic information for the practitioner caring for family members (Witts, 1937). For example, hereditary epistaxis [nosebleed] was evident in three successive generations with direct inheritance (Wordley, 1932). Another bleeding disorder something like hemophilia was noted to have a different hereditary pattern. Pseudo-hemophilia [Von Willebrand's disease] occurred in both sexes, and could, in fact, be more severe in affected females. Female to female transmission and affected identical twin sisters suggested that this might represent a Mendelian sex-linked dominant trait. Females with two X-chromosomes therefore could have a more serious disorder (Witts, 1932b; Davis, 1939). In other families, direct transmission to both sexes over three or four generations suggested a more typical dominant pattern for inheritance (Leak, 1934; Handley, R. and Nussbrecher, 1935).

A different bleeding disorder, characteristic of young children, exhibited another hereditary pattern. J.C. Hawksley from the Hospital for Sick Children noted erythroblastosis fetalis [severe hemolytic anemia in newborns] in several children born of first cousin parents. Collateral aunts and uncles had experienced the same disorder. Autosomal recessive inheritance could explain the pedigree (Hawksley and Lightwood, 1934).

Inherited fragility of the red blood cells that were damaged in episodic crises produced acholuric jaundice. Large pedigrees noted the character over several generations. One family with direct inheritance through four successive generations was reported from Australia (Cowen, 1936). F. Parkes Weber, physician to the German Hospital, also noted direct inheritance through four generations (Weber, 1931). Lord Dawson of Penn, President of the Royal College of Physicians and Physician to King George VI, encountered several affected families in his clinical practice. Direct heredity through two and four generations was observed (Dawson of Penn, 1931). Generally the sexes were equally affected (Evans, C., 1930; Hannay, 1937; Murray-Lyon, 1935; Barber, 1934; Joyce, 1933; Paxton, 1935). L.J. Witts concluded that a dominant pattern for inheritance was most likely (Witts, 1932a).

Hemochromatosis was recognized as an inborn error of iron metabolism in which the metal was deposited in the heart, liver and pancreas, producing damage to these organs during adulthood. Two brothers clearly had the same disorder. Three other brothers in the same family had milder symptoms and could be developing the syndrome. Two sisters appeared unaffected while the mother had mild symptoms as well. Robert D. Lawrence from King's College Hospital wondered whether this pattern for inheritance could be sex-linked, as in families with hemophilia (Lawrence, 1935).

Twenty-six families with varicose disease of the veins in the legs were examined. Direct heredity through four generations with both sexes affected suggested a dominant mechanism for inheritance (Ottley, 1934).

Bone and muscle diseases

New families affected with brachydactyly were reported with multiple affected generations. Karl Nissen, orthopedic surgeon from New Zealand, noted one such family that had emigrated from England in 1840. Six generations were affected with direct inheritance, consistent with a dominant trait (Burrows, 1938). Although such dominant inheritance was typical, Ruggles Gates observed an aberrant family. In this case unaffected parents were first cousins. About 25% of the children were affected, suggesting an unusual recessive form of brachydactyly (Gates, 1933).

A dominant pattern was also ascertained as the typical pattern for the inheritance of a number of other orthopedic anomalies. Webbing of the fingers [symphalangism] was noted in six successive generations from a Welsh family. Simple dominant heredity was most likely (Daniel, 1936). Scoliosis [curvature of the spine] was evident in females of three successive generations (Rutherfurd, 1934). A larger family showed direct heredity through five generations with equal numbers of men and women. A Mendelian dominant trait was recognized for this disorder (Garland, 1934). Direct transmission for clubbing of the fingers was also noted in several families (Kayne, 1933). Sexes were equally affected. F.L. Horsfall from Canada stated that the character was certainly not sex-linked, but he could not determine whether recessive or dominant inheritance was most likely (Horsfall, 1936). In another study, D.R. Sector concluded that clubbing was most likely a Mendelian dominant trait (Seaton, 1938).

Disorders of connective tissue—the tendons, ligaments and mesodermal elements that held other structures together—also were hereditary with similar patterns noted. Ehlers-Danlos syndrome involved unusual elasticity and fragility of the skin, and hyperextensability of the joints. Direct transmission through three and four generations was evident; the sexes were equally affected (Stuart, 1937; Wigley, 1938). Marfan's syndrome resulted in tall individuals with long digits, hyperextensability of the joints, fragility of major arteries and dislocation of the lenses in the eyes, all due to defective connective tissue. Direct inheritance with both sexes being affected was the common familial pattern (Ormond, 1930; King, 1934). F. Parkes Weber and R.W.B. Ellis agreed that a dominant trait was segregating in these affected families (Weber, 1933; Ellis, 1940).

Muscle disorders also frequently appeared to be directly transmitted from parent to child, as well. Myotonic dystrophy was commonly noted in several successive generations of affected families (Souter, 1933; Caughey, J.F., 1933; Caughey, J.E., 1933). O. Maas, neurologist to the National Hospital in London, collected 57 affected pedigrees. Direct inheritance was the rule. L.S. Penrose reviewed the material and agreed that a dominant character was segregating in these families (Maas, 1937). Another characteristic form of muscular dystrophy—the fascioscapulohumeral type—was evident in direct transmission through three and four successive generations. Dominant inheritance was consistent with the pedigree data (Pearson, 1933; Manson, 1935a). Stanley Barnes, neurologist at the University of Birmingham, discovered a unique familial myopathy. Six generations of 160 people in the family were investigated. Direct parent to child transmission was evident; the sexes were equally affected. About 50% of the offspring inherited the condition. All these features were consistent with a Mendelian dominant pattern for inheritance (Barnes, 1932).

Cancer

Family studies conducted at this time indicated the relevance of heredity as one important agent causing cancer. Macklin conducted an analysis of cancers in identical Canadian twins. She noted the same type of cancer tended to recur in the twins at a similar age (Macklin, 1935b). Unique families appeared to have a hereditary predisposition to developing various forms of cancer. In one example, a grandmother had gastric carcinoma, her daughter had liver cancer, and five granddaughters all suffered from breast cancer (Handley, W.S., 1938). Another example had a woman who stated that she was the thirteenth member of her family to develop cancer. Her daughter had breast cancer while her son developed gastric cancer (Evans, G., 1931).

Characteristic patterns for the inheritance of specific types of tumors were also recognized. Hereditary intestinal polyps were the source of many bowel cancers. Direct transmission from parent to children of both sexes being equally affected was the rule (Dukes, 1930). John Lockhart-Mummery, who had been reluctant to apply Mendelism to human heredity in previous years, now analyzed the inheritance of bowel cancer in ten families. Direct transmission was evident; in one family, affected fraternal twins were observed. He thought the character acted as a Mendelian dominant trait (Lockhart-Mummery and Dukes, 1939). Haldane evaluated the family histories of the ocular tumor retinoblastoma and concluded that a dominant character was evident as an etiologic agent in these cases as well (Haldane, 1933). Another eye tumor, pseudoglioma, was noted in two brothers with unaffected parents. A maternal uncle was also affected. Cockayne suggested a sex-linked recessive pattern for inheritance (Wilson, R., 1936).

Various skin tumors were also evident in multiple members of affected families. Granulosa rubra nasi [a tumor of the nose] appeared to be a dominant character (Hellier, 1937). John Ingram, from the Dermatology Department at the General Infirmary at Leeds, noted three generations of one family affected with sebaceous cysts. Direct transmission again was evident. He thought this was a dominant trait (Ingram and Oldfield, 1937). T.B. Munro from the Royal Eastern Counties Institution at Colchester reported another 20 affected people through four successive generations. His colleague L.S. Penrose reviewed the material and agreed that a Mendelian dominant factor was evident (Munro, T.B., 1937). Tumors of the peripheral nerves often formed in the neurocutaneous syndrome neurofibromatosis [Von Recklinghausen's disease]. Peter Gorer, from the Lister Institute in London, thought a dominant pattern for inheritance was most likely (Gorer, 1937). Another malignant skin tumor in children, xeroderma pigmentosum, appeared to be triggered by sun exposure. A family from Australia had three of eleven children affected (Belisario, 1935). Four of five boys were affected in another family from Uganda where inbreeding was a common ethnic character (Loewenthal and Trowell, 1938). Parents typically were normal. Gorer thought this was most consistent with inheritance of a recessive character (Gorer, 1937).

Eye Disorders

The application of Mendelian heredity to the understanding of the inheritance of eye diseases continued during this decade as well. W.R. Russell reported a family with Leber's disease [hereditary optic atrophy]. The unaffected parents were second cousins. A maternal cousin and three sons were affected. Two daughters and four other sons were normal-sighted. A sex-linked pattern of inheritance appeared to be at work in this case. Russell also noted that females could exhibit evidence of such disorders if they inherited two mutant X-chromosomes: one from the mother and one from the father (Russell, W.R., 1931). A family with affected dizygotic twins (one male and one female) provided an example of such a hereditary mechanism at work (King, 1939). Another family reported by A. Dorrell from the Royal Berkshire Hospital also had affected females. An affected woman produced four affected sons. Her daughter by a second marriage had normal vision, but then produced another affected female (Dorrell, 1932). However, evidence continued to accumulate suggesting that more than one form of optic atrophy existed. A large family segregated what appeared to be Leber's disease through six successive generations. Direct heredity was apparent; ten females and five males were affected (Thompson, A.H. and Willoughby Cushell, 1935). It was concluded that dominant, recessive and sex-linked forms of optic atrophy segregated in specific families.

Charles Usher reported a four-generation family with hereditary esotropia [turning inward of the eye]. Direct transmission produced 13 affected persons: three females and ten males (Usher, 1932). He also reviewed pedigrees from 22 families with epicanthus [an extra skin fold medial to the orbit]. Again, direct transmission was evident; both sexes were affected and could transmit the character to their offspring (Usher, 1935b). The epicanthic fold was sometimes inherited in conjunction with ptosis [drooping of the eyelid]. This usually appeared to be a separate syndrome, also directly inherited with sexes being equally affected in multigenerational families (McIlroy, 1930; Ross, 1932). In all these examples, no specific comments were made regarding the hereditary pattern observed. Finally in 1931,Cockayne reported a five-generation family with 13 affected and 14 normal offspring. He concluded that the trait segregated as a dominant (Cockayne, 1931).

Usher also examined the complex heredity of retinitis pigmentosa in two large families of six generations each. In both examples, direct transmission was evident; males and females were equally afflicted (Usher, 1930). An experimental therapy for retinitis pigmentosa was also reported at this time. Carotene (vitamin A) was administered to adults with early mild forms of the disease. The night blindness that was one of the earliest symptoms improved in many cases. In some subjects the night vision actually improved to a normal level after four months of treatment (Josephson and Freiburger, 1937). These findings generated optimism that hereditary diseases might actually be cured by medical intervention and were not invariably hopeless.

The members of the Ophthalmological Society frequently discussed hereditary aspects of the many different eye diseases. The example set by Nettleship earlier in the century encouraged this next generation of eye specialists to collect pedigrees in order to better understand the role of heredity in the etiology of such human disorders. Several lectures in 1933 summarized the state-of-the-art in this field. Van Duyse reviewed the various sex-linked, recessive and dominant disorders affecting the eye (Van Duyse, 1933). R.C. Punnett from Cambridge discussed the genetic mechanisms to explain the doctors' observations that the same apparent eye disorder could be inherited as a Mendelian dominant in one pedigree, but as a sex-linked trait in another family. Leber's disease and retinitis pigmentosa were the best-known examples of such phenomena. He proposed the existence of a second autosomal gene which acted as an inhibitor of expression of the sex-linked disorder. Segregation would thus appear as a dominant. In other cases, the suppressor gene could be absent, allowing apparent sex-linked heredity to be evident. A similar mechanism had been found to explain the inheritance of feather color in poultry (Punnett, 1933).

Charles Usher presented a discussion of "Heredity in Eye Diseases" in 1933 as well as the prestigious Bowman lecture "On a few Hereditary Eye Affections" to the Society in 1935. In both, he discussed how Mendelian heredity had allowed more accurate diagnosis of specific eye diseases. He used dominant, recessive and sex-linked terminology to outline the relationship between heredity and various specific eye disorders (Usher, 1933, 1935a).

Usher had been in clinical practice for more than 30 years and was quite aware of the important role heredity played in eye diseases. His experiences with Pearson reflected the frustrations of others who worked through the Galton Laboratory but were inhibited by the director in applying modern genetic principles to important human conditions. Usher had collaborated with Pearson as early as 1905 on hereditary aspects of human albinism (Pearson, 1905a). He worked with Nettleship and Pearson on *the Monograph on Albinism* project before the First World War (Pearson, Nettleship and Usher, 1911) and was familiar with developments in Mendelian heredity that were often discussed at the Ophthalmological Society. But his reports noted above in *Biometrika* and *Annals of Eugenics* on eye diseases could only report his observations. The editor, Karl Pearson, forbade any discussion of hereditary mechanisms. At the more accommodating forum of the Ophthalmological Society, of which he was the president, Usher could more openly discuss his interest in applying Mendelian heredity to better understand heredity and eye diseases.

The relevance of these issues soon made its way to the opposite side of the world. The long ocean voyage Bateson took to Australia in 1914 for the B.A.A.S. meeting helped make physicians in that area aware of the importance of Mendelian heredity and disease. For example, the island state of Tasmania had been founded as an English penal colony in 1803. By 1930 it had a population of about 220,000 people. D.J. Hamilton, a local ophthalmologist, surveyed the island's eye disease patients. About 38% of the blind appeared to have a genetic etiology for their condition. He found a large number of different eye diseases and identified characteristic familial patterns for their inheritance consistent with Mendelian recessive, dominant or sex-linked characters. His professional practice had convinced him,

> Since 1900 Mendel's laws have become widely appreciated, so that patients affected with hereditary diseases are now constantly seeking advice from their medical practitioners. Thus it behooves all medical men and especially ophthalmologists to be current with various types of transmission [of hereditary eye disease] (Hamilton, 1938).

Metabolic Disorders

Gout had been recognized for centuries as running through successive generations of certain families. L.L. Hill of the Devonshire Royal Hospital noted a positive family history in 45% of his cases. He explained the direct transmission of the character from parent to child over 400 years in one family as consistent with a dominant character (Hill, 1938).

The inheritance of diabetes was not so straightforward. Macklin in Canada noted both recessive and dominant pedigrees. This suggested to her that several genes were involved in causing this disorder of blood sugar regulation (Macklin, 1933b). Maddox reviewed pedigrees from 250 Australian families. Recessive hereditary was apparent in most cases (Maddox and Scott, 1935). Percy Cammidge collected data from 400 families in England. A recessive pattern for heredity was evident in 28% of families, while 20% had a dominant pattern. The recessive form was most common in cases diagnosed at a younger age. These patients typically required insulin to manage their disease. The dominant variant tended to develop symptoms later in adulthood. Dietary therapy was often adequate in those cases (Cammidge, 1934). Analysis of the pedigree therefore could aid the physician in prescribing treatment for each type of diabetes.

A form of familial hepatitis was presented to the Royal Society of Medicine in which affected children had parents who are unaffected. E.A. Cockayne suggested that the disorder might be a Mendelian recessive, as was Wilson's disease of the liver (Debre, 1939). Richard Ellis described another liver disorder characterized by glycogen storage (Von Gierke's disease). Parents were unaffected, and consanguinity was frequent. This disorder also appeared to be a recessive character (Ellis and Payne, 1936). Other hepatic storage disorders were inherited in the same fashion. Two variants of gargoylism with enlargement of the liver and spleen and unusual bone growth (Hunter and Hurler syndromes) resulted from the abnormal accumulation of lipoid material in the organs. Pedigree analysis was most consistent with recessive inheritance (Cockayne, 1936; Henderson, 1940).

Another inborn error of metabolism termed phenylketonuria was discovered in which affected individuals were unable to metabolize the amino acid phenylalanine derived from dietary protein. The accumulation of abnormal metabolites resulted in mental retardation (Braid and Hickman, 1929). Penrose found two cases in the Colchester study. Pedigree analysis showed normal parents, and he suggested a recessive form for inheritance (Penrose, 1935a). Another large consanguineous family provided further evidence for recessive inheritance. An unaffected woman had married twice. Her first husband was a first cousin. Together, they produced two children affected with phenylketonuria. Her second husband was unrelated, but their son married a maternal cousin. Offspring here also produced two affected children (Penrose, 1935b). The increased frequency of affected individuals within inbred families was quite consistent with a Mendelian recessive character.

NEUROLOGICAL DISEASES

The application of Mendelian analysis continued regarding diseases of the brain and nerves, but success was not so evident. The neurologist Thomas MacLachlan, from the Victoria Infirmary in Glasgow, reported a three-generation family segregating familial periodic paralysis. Direct parent to child inheritance was evident, but he concluded, "Transmission of the disease shows no characteristic feature" (MacLachlan, 1932). Charles Worster-Drought, neurologist to the Metropolitan Hospital, also had trouble identifying the hereditary mechanism involved in a syndrome of presenile dementia and spastic paralysis. Direct inheritance over three generations suggested to him that this was "a Mendelian recessive character" (Worster-Drought, C., 1940; Worster-Drought, L. and McMenery, 1933).

Similar direct inheritance over at least three generations was the rule for neurofibromatosis [Von Recklinghausen's disease] (Van der Hoeve, 1932; Stallard, 1938). Cockayne reviewed 111 affected pedigrees and concluded that dominant inheritance was likely in most families (Cockayne, 1933). Another disorder of the peripheral nervous system called progressive familial hypertrophic polyneuritis appeared to be inherited directly from parent to child through three and four generations. Both sexes were equally affected (Russell, W.R. and Garland, 1930; Cooper, 1936). Hugh Garland assembled thirteen different pedigrees and demonstrated that the character segregated in a Mendelian dominant fashion (Garland, 1936).

The neurocutaneous syndrome tuberous sclerosis [epiloia] was also evident in successive generations of affected families (Critchley and Earl, 1932). Gunther and Penrose analyzed twenty such pedigrees. Clinical symptoms of skin and neurologic disease varied widely within the same family. They concluded that tuberous sclerosis acted like an incomplete dominant character (Gunther and Penrose, 1935). Their sample revealed that about 25% of all cases appeared to be new mutations. The frequency of disease in southeastern England was estimated as 1 in 30,000 lives. Therefore, the mutation rate was expected to be 1 in 120,000 per generation (Penrose and Haldane, 1935).

The role of consanguinity in revealing the existence of recessive characters was evidenced in further analysis of families with neurologic disorders. Inbred families produced children with Tay-Sachs disease in several reports (Maitland-Jones, 1936). One family with related parents from Egypt produced five of eight children affected (Yacoub, 1938). Hogben's colleague, D. Slome from the Department of Social Biology at the University of London, reviewed 135 families with this disorder from the medical literature. Statistical analysis showed good agreement between the expected and actual number of affected children born into these families, assuming that Tay-Sachs disease was a recessive Mendelian character (Slome, 1933). A juvenile form of the same disease was recognized and also appeared to be inherited in a recessive fashion (Norman, 1935).

Consanguinity was another common feature in families with the disorder Gaucher's disease. R.H. Thompson of Guy's Hospital isolated a storage galactolipid from the spleens of affected children (Thompson, R.H.S. and Wright, 1937). The accumulation of such material over time damaged the organs, including the nerves and the brain. T.F. Bloehm from the University of Amsterdam reported a family with three affected siblings. A common grandfather had married twice and produced affected grandchildren in both lines of the family. The pattern of heredity was most consistent with a recessive trait (Bloehm, 1936).

Skin Disorders

Application of Mendelian heredity also assisted in defining various types of skin disease. Ectodermal dysplasia involved defective formation of teeth, hair and other organs in the skin. Those individuals with the anhydrotic variant lacked sweat glands. Males were typically severely affected, while females in the same family were normal or only mildly affected. The character was clearly transmitted through the female. In one pedigree, the fact that one female was mildly affected suggested that this trait was "not strictly sex-linked recessive type" (Rushton, 1934). C.C. de Silva collected six affected families in Ceylon. His cases were typically sex-linked with female carriers. He reviewed his cases with the London skin specialists Cockayne and Parkes Weber (de Silva, 1937; de Silva, 1939). The other variety of ectodermal dysplasia did not have defective sweat glands. Reginald Brain, dermatologist from the Hospital for Sick Children, described this variant which bred true in affected families, being passed directly from parent to child. It acted as a Mendelian dominant trait (Brain, 1937). Another affected French-Canadian family from Quebec appeared to have descended from a common ancestor with the mutation. Dominant inheritance with males and females equally affected was evident (Clouston, 1939).

Bullous eruption of the feet also appeared in successive three and four generation families. Both sexes were affected, and direct transmission was the rule. Cockayne labeled it as a dominant trait (Cockayne, 1938b).

Abnormalities of the nails and hair typically followed Mendelian patterns for inheritance. Multigeneration pedigrees demonstrated the direct transmission of nail dystrophy, characteristic of a dominant trait (Susman, 1934; Templeton, 1936). The analysis of two piebald families in *Biometrika* after R.A. Fisher became the editor reflected the change in scientific orientation for that publication. Cockayne and Nussey reported affected families with direct transmission through five successive generations. Both sexes were affected. The authors were now allowed to state that this pattern for inheritance was consistent with a Mendelian dominant trait (Cockayne, 1935b; Nussey, 1938).

Miscellaneous Conditions

Mendelism appeared beneficial in understanding mechanisms of disease in some cases, but not in others. Premature deafness in adults due to changes in the ear ossicles [otosclerosis] was clearly different from hereditary deafness present at birth. This character segregated with direct transmission through at least three generations, but the physician reporting the analysis did not believe that Mendelian principles would help to explain the inheritance of this disorder (Gray, 1936). The aural surgeon A.B. Smith of Edinburgh noted segregation of unilateral deafness, another specific hereditary trait, through four successive generations. Direct parent to child inheritance was the rule. As late as 1939, the author thought it was "beyond the scope of the paper to discuss the factors of Mendelian inheritance..." (Smith, 1939).

Polycystic kidney disease often affected one parent and subsequent children in certain families. Direct inheritance was typical (Burns, 1933). C.H. Reason from London noted the disorder in fraternal twins, as well as in one parent and other children in a family. This was also consistent with a dominant trait (Reason, 1933).

The hereditary pattern for situs inversus[15] was different. Parents were usually normal, while several children in one generation were affected. The character appeared to be a recessive trait (Manson, 1935b). One family with first cousin parents had three affected and nine normal offspring, again consistent with heterozygous parents and recessive heredity (Feldman, 1935). Cockayne subsequently collected 53 families with situs inversus. About 11% were consanguineous. The typical London consanguinity frequency at that time was close to 1%. The sexes were equally affected. He found monozygotic affected twins. All this was consistent with recessive heredity (Cockayne, 1938a).

Allergic symptoms also were found among members of several generations in specific families. G.W. Bray from the Hospital for Sick Children surveyed 200 family histories for asthma, seasonal allergies and eczema. Other family members were affected in 68% of cases. He could not discern whether the allergy tendency segregated as a Mendelian recessive or dominant character (Bray, 1930). A large family in another report demonstrated direct transmission of the allergic trait from parent to children over five successive generations. Sexes were about equally affected, but no specific hereditary mechanism could be described (Crawford, 1936). But, H. Gruneberg from University College London described chronic sinusitis, another allergic trait, that affected members of a family in three successive generations. Both sexes were equally affected. He described this character as consistent with a Mendelian dominant (Gruneberg, 1934).

The International Genetical Congress

Discussions of medical topics, presented by medical personnel, figured prominently at the Seventh International Genetical Congress that opened in Edinburgh on 23 August 1939. The physician F.A.E. Crew from the Animal Research Institute in Edinburgh was named President of the event. A selection of the 60 lectures relevant to human genetics presented at the conference is listed in Table 14.1.

Twin studies were used to examine the hereditary factors in the mental illness schizophrenia. Monozygotic twins were concordant in 82% of cases, while dizygotic twins both were affected only 12% of the time. This suggested that a strong hereditary predisposition existed for this disorder. Pedigree analysis showed its inheritance as a recessive trait (Hurst, 1940). Madge Macklin reported further analysis of twins and the occurrence of specific human cancers. This class of disease was likewise much more common in identical vs. fraternal twin siblings ("Human Genetics," 1939b), again suggesting a genetic predisposition to cancer.

Cytological evidence was described in which human cells appeared to have 48 chromosomes. Males were XY and females were XX with distinctive morphological differences between the sex chromosomes that had been identified microscopically

(Kemp, T., 1941). Penrose reviewed the genetic aspects of Down syndrome and concluded that it might have its origin as a chromosome anomaly (Penrose, 1941). In another presentation, the genetics of situs inversus was examined using 119 pedigrees. Parents were consanguineous in 11% of cases. Affected children were present in 25% of the offspring. This finding was most consistent with a recessive character (Feldman, 1941). The segregation pattern for phenylketonuria [PKU] was studied in 43 families. Consanguinity was noted in 12% of the cases. Collateral relatives such as aunts, uncles and cousins were also affected. PKU also appeared to be inherited as a recessive trait (Munro, T.A., 1941). The abnormal formation of the skull bones [oxycephaly] was studied in children from 19 family pedigrees. Some variability of expression was noted, but the inheritance pattern was most consistent with a dominant disorder (Feriman, 1941).

Several attempts to demonstrate human genetic linkage were also discussed at the meetings. Barbara Banks from the Cold Spring Harbor Laboratory in the U.S. reported correlations between hair color and deficiency of tooth development ("Human Genetics," 1939). Robert Race from the Galton Laboratory studied the potential linkage relationships between the hereditary anemia termed acholuric jaundice, PTC tasting, attached ear lobe, eye and hair color, and the ABO and MN blood groups. No linkage relationships were identified (Race, Taylor and Vaughan, 1941). J.A. Munro and L.S. Penrose examined the correlation between ABO status and PKU inheritance in 25 families. One possible linkage was observed (Munro, T.A., Penrose and Taylor, 1941). David Finney examined prior work done on allergy predisposition and the blood groups. He also thought there was some evidence of linkage (Finney, 1940, 1941).

Redcliffe Salaman, the general practitioner from Barley near Cambridge, was there as well. He had followed Bateson's 1906 advice to plant potatoes as a way of learning the Mendelian laws for heredity. He had continued this work over the next 35 years and was recognized as a world authority on potato genetics. He now reported his results on breeding potatoes resistant to the infamous 1845 Irish blight (Salaman, 1941).

Table 14.1
Program of the Seventh International Genetical Congress
Edinburgh, Scotland
August 1939

Subject	Speaker
Heredity of manic-depressive disease in Ireland	Tomason
Schizophrenia	Patzig
	Hurst
Human chromosomes	Kemp
Transposition of viscera	Feldman
Acholuric jaundice	Race
External ear disorders	Quelprud
Maternal age and heredity	Penrose
Linkage studies	Banks
	Munro
	Finney
	Penrose
	Taylor
Phenylketonuria	Munro
Anemias	Lundholm
Pick's disease	Sanders
Oxycephaly	Feriman
Intelligence	Hogben
Mental deficiency	Roberts
Cancers in twins	Macklin
Potato blight resistance	Salaman

Reference: Punnett, 1941

The topics on the program for the 1939 Congress in Edinburgh were identical with those of any more recent genetic meeting. Twin studies to assess the role of heredity in a character, human chromosome studies to understand anomalies such as Down syndrome, characterization of new dominant and recessive disorders, and linkage studies to define the human genetic chromosome map were current then and still encompass the work of the modern medical geneticist. An editorial in the *Lancet* pointed out that the 1939 Congress had clearly documented that there was a difference between medical genetics, and plant and animal studies ("Something better," 1939). Medical genetics had now been recognized as a distinct category of medical science and practice.

Fifteen

On the Success and Failure of Competing Theories of Human Genetics

"... by means of thought, Einstein, speculation, mathematics, the Mendelian theory..."
(*Mrs. Dalloway* by Virginia Woolf).

Virginia Woolf's epigram for the modern era from 1925 coalesced the thinking that Mendel's work had come to fruition. It had become an accepted aspect of contemporary European thought. The biometric theory had been subsumed into the expanded Mendelian theory by World War II, as the two competing approaches had been shown not to be at odds with each other, but in fact, coincident and mathematically compatible.

Pearson had earlier published a 1911 treatise titled *The Grammar of Science* that set forth his vision for modern society.

> I assert that the encouragement of scientific investigation and the spread of scientific knowledge by largely inculcating scientific habits of mind will lead to more efficient citizenship and so to increased social stability. Minds trained to scientific methods are less likely to be led by mere appeal to the passions or by blind emotional excitement to constrain certain acts which in the end may lead to social disaster (Pearson, 1911).

Encouraging people to think scientifically then would surely guide them to choose correctly for the future good of civilization. But in his own campaign to encourage consideration of the biometric theory for heredity by the public in general, and the medical community in England in particular, Pearson expressed fear that there was no longer a level playing field. He complained, "Mendelism is at present the mode—no other conception of heredity can even obtain a hearing..." (Pearson, Nettleship and Usher, 1913). Over the years he had collaborated with a large number of physicians on specific projects such as the albinism memoir. He acted as general clerk of the works, arranging tasks to be completed by the physicians. But when he lost interest in the project, it was not even completed.

Pearson's worst fears were, in fact, realized in the publications from his own institution, the Eugenics Record Office. He had declared that issues of *Biometrika*, the *Annals of Eugenics* and the memoir series *Treasury of Human Inheritance* published after 1910 would be free of theorizing. Facts alone would be presented for other scientific investigators to utilize in the future. This goal largely succeeded. The positive (white bar) and the negative (black bar) articles about Mendelism that appeared in the Galton

Laboratory's publications before 1940 are presented in Figure 15.1. Only two positive analyses slipped through Pearson's editorial hand in the twenty years before his retirement in 1933. But once R.A. Fisher took over as editor, numerous articles discussing Mendelian theory and human heredity again appeared from the Laboratory. To Pearson's dismay, without exception, the articles utilized Mendelism to explain, in modern statistical terms, the heredity of both normal and abnormal human characters. No mention of the biometric approach that he had developed again appeared in those pages before World War II.

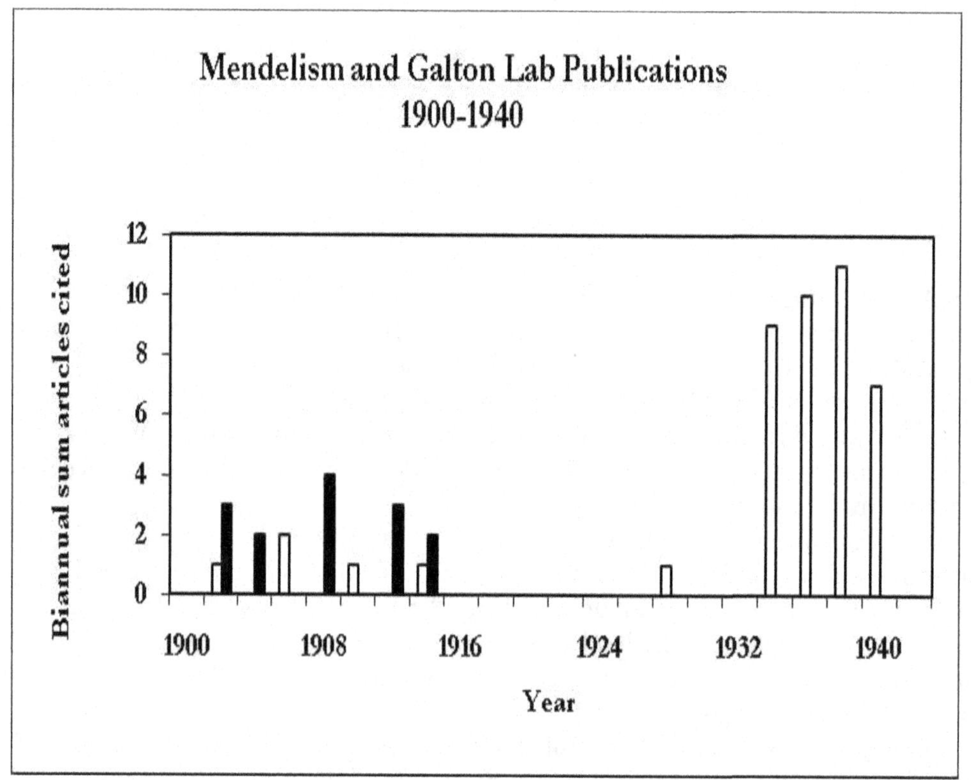

Figure 15.1

It appears that consciously or not, Pearson did everything he could to ensure that the biometric theory would fail to be accepted by British medical personnel of his day. Every new theory needs a champion, some prominent individual in the community of scientists to act as spokesperson for the new idea (Rushton, 1994). Scientific ideas compete in an open market place. Each offers the possibility of a plausible solution to what might be a potentially significant problem. In its promise, an idea will attract other scientists—fellow explorers, who will criticize and ultimately determine the idea's usefulness in the real world. While these explorers can breathe life into an idea, their absence or defection leads to its death (Krantz and Wiggins, 1973).

Pearson did champion biometry in the first decade of the new century. But, the 1904 Oxford B.A.A.S. meeting, the Royal Society of Medicine meetings in 1908, and his own conclusion that biometry and Mendelism were not incompatible in 1909 deflated his enthusiasm for his own theory. He was unable to admit that he was wrong to claim that Mendelism had not been shown to successfully explain the transmission of any human hereditary condition (Pearson, 1909). The biometric theory died because of lack of interest by the British medical community. In the scientific community at large, "The greatest danger of any new idea is for it to be ignored" (Hukk, 1988). Pearson declared his research group to be "theory-free" in 1910 and never spoke before another audience on the role of his views on genetics and medical practice after 1912.

A scientific theory may appear brilliant to its creator but if it cannot be used to explain natural phenomena, it will not be accepted by other practitioners. One model for a successful scientific theory requires that the new idea must:

1. Provide a model for problem solving;
2. Have both theoretical and practical features;
3. Be shared by a community of practitioners involved in problem solving;
4. And be accepted in time by a wider community of practitioners and eventually the general public (Greenblatt, 2003).

Pearson's management of his theory of heredity may be contrasted with the work of another prominent scientist of the same era. Albert Einstein argued that any scientific theory had to reflect the essential harmony that he believed existed in nature (Levenson, 2003a). He was personally invested in his theories, too. By 1913 he had developed a theory of general relativity that was both mathematically elegant and also made specific predictions that could be tested in the real world (Levenson, 2003b). A team from the Royal Society examined data on the bending of light during a solar eclipse in 1919. The results were precisely as Einstein had predicted. His graceful theory had successfully captured nature at work. Einstein was delighted. He noted, "I knew I was right" (Levenson, 2003c).

But Einstein did not fear discussion of his ideas with other scientists. As early as 1911, he began to attend conferences where his theories could be criticized by his colleagues. After World War I, he traveled to England, France, Japan, Israel and the United States to both popularize his theories and to listen to comments from other workers in the field of theoretical physics (Levenson, 2003d).

Although he felt personally attached to his own theories, Einstein was able to propose an idea, seek its validation in nature and then reject a theory if it did not explain natural phenomêna. In 1929 he published a unified field theory that was elegant and, he thought, complete. To his mind the "...results [were] so beautiful that I have every confidence" that they were correct (Levenson, 2003e). But the theory could not be tested; it made no predictions that could be tried experimentally. Two years later Einstein agreed that the equations reflected nothing about reality and hence were worthless for constructing a scientific theory (Levenson, 2003f).

In contrast with Pearson, Bateson collaborated with British physicians, acting as a mentor, helping them learn about heredity by analyzing the family data they gathered in ways that would prove useful in the daily practice of medicine. The understanding of how specific diseases were inherited in particular families allowed physicians to explain the causes of many disorders and to guide families in reproductive plans for the future. He, too, did not appear before many medical audiences after 1913. But unlike Pearson, Bateson had medical colleagues who had learned from their interaction with him and then could both apply the Mendelian theory to pedigree data and explain to their own colleagues the relevance of the new theory of heredity to medical practice. The numbers of articles on Mendelism in the British medical literature from 1910 to 1940 is presented in Figure 15.2. The interest in Mendelism peaked during the first decade of the century when the new theory was being discussed and then initially applied to human characters. Interest waned during World War I, and then rose in the 1920s before surging in the 1930s as new techniques began to develop a genetic map for human beings.

New ideas always conflict with accepted facts in any profession. New theories are not always applicable to any particular scientific field just because they are novel. The physician in the early twentieth-century was in an intellectual transition between the classical gentleman and the scientist-clinician of the modern era. Scientific observations, experiments, reasoning and innovations in medical theories always clashed with the conservative culture of accepted wisdom based on clinical experience—the art of medical practice (Youngson, 1979).

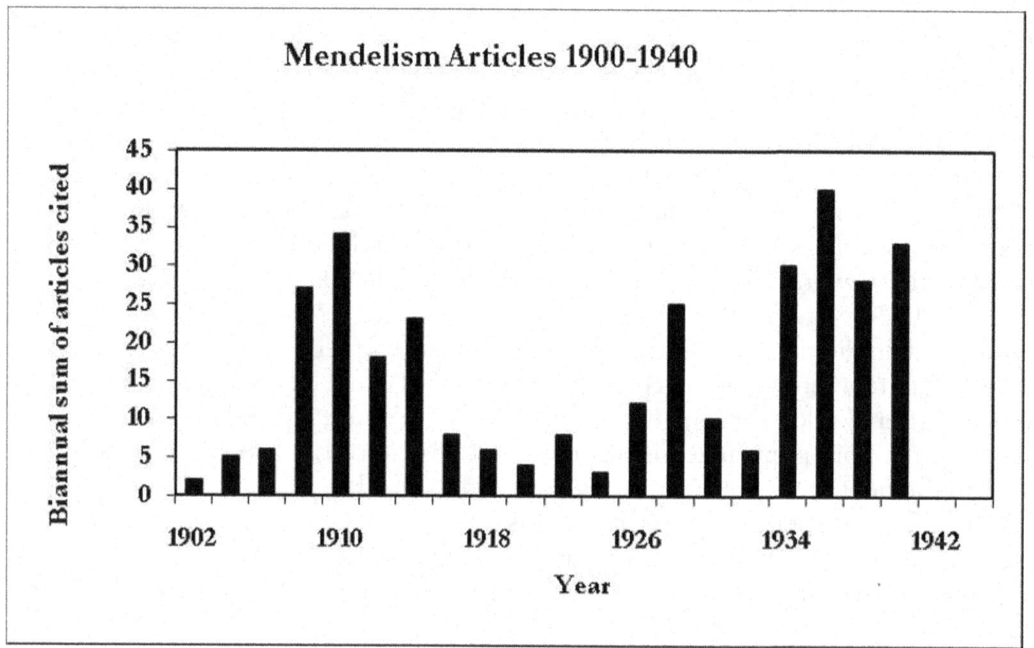

Figure 15.2

The publications on Mendelism during this period of time written by Fellows of the Royal Colleges of Physicians and Surgeons are examined in Figure 15.3. The black bars represent the works published between 1902 and 1916, while the white bars represent later works from 1927 to 1940. During the earlier period, younger men certainly did publish on the topic of Mendelism and medicine, but the majority of material was presented by senior men. By the later period, just before World War II, the next generation of physicians had emerged and had become familiar with the role of Mendelism at a much younger age. In this case, the majority of publications were prepared by the younger men with the senior Fellows still actively involved.

This analysis is not meant to assess the intelligence or perspicacity of British physicians in general. Rather, it is intended to be a crude index of orthodoxy in medical thought. Those men and women who became Fellows of the several colleges were accepted as middle of the road, as safe practitioners by the medical community. If they accepted Mendelism as established young physicians and surgeons, this would certainly indicate that the theory had become the norm for the medical establishment in Britain.

NEW PATHS IN GENETICS

The Second World War once again curtailed development of medical genetics in the British medical community. J.B.S. Haldane presented a lecture with this title at the University of Groningen in Holland during March 1940. He summarized the state of the field before barely escaping the German invasion of the Netherlands by sneaking

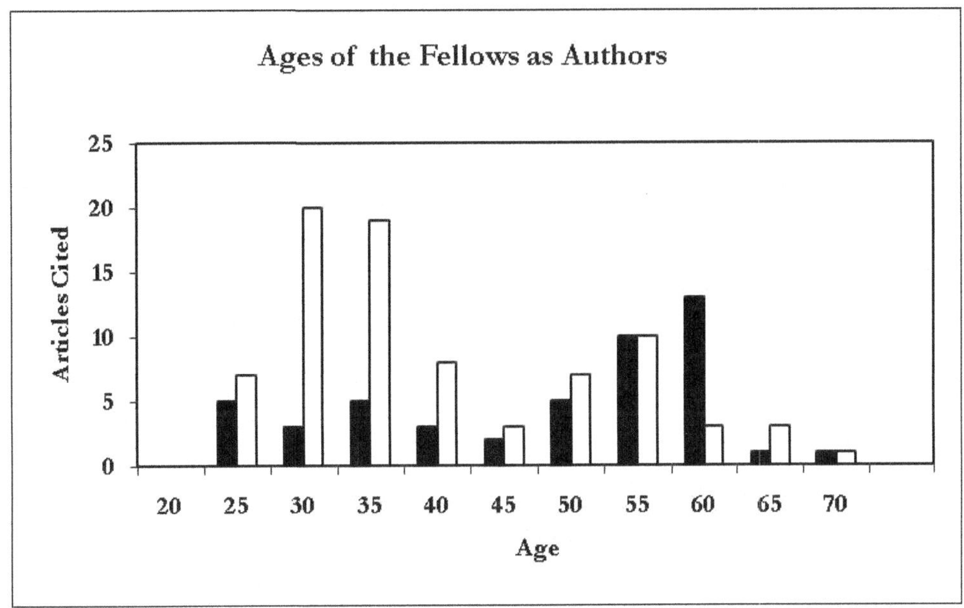

Figure 15.3

through Scandinavia before returning to England (Haldane, 1942). Ruggles Gates spent the war years in the United States revising his 1929 book *Heredity in Man* into a two-volume work titled *Human Genetics*, comprising 1518 pages when it finally appeared in 1946 (Gates, 1929, 1946).

By then Mendelism had come into its own. After the War, the Galton Laboratory was recognized as an international center for the training of physicians and scientists on the latest teachings in both theoretical and practical human genetics. Speculation about human heredity finally had a solid theoretical base. This occurred because its concepts functioned in the real world of medical practice. William Harvey had suggested the same test of a scientific approach in 1651:

> Nor is any long refutation necessary where the truth can be seen with one's proper eyes; where the inquirer by simple inspection finds everything in conformity with reason; and where at the same time he is made to understand how unsafe, how base a thing it is to receive instruction from other's comments without careful examination of the objects themselves, the rather as the book of Nature lies open and is so easy of consultation (Meyer, 1936).

The physicians of the modern era did examine their pedigree data and found the application of the Mendelian theory of genetics most useful in the contemporary practice of medicine.

Appendix

Appendix

The Hereditary Disease Database (H.D.D.) was developed over several years by a detailed reading of the *Index Medicus* which began publication in 1879 under the sponsorship of the Surgeon General of the United States. The *Index* was a monthly author and subject compilation of all the world's medical literature, truly an immense undertaking in the years before computerization. The Table lists the subject headings reviewed in each issue for the compilation of the H.D.D. The *Index Medicus* ceased publication in mid-1898 due to financial constraints. Another publication, *Bibliographica Medica*, began publication the following year in Paris. It used a different indexing system and was not as comprehensive. This endeavor lasted only two years. The *Index Medicus* resumed publication in 1903 and continued in the same format until 1927. Thereafter, it was recast as a quarterly publication with a revised subject-heading list. For statistical purposes in this book, the periods before and after 1927 have been considered separately. More than 6000 references were examined in the course of building the H.D.D. on which this work is grounded.

H.D.D. Subject Headings
Index Medicus 1879-1927

Abnormalities and deformities
Achondroplasia
Acrocephaly
Albinism
Alopecia, hereditary
Anemia, sickle cell
Anemia, splenic
Asthma, hereditary
Ataxia
Atrophy, muscular
Blood groups
Bones, fragility and growth
Brain, disease
Cancer, cells and heredity
Cerebellum, diseases and tumors
Chorea, hereditary
Chromosomes
Colorblindness
Constitution
Cornea, abnormalities and diseases
Cretinism
Deafness, hereditary
Dementia praecox, hereditary
Diabestes insipidus
Diabetes mellitus, hereditary
Diathesis
Dwarfism
Dystrophy, muscular
Ectodermal defects
Edema, hereditary
Epidermolysis
Epilepsy, hereditary
Eugenics
Exostoses
Eyelids, ptosis
Eyes, abnormalities
Eye diseases
Feeblemindedness, hereditary
Fingers and toes, abnormalities
Foot, deformities
Glaucoma, etiology
Gout
Hair, diseases and growth
Hand, deformities
Harelip
Heart, deformities
Hemeralopia
Hemochromatosis
Hemophilia
Heredity
Hernia, inguinal
Hydrocephalus
Hypertelorism
Hypospadius
Ichthyosis
Idiocy, amaurotic and mongolian
Iris, abnormalities
Jaundice, hemolytic
Keratosis
Kidneys, cysts
Lens, crystalline, abnormalties
Lenticular nucleus, degeneration
Liver, cysts
Marriage
Mental diseases, hereditary
Microcephaly
Migraine, hereditary
Myatonia congenita
Myopia
Myotonia congenita
Nails, abnormalities
Nephritis, etiology
Neuritis, multiple
Neurofibromatosis
Niemann's disease
Nose, deformities
Nystagmus
Ochronosis
Palate, cleft

H.D.D. Subject Headings, *Continued*
***Index Medicus* 1879-1927**

Parkinsonism
Patella, deformities
Peptic ulcer, hereditary
Polydactyly
Psoriasis, hereditary
Pupils, abnormalities
Pyramidal tract, diseases
Retina, abnormalities and tumors
Retinitis pigmentosa
Sclera, blue
Sclerosis, amyotrophic lateral
Siderosis
Skin diseases, hereditary
Skin tumors, hereditary
Spasm
Spine, curvature
Splenomegaly
Strabismus
Syphilis, congenital
Syringomyelia, hereditary
Teeth, abnormalities
Telangiectasis
Tremor
Tuberculosis, hereditary
Tumors, hereditary
Twins
Urine, alkapton and pentose
Vasomotor system
Xanthoma
Xeroderma pigmentosum

Notes

Notes

1. Apparitions.
2. Yolk of the egg.
3. Asserting one particular church's beliefs.
4. Serious nose bleeds.
5. Mercury.
6. Attributes.
7. Ballooning of the aorta.
8. Interesting that certain facts of medical practice never change!
9. Shortly before his death in 1926, Bateson presented a lecture on recent developments in human genetics before the University College Medical Society in London (Bateson, W. (1925) Lecture notes. 17 November 1925 (B G8C-18)).
10. The Pearson papers at the University College London also contain no drafts of the manuscript for Part III of the monograph (Higgit, R. (1998) Personal communication from the Manuscripts and Rare Book Division, University College London Library. 5 January 1998).
11. In sex-linked disorders, the pedigree charts typically showed an affected father, then an unaffected carrier daughter in the next generation, followed by an affected grandson in the most recent generation. This skipping pattern has been likened to the jumping course of the knight's moves in the game of chess. See Figure 13.1.
12. Difficulty focusing on distant objects .
13. Fisher, R.A. (1934-1935) The detection of linkage with "dominant" abnormalities. Annals of Eugenics 6:187-201.

———. (1934-1935) The detection of linkage in recessive abnormalities. Annals of Eugenics 6:339-351.

———. (1934) The amount of information supplied by families as a factor of linkage in the population sampled. Annals of Eugenics 6:66-70.

Haldane, J.B.S. (1932) A method for investigating recessive characters in man. Journal of Genetics 25:251-255.

———. (1934-1935) Methods for the detection of autosomal linkage in man. Annals of Eugenics 6:26-65.

———. (1937-1938) The estimation of the frequencies of recessive conditions in man. Annals of Eugenics 8:255-262.

Haldane JBS, P. Moshinsky. (1939) Inbreeding in Mendelian populations with special reference to cousin marriages. Annals of Eugenics 9:321-340.

Hogben L.T. (1931) The genetic analysis of familial traits. Journal of Genetics 25:97-112.

———. (1932) The genetic analysis of familial traits. Journal of Genetics 25:211-240.

———. (1932) Filial and fraternal correlations of sex-linked inheritance. Proceedings of the Royal Society of Edinburgh 52:331-336.

———. (1932) The correlation of relatives on the supposition of sex-linked transmission. Journal of Genetics 26:417-432.

———. The effect of consanguineous parentage upon metrical characters in the offspring. Proceedings of the Royal Society of Edinburgh 53:233-251.

———. (1934) The detection of linkage in human families I. Both heterozygous genotypes indeterminate. Proceedings of the Royal Society London 114B:340-353.

13, *continued.* ———. (1934) The detection of linkage in human families III. One heterozygous genotype indeterminate. Proceedings of the Royal Society London 114B:353-364.

Penrose L.S. (1934-1935) The detection of autosomal linkage data which consist of pairs of brothers and sisters with unspecified parentage. Annals of Eugenics 6:133-137.

———. (1937-1938) Genetic linkage in graded human characters. Annals of Eugenics 8:233-237.

14. Kevles, D.J. (1985) In the Name of Eugenics. New York: Knopf.

Farrall, L.A. (1985) The Origins and Growth of the English Eugenics Movement 1865-1925. New York: Garland Publishing.

Mazumdar, P.M.H. (1992) Eugenics, Human Genetics and Human Failings. London: Routledge.

15. Transposition of the internal thoracic and abdominal organs.

References

References

General biographical data was obtained from:

Thorne, J.D., J.C. Collocott. (1984). Chambers Biographical Dictionary. Edinburgh: W. and R. Chambers.
Who's Who 1897-1998. (1998). CD-ROM. Oxford: Oxford University Press.
Dictionary of National Biography. (1995) CD-ROM. Oxford, Oxford University Press.

The general source on British history was:

Kenyon, J.P. (1992). A Dictionary of British History. Chatham: Mackays.

The following abbreviations are used to designate unpublished manuscript material:

APS	American Philosophical Society Philadelphia, PA	Letters of William Bateson Letters of Charles Darwin
P	Special Collections Division University College Library London, England	Manuscripts from Karl Pearson Collection
B	John Innes Archives, courtesy of John Innes Foundation Norwich Bioscience Institute Norwich, England	Manuscripts from William Bateson Collection
C	Scientific Manuscripts Collection Syndics of Cambridge University Library Cambridge, England	Letters of William Bateson Letters of Charles Darwin

PREFACE

Baltzer, F. (1964) Theodor Boveri. Science 144:809-815.
———. (1967) Theodor Boveri: The Life of a Great Biologist 1862-1915. Berekeley: University of California Press.
Bateson, B. (1928) William Bateson, F.R.S. Naturalist: His Essays and Addresses. Cambridge: Cambridge University Press, p. 93.
Bateson, W. (1900) Problems of heredity as a subject for horticultural investigation. Journal of the Royal Horticultural Society 25:1-8.
Churchill, F.B. (1987) From heredity theory to Vererbung: The transmission problem 1850-1915. Isis 78:336-364.
Correns, C. (1900) G. Mendel's Regel uber das Verhalten der Nachkommenschaft der Rassenbastarde. Berichte der Deutscher botanischer Gesellschaft 18:158-168.
De Vries, H. (1900a) Sur la loi de disjunction des hibrides. Comptes Rendus de l'Academie des Science 130:845-847.
———. (1900b) Das Spaltungsgesetz der Bastarde. Berichte der Deutscher botanischer Gesellschaft 18:83-90.
Dunn, L.C. (1991a) A Short History of Genetics. Ames, Iowa: Iowa State University Press, pp. 4-5.
———. (1991b) A Short History of Genetics, p. 113.
Mayr, E. (1982a) The Growth of Biologic Thought. Cambridge: Harvard University, p. 729.
———. (1982b) The Growth of Biologic Thought, pp. 748-749.
Muller-Wille, S. (2007) Figures of Inheritance, 1650-1850. In S. Muller-Wille and H.J. Rheinberger (eds): Heredity Produced—At the Crossroads of Biology, Politics and Culture. Cambridge, MA: MIT Press, pp. 177-204.
Olby, R. (1985) Origins of Mendelism, 2nd ed. Chicago: University of Chicago, p. 136.
———. (1987) William Bateson's introduction of Mendelism to England: A reassessment. British Journal for the History of Science 30:399-420.
Rheinberger, H.J. (1995) When did Correns read Gregor Mendel's paper? Isis 86:612-616.
Stamhuis, I., O.G. Meijer, and E.J.A. Zevenhuizen (1999) Hugo de Vries on heredity. Isis 90:238-267.
Sutton, W.S. (1902) On the morphology of the chromosome group in *Brachylata mogra.* Biological Bulletin 4:124-139.
Von Tschermak, E. (1900) Uber kunstliche Kreuzung bei *Pisum sativum.* Berichte der Deutscher botanischer Gesellschaft 18:232-239.
Von Tschermak-Seysenegg, E. (1951) The rediscovery of Gregor Mendel's work. Journal of Heredity 42:163-171.
Wilson, E.B. (1895) An Atlas of the Fertilization and Karyokinesis of the Ovum. New York: Macmillan, p. 4.
———. (1900a) The Cell in Development and Inheritance, 2nd ed. New York: Macmillan, pp. 244-245.
———. (1900b) The Cell in Development and Inheritance, pp. 351-352.
———. (1902) Mendel's principles of heredity and the maturation of germ cells. Science 16:991-993.
Zirkle, C. (1964) Some oddities in the delayed discovery of Mendelism. Journal of Heredity 55:65-72.

CHAPTER ONE

Bodemer, G.W. (1974) Materialistic and neoplatonic influences in embryology. In A.G. Debus (ed): Medicine in Seventeenth Century England. Berkeley: University of California, p. 183.

Booth, C.C. (1979) The development of clinical science in Britain. British Medical Journal 1:1469-1473.

Conrad, L.I., M. Neve, V. Nutton, et al, (eds). (1995a) The Western Medical Tradition. Cambridge: Cambridge University Press, p. 254.

———. (1995b) The Western Medical Tradition, pp. 330-337.

———. (1995c) The Western Medical Tradition, p. 291.

———. (1995d) The Western Medical Tradition, pp. 330-340.

Frank, R.G. (1980a) Harvey and the Oxford Physiologists. Berkeley: University of California, p. 16.

———. (1980b) Harvey and the Oxford Physiologists, pp. 25-28.

———. (1980c) Harvey and the Oxford Physiologists, p. 26.

———. (1980d) Harvey and the Oxford Physiologists, p. 27.

Gould, S.J. (2000) Francis Bacon and the instrument of Instauration. Science 287:254-255.

Guyton, A.G. (1989) William Harvey, His Times, and Achievements. In R. Willis (ed): The Works of William Harvey. Philadelphia: University of Pennsylvania.

Harrison, P. (2001) Curiosity, forbidden knowledge and the Reformation of natural philosophy in early modern England. Isis 92:265-290.

Harvey, W. (1651a) Exercitationes de Generatione Animalium. London: Syndenham Society, 1847 edition, p. xi.

———. (1651b) Exercitationes de Generatione Animalium, p. 151.

———. (1651c) Exercitationes de Generatione Animalium, p. 157.

———. (1651d) Exercitationes de Generatione Animalium, p. 336.

———. (1651e) Exercitationes de Generatione Animalium, p. 338.

———. (1651f) Exercitationes de Generatione Animalium, p. 356.

———. (1651g) Exercitationes de Generatione Animalium, p. 74.

———. (1651h) Exercitationes de Generatione Animalium, p. 575.

Hesse, M. (1970) Francis Bacon. In C.C. Gillispie (ed): Dictionary of Scientific Biography, Vol. 1. New York: Scribners, pp. 372-377.

Keele, K.D. (1974) Physiology. In A.G. Debus (ed): Medicine in Seventeenth Century England. Berkeley: University of California, p. 152.

Keynes, G. (1966) The Life of William Harvey. Oxford: Oxford University Press, pp. 9-11.

Knobil, E. (1981) William Harvey and the physiology of reproduction. Physiologist 24:3-7.

Lopez-Beltran, C. (2007) The Medical Origins of Heredity. In S. Muller-Wille and H.J. Rheinberger (eds): Heredity Produced—At the Crossroads of Biology, Politics and Culture. Cambridge, MA: MIT Press, p. 108.

Meyer, A.W. (1936) An analysis of De Generatione Animalium of William Harvey. Stanford, CA: Stanford University Press, pp. 20-21.

Muller-Wille, S. (2007) Figures of Inheritance, 1650-1850. In S. Muller-Wille and H.J. Rheinberger (eds): Heredity Produced—At the Crossroads of Biology, Politics and Culture. Cambridge, MA: MIT Press, pp. 177-204.

Muller-Wille, S. and H.J. Rheinberger. (2007) Heredity—The Formation of an Epistemic Space. In S. Muller-Wille and H.J. Rheinberger (eds): Heredity Produced—At the Crossroads of Biology, Politics and Culture. Cambridge, MA: MIT Press, p. 3.
Ravetz, J.R. (1972) Francis Bacon and the reform of philosophy. In A.G. Debus (ed): Science, Medicine and Society in the Renaissance, Vol. 2. New York: Neale Watson, p. 100.
Sloan R. (1996) English Medicine in the Seventeenth Century. Durham: Durham Academic Press, p. 82.
Warhaft, S. (ed). (1965a) Francis Bacon—A Selection of his Works. Indianapolis: Odyssey Press, p. 328.
———. (1965b) Francis Bacon—A Selection of his Works, p. 332.
———. (1965c) Francis Bacon—A Selection of his Works, pp. 305-306.
———. (1965d) Francis Bacon—A Selection of his Works, p. 333.
———. (19653) Francis Bacon—A Selection of his Works, p. 299.
———. (1965f) Francis Bacon—A Selection of his Works, p. 364.
———. (1965g) Francis Bacon—A Selection of his Works, p. 320.
Wear, A. (1995a) Medicine in early modern Europe 1500-1700. In L.I. Conrad (ed): The Western Medical Tradition. Cambridge: Cambridge University Press, pp. 334-335.
———. (1995b) Medicine in early Modern Europe 1500-1700, p. 337.
Willius, F.A. and T.E. Keys. (1941) Classics of Cardiology. New York: Dover, p. 15.

Chapter Two

Browne, T. (1672) Pseudodoxia Epidemica, 6th ed. London: J.R. for Nath. Ekins, p. 7.
Digby, K. (1645) Two Treatises: In the One of Which, the Nature of Bodies, in the Other, In Way of Discovery of the Immortality of Reasonable Souls. London: John Williams, p. 266.
Floyer, J. (1698) Treatise of the Asthma. London: Wilkins, p. 20.
Frank, R.G. (1980a) Harvey and the Oxford Physiologists. Berkeley: University of California, p. 46.
———. (1980b) Harvey and the Oxford Physiologists, pp. 48-50.
———. (1980c) Harvey and the Oxford Physiologists, pp. 52-89.
———. (1980d) Harvey and the Oxford Physiologists, pp. 23-30.
———. (1980e) Harvey and the Oxford Physiologists, p. 36.
Fulton, J.F. (1937) Sir Kenelm Digby. New York: Oliver.
Gayton, E. (1654) Pleasant notes upon Don Quixot. Quoted in Compact Edition of the Oxford English Dictionary 1971 edition. Oxford: Oxford University Press, p. 237
Glanvill, J. (1676) Letters and Poems in Honour of the Incomparable Princess, Margaret, Dutchess of Newcastle. London: Newcombe, p. 124.
Glisson, F. (1668) A Treatise of the Rickets. London: Streater, pp. 151-152.
Godon, J.E. (1966) Nathaniel Highmore. Practitioner 196:851-858.
———. (1972) Nathaniel Highmore. In C.C. Gillispie (ed): Dictionary of Scientific Biography, Vol. 6. New York: Scribners, pp. 386-387.
Grell, O.P. and A. Cunningham. (1996a) Religio Medici—Medicine and Religion in Seventeenth Century England. Hants, England: Scolar Press, pp. 44-45.
———. (1996b) Religio Medici—Medicine and Religion, pp. 2-3.

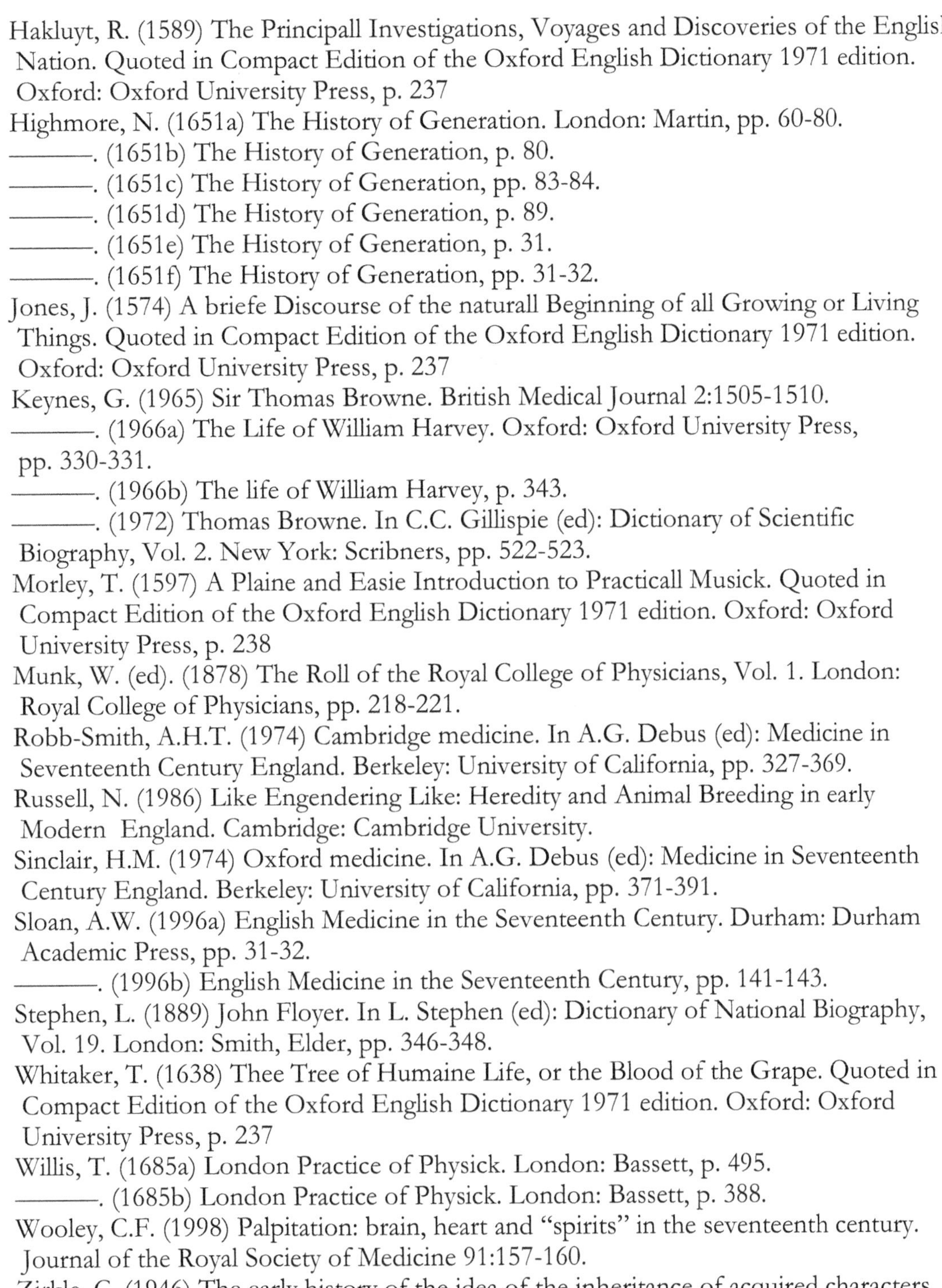

Hakluyt, R. (1589) The Principall Investigations, Voyages and Discoveries of the English Nation. Quoted in Compact Edition of the Oxford English Dictionary 1971 edition. Oxford: Oxford University Press, p. 237

Highmore, N. (1651a) The History of Generation. London: Martin, pp. 60-80.

———. (1651b) The History of Generation, p. 80.

———. (1651c) The History of Generation, pp. 83-84.

———. (1651d) The History of Generation, p. 89.

———. (1651e) The History of Generation, p. 31.

———. (1651f) The History of Generation, pp. 31-32.

Jones, J. (1574) A briefe Discourse of the naturall Beginning of all Growing or Living Things. Quoted in Compact Edition of the Oxford English Dictionary 1971 edition. Oxford: Oxford University Press, p. 237

Keynes, G. (1965) Sir Thomas Browne. British Medical Journal 2:1505-1510.

———. (1966a) The Life of William Harvey. Oxford: Oxford University Press, pp. 330-331.

———. (1966b) The life of William Harvey, p. 343.

———. (1972) Thomas Browne. In C.C. Gillispie (ed): Dictionary of Scientific Biography, Vol. 2. New York: Scribners, pp. 522-523.

Morley, T. (1597) A Plaine and Easie Introduction to Practicall Musick. Quoted in Compact Edition of the Oxford English Dictionary 1971 edition. Oxford: Oxford University Press, p. 238

Munk, W. (ed). (1878) The Roll of the Royal College of Physicians, Vol. 1. London: Royal College of Physicians, pp. 218-221.

Robb-Smith, A.H.T. (1974) Cambridge medicine. In A.G. Debus (ed): Medicine in Seventeenth Century England. Berkeley: University of California, pp. 327-369.

Russell, N. (1986) Like Engendering Like: Heredity and Animal Breeding in early Modern England. Cambridge: Cambridge University.

Sinclair, H.M. (1974) Oxford medicine. In A.G. Debus (ed): Medicine in Seventeenth Century England. Berkeley: University of California, pp. 371-391.

Sloan, A.W. (1996a) English Medicine in the Seventeenth Century. Durham: Durham Academic Press, pp. 31-32.

———. (1996b) English Medicine in the Seventeenth Century, pp. 141-143.

Stephen, L. (1889) John Floyer. In L. Stephen (ed): Dictionary of National Biography, Vol. 19. London: Smith, Elder, pp. 346-348.

Whitaker, T. (1638) Thee Tree of Humaine Life, or the Blood of the Grape. Quoted in Compact Edition of the Oxford English Dictionary 1971 edition. Oxford: Oxford University Press, p. 237

Willis, T. (1685a) London Practice of Physick. London: Bassett, p. 495.

———. (1685b) London Practice of Physick. London: Bassett, p. 388.

Wooley, C.F. (1998) Palpitation: brain, heart and "spirits" in the seventeenth century. Journal of the Royal Society of Medicine 91:157-160.

Zirkle, C. (1946) The early history of the idea of the inheritance of acquired characters and of pangenesis. Transactions of the American Philosophical Society 35:101.

CHAPTER THREE

Akenside, M. (1768) Observations on cancers. Medical Transactions 1:64-69.
Baker, H. (1755) A supplement to the account of a distempered skin. Philosophical Transactions 49:21-24.
Bate, J. (1759-1760) An account of the remarkable alteration of colour in a Negro woman. Philosophical Transactions 51:175-178.
Braudel, F. (1981) The Structures of Everyday Life, Vol. 1. New York: Harper and Row, pp. 528-548.
Byrd, W. (1697) An account of a Negro boy that is dappled in several places of his body with white spots. Philosophical Transactions 19:781-782.
Cooke, B. (1749) A child born with jaundice upon it, received from its father, and of the mother taking the same abstemper from her husband, the next time being with child. Philosophical Transactions 46:205-207.
Cyprianus (1695) An account of a child born with a large wound in the breast, supposed to proceed from the force of imagination. Philosophical Transactions 19:291-292.
Darwin, C. (1868) The Variation of Animals and Plants under Domestication, Vol. 2. London: John Murray. Chapter 27.
Elliotson, J. (1831) Ichthyosis. London Medical Gazette 7:636-637.
Frank, R.G. (1980a) Harvey and the Oxford Physiologists. Berkeley: University of California, pp. 43-57.
———. (1980b) Harvey and the Oxford Physiologists, p. 25.
Freke, J. (1739-1741) A case of extraordinary exostoses on the back of a boy. Philosophical Transactions 41:369-370.
Galbraith, D. (2001) The Rising Sun. New York: Grove Press, pp. 155-157.
Girdlestone, T. (1802) Letter. Medical and Physical Journal 8:508.
Gregory, W. (1739) An account of a monstrous fetus, resembling a hooded monkey. Philosophical Transactions 41:764-766.
"Gresham College history" (2006). http://www.gresham.ac.uk/newpage1.htm. Accessed 25 April 2006.
Hall, A.R. (1974) Medicine and the Royal Society. In A.G. Debus (ed): Medicine in Seventeenth Century England. Berkeley: University of California, p. 425.
Harrison, P. (2001) Curiosity, forbidden knowledge and the Reformation of natural philosophy in early modern England. Isis 92:265-290.
Hesse, M. (1970) Francis Bacon. In C.C. Gillispie (ed): Dictionary of Scientific Biography, Vol. 1. New York: Scribners, pp. 372-377.
Huddart, J. (1777) An account of persons who could not distinguish colors. Philosophical Transactions 67:260-265.
Hunter, J. (1780) Account of a woman who had smallpox during pregnancy, and who seemed to have communicated the same disease to the fetus. Philosophical Transactions 70:128-142.
Hunter, M. (1981) Science and Society in Restoration England. London: Cambridge University Press, p. 8.
Keele, K.D. (1974) Physiology. In A.G. Debus (ed): Medicine in Seventeenth Century England. Berkeley: University of California, p. 163.
Kenyon, J.P. (ed). (1992) A Dictionary of British History. Ware: Wordsworth, p. 158.
Laslett, T.P.R. (1960) The foundation of the Royal Society and the medical profession in England. British Medical Journal 2:165-169.

Lort, M. (1778) An account of a remarkable imperfection of sight. Philosophical Transactions 68:611-614.
Lyons, H. (1944a) The Royal Society 1660-1940. Cambridge: Cambridge University Press, p. 27.
———. (1944b) The Royal Society 1660-1940, p. 17.
———. (1944c) The Royal Society 1660-1940, pp. 341-342.
Machin, J. (1731-1732) An uncommon case of distempered skin. Philosophical Transactions 37:299-300.
Martin, P.J. (1818) Case of hereditary ichthyosis. Medico-Chirurgical Transactions 9:52-55.
Morgan, K.V. (ed). (1997a) The Oxford Illustrated History of Britain. Oxford: Oxford University Press, p. 293.
———. (1997b) The Oxford Illustrated History of Britain, p. 351.
Mortimer, C. (1749) The case of a lady, who was delivered of a child, which had the smallpox appeared in a day or two after its birth. Philosophical Transactions 46:233-234.
Munk, W. (ed). (1878) The Roll of the Royal College of Physicians, Vol. 1. London: Royal College of Physicians, pp. 218-221.
"The New World voyages of William Dampier" (1999). Athena Review 1:1-4.
Parsons, J. (1765) An account of the white Negro shown before the Royal Society. Philosophical Transactions 55:45-53.
Pearson, K., E. Nettleship, and C.H. Usher. (1911-1913) A Monograph on Albinism in Man. London: Dulau.
Penrose, L. and C. Stern (1958) Reconsideration of the Lambert pedigree (ichthyosis hystrix gravior). Annals of Human Genetics 22:258-283.
Porter, R. (1989) The early Royal Society and the spread of medical knowledge. In R. French and A. Wear (eds): The Medical Revolution of the Seventeenth Century. Cambridge: Cambridge University Press, pp. 272-293.
Prest, W. (1998) Albion Ascendent—English History 1660-1815. Oxford: Oxford University Press, p. 26.
"The Royal Society" (2006). http://www.english.upenn.edu. jlynch/FrankDemo/Contexts/rs.html. Accessed 5 April 2004.
Sedgwick, W. (1861) On sexual limitation in hereditary disease. British and Foreign Medico-Chirurgical Review 27:477-489.
Sinclair, H.M. (1974) Oxford medicine. In A.G. Debus (ed): Medicine in Seventeenth Century England. Berkeley: University of California, pp. 371-391.
Sloan, A.W. (1996) English Medicine in the Seventeenth Century. Durham: Durham Academic Press, p. 170.
Stimson, D. (1948a) Scientists and Amateurs—A History of the Royal Society. New York: Schuman, pp. 37-45.
———. (1948b) Scientists and Amateurs—A History of the Royal Society, pp. 46-50.
Wafer, L. (1699) A New Voyage and Description of the Isthmus of America. London: James Knopton, pp. 134-138.
Wallis, J. (1700) "Account of some Passages of his Life." http://www.fordham.edu/halsdall/med/1662royalsociety.html. Accessed 4 April 2004.
Watson, W. (1749) Some accounts of the fetus in utero being differently affected by smallpox. Philosophical Transactions 46:235-237.
Wear, A. (1995a) Medicine in early modern Europe 1500-1700. In L.I. Conrad (ed): The Western Medical Tradition. Cambridge: Cambridge University Press, pp. 215-361.

———. (1995b) Medicine in early modern Europe 1500-1700. In L.I. Conrad (ed): The Western Medical Tradition, p. 341.
Webster, C. (1967) The College of Physicians: "Solomon's House" in Commonwealth England. Bulletin of the History of Medicine 49:393-412.

CHAPTER FOUR

Ackerknecht, E.H. (1982) Diathesis: The word and the concept in medical history. Bulletin of the History of Medicine 56:317-325.
Armstrong, G. (1777) An Account of the Diseases most Incident to Children from Birth till the Age of Puberty. London: T. Cadell.
Barrett, C. (1904) Diary and Letters of Madame D'Arbley. London: Macmillan.
Booth, C.C. (1979) The development of clinical science in Britain. British Medical Journal 1:1469-1473.
Browne, E.J. (1995) Charles Darwin Voyaging. Princeton: Princeton University Press, p. 37.
Bynum, W.F. (1980) Health, disease and medical care. In G.S. Rousseau and R. Porter (eds): The Ferment of Knowledge. Cambridge: Cambridge University Press, pp. 211-253.
Cook, H.J. (2000a) Boerhaave and the flight from reason. Bulletin of the History of Medicine 74:234.
———. (2000b) Boerhaave and the flight from reason. Bulletin of the History of Medicine 74:236.
Corfield, P.J. (1995) Power and the Professions in Britain 1700-1850. London: Routledge, p. 138.
Cross, S.J. (1981a) John Hunter, the Animal Oeconomy and late eighteenth century physiological discourse. Studies in the History of Biology 5:1-110.
———. (1981b) John Hunter, the Animal Oeconomy and late eighteenth century physiological discourse. Studies in the History of Biology 5:31.
———. (1981c) John Hunter, the Animal Oeconomy and late eighteenth century physiological discourse. Studies in the History of Biology 5:35.
Dalton, J. (1794) Extraordinary facts relating to the vision of colours. Memoirs and Proceedings of the Manchester Literary and Philosophical Society 5:28-45.
Darwin, E. (1800a) Phytologia. London: T. Bensley, p. 115.
———. (1800b) Phytologia, p. 130.
———. (1801a) Zoonomia, or the Laws of Organic Life, 3rd ed., Vol. 2. London: J. Johnson, pp. 296-297.
———. (1801b) Zoonomia, p. 296.
———. (1801c) Zoonomia, p. 311.
———. (1801d) Zoonomia, p. 178.
———. (1801e) Zoonomia, p. 179.
———. (1803) Zoonomia; or the Laws of Organic Life, Second American ed., Vol. 1. Boston: Thomas and Andrews, p. 394.
———. (1804a) The Temple of Nature. New York: Sword, p. 139.
———. (1804b) The Temple of Nature, p. 175.
———. (1804c) The Temple of Nature, p. 177.
———. (1804d) The Temple of Nature, p. 178.
Digby, A. (1994) Making a Medical Living. Cambridge: Cambridge University Press.
Duddell, B. (1736) Treatise of the Diseases of the Horny Coat of the Eye and the Various Kinds of Cataract. London: Lark.
"Editorial" (1757). Medical Observations and Inquiries 1:iii-xii.

"Editorial" (1768). Medical Transactions 1:ii-iii.

"Editorial" (1773). Memoirs of the Medical Society of London 1:iii-iv.

"Editorial" (1784). Medical Communication of the Society for Promoting Medical Knowledge 1:iii-vi.

Farar, S. (1790) An account of a very uncommon blindness in the Eyes of newly born children. Medical Communication of the Society for Promoting Medical Knowledge 2:463-465.

Fordyce, W. (1784) Fragmenta Chirurgica et Medica. London: T. Codell, p. 41.

Franklin, A.W. (1974a) Clinical medicine. In A.G. Debus (ed): Medicine in Seventeenth Century England. Berkeley: University of California, pp. 113-145.

———. (1974b) Clinical medicine. In A.G. Debus (ed): Medicine in Seventeenth Century England, p. 123.

———. (1974c) Clinical medicine. In A.G. Debus (ed): Medicine in Seventeenth Century England, p. 131.

———. (1974d) Clinical medicine. In A.G. Debus (ed): Medicine in Seventeenth Century England, p. 119.

———. (1974e) Clinical medicine. In A.G. Debus (ed): Medicine in Seventeenth Century England, pp. 134-136.

Goldsmith, O. (1774) History of the Earth, vol. 2, p. 238. Quoted in Zirkle, C. (1946) The early history of the idea of the inheritance of acquired characters and of pangenesis. Transactions of the American Philosophical Society 35:91-151.

Granshaw, L. (1992) The rise of the modern hospital in Britain. In A. Wear (ed): Medicine in Society. Cambridge: Cambridge University Press, pp. 197-218.

Gregory, J. (1788) A Comparative View of the State and Faculties of Man with those of the Animal World, p. 17. Quoted in Zirkle, C. (1946) The early history of the idea of the inheritance of acquired characters and of pangenesis. Transactions of the American Philosophical Society 35:91-151

Heberden, W. (1768) On the chicken pox. Medical Transactions 1:427-436.

——— (1785) On the measles. Medical Transactions 3:389-406.

Hunter, J. (1775) Disputatio Inauguralis Quaedam de Hominum Varietibus et Harum Causis, Exponens, p. 386. Quoted in Zirkle, C. (1946) The early history of the idea of the inheritance of acquired characters and of pangenesis. Transactions of the American Philosophical Society 35:91-151

Hunter, J. (1780) Account of a woman who had smallpox during pregnancy, and who seemed to have communicated the same disease to the fetus. Philosophical Transactions 70:128-142.

King, L.S. (1958) The Medical World of the Eighteenth Century. Chicago: University of Chicago.

King-Hele, D. (1999a) Erasmus Darwin—A Life of Unequalled Achievement. London: Giles de la Mare, p. 88.

———. (1999b) Erasmus Darwin—A Life of Unequalled Achievement, p. 44.

Kite, C. (1795) Cases of several women who had smallpox during pregnancy. Memoirs of the Medical Society of London 4:295-320.

Langford, P. (1992) A Polite and Commercial People—England 1727-1783. Oxford: Oxford University Press.

Lawrence, C. (1994a) Medicine in the Making of Modern Britain 1700-1921. London: Routledge.

———. (1994b) Medicine in the Making of Modern Britain 1700-1921, p. 15.

Lawrence, S.C. (1995) Anatomy and address: Creating medical gentlemen in eighteenth-century London. In V. Nutton and R. Porter (eds): The History of Medical Education in Britain. Amsterdam: Rodopi, pp. 199-228.

———. (1996a) Charitable Knowledge: Hospital Pupils and Practitioners in Eighteenth Century London. Cambridge: Cambridge University Press.
———. (1996b) Charitable Knowledge, p. 234.
———. (1996c) Charitable knowledge:, p. 261.
Lopez-Beltran, C. (2007a) The Medical Origins of Heredity. In S. Muller-Wille and H.J. Rheinberger (eds): Heredity Produced—At the Crossroads of Biology, Politics and Culture. Cambridge, MA: MIT Press, pp. 111-112.
———. (2007b) The Medical Origins of Heredity. In S. Muller-Wille and H.J. Rheinberger (eds): Heredity Produced—At the Crossroads of Biology, Politics and Culture, p. 109.
Loudon, I. (1986) Medical Care and the General Practitioner 1750-1850. Oxford: Clarendon Press.
Lucas, J. (1795) Remarks upon peculiarities in the human system apparently arising from disease before birth. Memoirs of the Medical Society of London 4:94-102.
Neitz, M. and J. Neitz (1995) Numbers and ratios of visual pigment genes for normal red-green color vision. Science 267:1013-1016.
Owen, J.B. (1974) The Eighteenth Century 1714-1815. New York: Norton.
Pearson, J. (1793) Practical Observations on Cancerous Complaints. London: Johnson.
Perceval, C. (1790) Letter to Robert Perceval. Transactions of the Royal Irish Academy 4:97-98.
Porter, R. (1995a) Disease, Medicine and Society. Cambridge: Cambridge University Press, p. 21.
———. (1995b) The Eighteenth Century. In L.I. Conrad (ed): The Western Medical Tradition. Cambridge: Cambridge University Press, pp. 371-475.
———. (1995c) The Eighteenth Century. In L.I. Conrad (ed): The Western Medical Tradition, p. 404.
———. (1995d) The Eighteenth Century. In L.I. Conrad (ed): The Western Medical Tradition, pp. 379-380.
Porter, R. and D. Porter (eds). (1988a) In Sickness and in Health: The British Experience 1650-1850. New York: Basil Blackwell.
———. (1988b) In Sickness and in Health: The British Experience 1650-1850, p. 160.
Rather, L.J. (1974a) Pathology in Mid-Century. In A.G. Debus (ed): Medicine in Seventeenth Century England. Berkeley: University of California, p. 86.
———. (1974b) Pathology in Mid-Century. In A.G. Debus (ed): Medicine in Seventeenth Century England, p. 99.
Risse, G. (1992a) Medicine in the age of enlightenment. In A. Wear (ed): Medicine in Society. Cambridge: Cambridge University Press, pp. 149-195.
———. (1992b) Medicine in the age of enlightenment. In A. Wear (ed): Medicine in Society, p. 171.
———. (1992c) Medicine in the age of enlightenment. In A. Wear (ed): Medicine in Society, p. 170.
Rowley, W. (1790) A Treatise on One Hundred Eighteen Principle Diseases of the Eyes and Eyelids. London: Wingrove.
Rushton, A.R. (2008) Royal Maladies: Inherited Diseases in the Ruling Houses of Europe. Victoria, British Columbia: Trafford.
Turnbull, W. (1795) A case where smallpox was communicated from the mother to the child in utero. Memoirs of the Medical Society of London 4:364-367.
Wafer, L. (1699) A New Voyage and Description of the Isthmus of America. London: James Knopton.
Walker, R.M. (1965) Medical Education in Britain. London: Whitefriars.
Waller, J.C. (2002a) The illusion of an explanation: The concept of hereditary disease. Journal of the History of Medicine 57:427.

———. (2002b) The illusion of an explanation: The concept of hereditary disease. Journal of the History of Medicine 57:419.
———. (2002c) The illusion of an explanation: The concept of hereditary disease. Journal of the History of Medicine 57:418-419.
Watson, W. (1749) Some accounts of the fetus in utero being differently affected by smallpox. Philosophical Transactions 46:235-237.
Wear, A. (1989) Medical practice in late seventeenth and early eighteenth century England. In R. French and A. Wear (eds): The Medical Revolution of the Seventeenth Century. Cambridge: Cambridge University Press, p. 295
———. (1992) Making sense of health and the environment in early modern England. In A. Wear (ed): Medicine in Society. Cambridge: Cambridge University, pp. 119-147.
Wilson, P.K. (2003) Erasmus Darwin on hereditary disease: Conceptualizing heredity in Enlightenment English medical writings. In J.H. Rheinberger and W. Muller S (eds): A Cultural History of Heredity II: 18th and 19th Centuries. Berlin: Max Planck Institut fur Wissenschaftsgeschichte, p. 116.

Chapter Five

Beales, D. (1969a) From Castlereagh to Gladstone 1815-1885. New York: Norton, p. 88.
———. (1969b) From Castlereagh to Gladstone 1815-1885, p. 108.
———. (1969c) From Castlereagh to Gladstone 1815-1885, p. 175.
———. (1969d) From Castlereagh to Gladstone 1815-1885, pp. 180-181.
Beaglehole, J.G. (1974) The Life of Captain James Cook. Stanford CA: Stanford University Press, pp. 506-507.
———. (1966) The Exploration of the Pacific. Stanford CA: Stanford University Press, pp. 229-311.
Bynum, W.F. (1980) Health, disease and medical care. In G.S. Rousseau and R. Porter (eds): The Ferment of Knowledge. Cambridge: Cambridge University Press, pp. 246-247.
Corfield, P.J. (1995) Power and the Professions in Britain 1700-1850. London: Routledge.
Desmond, A. (1989) The Politics of Evolution. Chicago: University of Chicago Press, p. 101.
Durey, M. (1983) Medical elites, the general practitioner and patient power during the cholera epidemic of 1831-2. In I. Inkster and J. Jarrell (eds): Metropolis and Province, Science in British culture, 1780-1850. Philadelphia: University of Pennsylvania Press, pp. 257-278.
Fee, E. and D. Porter. (1992) Public health, preventive medicine and professionalization: England and America in the nineteenth century. In A. Wear (ed): Medicine in Society. Cambridge: Cambridge University Press, pp. 249-275.
Foole, G.A. (1954) Science and its function in early nineteenth century England. Osiris 11:438-454.
Haigh, E. (1991) William Brande and the chemical education of medical students. In R. French and A. Wear (eds): British Medicine in an Age of Reform. London: Routledge, pp. 186-202.
Hibbert, C. (1987a) The English: A Social History. New York: Norton, p. 601.
———. (1987b) The English: A Social History, p. 603.
———. (1987c) The English: A Social History, p. 605.

Hill, J. (1985) The new man of science in nineteenth century Britain. Perspectives in Biology and Medicine 28:581-586.
Hope, J. (1839) A Treatise on the Diseases of the Heart and Great Vessels, 3rd ed. London: Churchill.
Langford, P. (1992a) A Polite and Commercial People—England 1727-1783. Oxford: Oxford University Press, pp. 13-14.
———. (1992b) A Polite and Commercial People—England 1727-1783, p. 291.
———. (1992c) A Polite and Commercial People—England 1727-1783, pp. 66-67.
———. (1992d) A Polite and Commercial People—England 1727-1783, pp. 660-663.
Lawrence, C. (1994) Medicine in the Making of Modern Britain 1700-1921. London: Routledge.
Lawrence, S.C. (1996) Charitable Knowledge: Hospital Pupils and Practitioners in Eighteenth Century London. Cambridge: Cambridge University Press, p. 310.
Loudon, I. (1984) The concept of the family doctor. Bulletin of the History of Medicine 58:347-362.
———. (1992) Medical practitioners 1750-1850 and the period of medical reform in Britain. In A. Wear (ed): Medicine in Society. Cambridge: Cambridge University Press, pp. 219-247.
MacLeod, R.M. (1983a) Whigs and savants: reflections on the reform movement in the Royal Society, 1830-1848. In I. Inkster and J. Jarrell (eds): Metropolis and Province, Science in British Culture, 1780-1850. Philadelphia: University of Pennsylvania Press, pp. 60-63.
———. (1983b) Whigs and savants: reflections on the reform movement in the Royal Society, 1830-1848. In I. Inkster and J. Jarrell (eds): Metropolis and Province, Science in British Culture, 1780-1850. Philadelphia: University of Pennsylvania Press, pp. 64-66.
———. (1983c) Whigs and savants: reflections on the reform movement in the Royal Society, 1830-1848. In I. Inkster and J. Jarrell (eds): Metropolis and Province, Science in British Culture, 1780-1850. Philadelphia: University of Pennsylvania Press, p. 71.
———. (1983d) Whigs and savants: reflections on the reform movement in the Royal Society, 1830-1848. In I. Inkster and J. Jarrell (eds): Metropolis and Province, Science in British Culture, 1780-1850. Philadelphia: University of Pennsylvania Press, p. 57.
———. (1983e) Whigs and savants: reflections on the reform movement in the Royal Society, 1830-1848. In I. Inkster and J. Jarrell (eds): Metropolis and Province, Science in British Culture, 1780-1850. Philadelphia: University of Pennsylvania Press, pp. 76-78.
———. (1983f) Whigs and savants: reflections on the reform movement in the Royal Society, 1830-1848. In I. Inkster and J. Jarrell (eds): Metropolis and Province, Science in British Culture, 1780-1850. Philadelphia: University of Pennsylvania Press, p. 56.
———. (1983g) Whigs and savants: reflections on the reform movement in the Royal Society, 1830-1848. In I. Inkster and J. Jarrell (eds): Metropolis and Province, Science in British Culture, 1780-1850. Philadelphia: University of Pennsylvania Press, pp. 79-80.
Matthew, C. (2000a) The Nineteenth Century. Oxford: Oxford University Press, p. 55.
———. (2000b) The Nineteenth Century, p. 42.

Orange, A.D. (1972a) The origins of the British Association for the Advancement of Science. British Journal for the History of Science 6:152-176.
———. (1972b) The origins of the British Association for the Advancement of Science. British Journal for the History of Science 6:156-157.
———. (1972c) The origins of the British Association for the Advancement of Science. British Journal for the History of Science 6:169.
Owen, J.B. (1974a) The Eighteenth Century 1714-1815. New York: Norton, pp. 124-125.
———. (1974b) The Eighteenth Century 1714-1815, pp. 296-297.
———. (1974c) The Eighteenth Century 1714-1815, pp. 153-157.
Poynter, F.N.L. (1961) The influence of government legislation on medical practice. In F.N.L. Poynter (ed): The Evolution of Medical Practice in Britain. London: Pitman, pp. 5-16.
———. (1966) Education and the General Medical Council. In F.N.L. Poynter (ed): The Evolution of Medical Education in Britain. London: Pitman, p. 201.
Rohl, J.C.G., M. Warren, and D. Hunt. (1999) Purple Secret—Genes, 'Madness,' and the Royal Houses of Europe. London: Bantam, pp. 134-135.
Shortt, S.E.D. (1983) Physicians, science and status: Issues in the professionalization of Anglo-American medicine in the nineteenth century. Medical History 27:51-68.
Tansey, E.M. (1994) The funding of medical research before the Medical Research Council. Proceedings of the Royal Society of Medicine 87:546-548.
Trohler, U. (2000a) "To Improve the Evidence of Medicine" The 18th Century British Origins of a Critical Approach. Edinburgh: Royal College of Physicians of Edinburgh, p. xi.
———. (2000b) "To Improve the Evidence of Medicine" The 18th Century British Origins of a Critical Approach, p. 3.
———. (2000c) "To Improve the Evidence of Medicine" The 18th Century British Origins of a Critical Approach, p. 9.
———. (2000d) "To Improve the Evidence of Medicine" The 18th Century British Origins of a Critical Approach, p. 32.
———. (2000e) "To Improve the Evidence of Medicine" The 18th Century British Origins of a Critical Approach, p. 35.
———. (2000f) "To Improve the Evidence of Medicine" The 18th Century British Origins of a Critical Approach, p. 83.
———. (2000g) "To Improve the Evidence of Medicine" The 18th Century British Origins of a Critical Approach, p. 70.
———. (2000h) "To Improve the Evidence of Medicine" The 18th Century British Origins of a Critical Approach, p. 126.
Waddington, I. (1977) General practitioners and consultants in early nineteenth century England: The sociology of an intra-professional conflict. In J. Woodward and D. Richards (eds): Health Care and Popular Medicine in Nineteenth Century England. New York: Holmes and Meier, pp. 164-188.
———. (1984a) The Medical Profession in the Industrial Revolution. Atlantic Highlands, NJ: Humanities Press, pp. 17-18.
———. (1984b) The Medical Profession in the Industrial Revolution, pp. 3-4.
———. (1984c) The Medical Profession in the Industrial Revolution, p. 11.
———. (1984d) The Medical Profession in the Industrial Revolution, pp. 3-4.
Walker, R.M. (1965) Medical Education in Britain. London: Whitefriars.

Warner, J.H. (1991a) The idea of science in English medicine: The 'decline of science' and the rhetoric of reform, 1815-45. In R. French and A. Wear (eds): British Medicine in an Age of Reform. London: Routledge, pp. 136-164.
———. (1991b) The idea of science in English medicine: The 'decline of science' and the rhetoric of reform, 1815-45. In R. French and A. Wear (eds): British Medicine in an Age of Reform. London: Routledge, p. 147.
Weisz, G. (2001) Reconstructing Paris medicine. Bulletin of the History of Medicine 75:105-119.
Williams, L.P. (1961) The Royal Society and the founding of the British Association for the Advancement of Science. Notes and Records of the Royal Society of London 16:221-233.
Woodward, J. (1961) Medicine and the city in the nineteenth-century experience. In F.N.L. Poynter (ed): The Evolution of Medical Practice in Britain. London: Pitman, p. 69.
Youngson, A.J. (1979) The Scientific Revolution of Victorian Medicine. London: Helm.

CHAPTER SIX

Adams, J. (1814a) A Treatise on the Supposed Hereditary Properties of Diseases. London: Callow, p. 11.
———. (1814b) A Treatise on the Supposed Hereditary Properties of Diseases, p. 12.
———. (1814c) A Treatise on the Supposed Hereditary Properties of Diseases, p. 13
———. (1814d) A Treatise on the Supposed Hereditary Properties of Diseases, p. 14.
———. (1814e) A Treatise on the Supposed Hereditary Properties of Diseases, pp. 16-17.
———. (1814f) A Treatise on the Supposed Hereditary Properties of Diseases, p. 18.
———. (1814g) A Treatise on the Supposed Hereditary Properties of Diseases, pp. 19-21.
———. (1814h) A Treatise on the Supposed Hereditary Properties of Diseases, pp. 25-32.
———. (1814i) A Treatise on the Supposed Hereditary Properties of Diseases, pp. 33-34.
———. (1814j) A Treatise on the Supposed Hereditary Properties of Diseases, pp. 87-89.
———. (1814k) A Treatise on the Supposed Hereditary Properties of Diseases, pp. 41.
Adams, W. (1812) Practical Observations on Ectropium. London: Callow, pp. 103-104.
———. (1817) Practical Inquiry into the Causes of frequent Failure of the Operation of Depression and Extraction of Cataract. London: Baldwin.
Arnott, A. (1833) Thirty one fractures in one and the same individual. London Medical Gazette 12:366.
Bach, J.R. (2000) The Duchenne de Boulogne-Meryon controversy and pseudohypertrophic muscular dystrophy. Journal of the History of Medicine 55:158- 178.
Barry, M. (1843) Observation. Philosophical Transactions 133:33.
Bellingham, O. (1855) Cases of harelip. Dublin Medical Press 33:161-163.
Bondeson, J. (1996) The hairy family of Burma. Journal of the Royal Society of Medicine 89:403-408.
Bronner, E. (1856) Cases of colour blindness. Medical Times and Gazette 14:359-361.

Buckle, H.T. (1857) History of Civilisation in England, Vol. 1. London: Routledge, p.162
Burnes, D. (1840) Hemorrhagic diathesis. Lancet 1:404-406.
Burns, A. (1809) Observations on Some of the Most Frequent and Important Diseases of the Heart. Edinburgh: Muirhead.
Buxton, D. (1859) On the affect of maternal impressions during gestation in producing the deafness of children. Liverpool Medico-Chirurgical Journal 3:29-34.
Carlisle, A. (1814) An account of a family having hands and feet with supernumerary fingers and toes. Philosophical Transactions 104:94-101.
Cartron, L. (2003) Pathological heredity as a bid for greater recognition of medical authority in France, 1800-1830. In J.H. Rheinberger and S. Muller-Wille (eds): A Cultural History of Heredity II: 18th and 19th Centuries. Berlin: Max Planck Institut fur Wissenschaftsgeschichte, pp. 123-124.
———. (2007) Degeneration and "Alienism" in early nineteenth-century France. In S. Muller-Wille and J.H. Rheinberger (eds): Heredity Produced— At the Crossroads of Biology, Politics and Culture, 1500-1870. Cambridge: MIT Press, pp. 166-167.
Cochrane, J. (1841) On the hemorrhagic diathesis. Lancet 2:147.
Combe, G. (1825) System of Phrenology, Vol. 2. Edinburgh: J. Anderson, pp. 481-483.
Cooper, W. (1857) Microphthalmos. Royal London Ophthalmic Hospital Reports 1:110-116.
Curling, T. (1851) Cases of exostosis. Lancet 2:529-530.
Davis, R. (1850) Lamentable effects of the mental emotion of the mother on the fetus in utero. Lancet 2:466.
Davis, T. (1826) Case of hereditary hemorrhea. Edinburgh Medical and Surgical Journal 25:291-293.
Dieffenbach, E. (1841) An account of the Chatham Islands. Journal of the Royal Geographic Society 11:195-215.
Dyer, S.S. (1846) Case of cataract in both eyes, occurrence of the affection in the males of three generations. Provincial Medical and Surgical Journal:383-384.
Elliotson, J. (1831) Ichthyosis. London Medical Gazette 7:636-637.
———. (1840a) Human Physiology, 5th ed., Vol. 2. London: Longman, pp. 1095-1096.
———. (1840b) Human Physiology, 5th ed., Vol. 2. London: Longman, p. 1103.
Emery, A.E. (1989) Joseph Adams (1756-1818). Journal of Medical Genetics 26:116-118.
Emery, A.E.H. and M.L.H. Emery. (1995a) The History of a Genetic Disease. London: Royal Society of Medicine, pp. 28-29.
———. (1995b) The History of a Genetic Disease, pp. 36-38.
Garrod, A. (1859) Nature and Treatment of Gout. London: Walton, pp. 250-255.
Goss, J. (1822) On the variation in the colour of peas, occasioned by cross-impregnation. Transactions of the Horticultural Society of London 5:234-237.
Green, M. (1824) Surgical lecture. Lancet 2:254.
Hamilton, A. (1827) Hairy men; white Negroes. London Medical Repository and Review 5:266-267.
"Hereditary tendency to hemorrhage." (1826) Edinburgh Medical and Surgical Journal 25:455-456.
Holland, H. (1857) Medical Notes and Reflections. Philadelphia: Lea and Blanchard.
Home, E. (1828a) Lectures on Comparative Anatomy, Vol. 5. London: Nicol, pp. 186-87.
———. (1828b) Lectures on Comparative Anatomy, Vol. 5, pp. 190-192.
Houston, J. (1842) Cases of harelip. Dublin Medical Press 7:129-131.

Humphreys, D. (1813) On a new variety in the breeds of sheep. Philosophical Transactions 103:88-95.
Hurst, A.F. (1927) The Constitutional Factor in Disease. London: Kegan Paul, Trench, Trubner, p. 9.
Hutchinson, H. (1946) Jonathan Hutchinson. London: Heinemann, p. 217.
Hutchinson, J. (1857) Hereditary influence. Journal of Psychological Medicine 10:384-402.
"Institution for investigating the nature of cancer." (1806) Edinburgh Medical and Surgical Journal 2:382-389.
"Intermarriage." (1839) British and Foreign Medical Review 7:370-385.
Kellie, A. (1808) Letter. Edinburgh Medical and Surgical Journal 4:252-253.
King, L.J. (1970) Alexander Walker. In C.C. Gillispie (ed): Dictionary of Scientific Biography, Vol. 14. New York: Scribners, pp. 128-131.
Knight, T.A. (1823) Some remarks on the supposed influence of the pollen in crossbreeding. Transactions of the Horticultural Society of London 5:377-380.
Lane, S. (1840) Haemorrhagic diathesis—successful transfusion of blood. Lancet 1:185-188.
Langworthy, W.S. (1850) Singular congenital malformation. Lancet 1:146.
Latham, R.M. (1846) On Diseases of the Heart, Vol. 2. London: Longman.
Lawrence, M. (1827) On cataracts. Lancet 10:678.
"A letter to Dr. Keller." (1808) Edinburgh Medical and Surgical Journal 4:252-253
Lewes, G.H. (1859a) The Physiology of Common Life, Vol. 2. Edinburgh: W. Blackwood, pp. 376-377.
———. (1859b) The Physiology of Common Life, Vol. 1, pp. 375-409.
Lomax, E. (1977) Hereditary or acquired disease? Early nineteenth century debates on the cause of infantile scrofula and tuberculosis. Journal of the History of Medicine 32:356-374.
Lopez-Beltran, C. (2003a) Heredity old and new: French physicians and l'heredite naturelle in early 19th century. In J.H. Rheinberger and W. Muller S (eds): A Cultural History of Heredity II: 18th and 19th Centuries. Berlin: Max Planck Institut fur Wissenschaftsgeschichte, pp. 10-13.
———. (2003b) Heredity old and new: French physicians and l'heredite naturelle in early 19th century. In J.H. Rheinberger and W. Muller S (eds): A Cultural History of Heredity II: 18th and 19th Centuries. Berlin: Max Planck Institut fur Wissenschaftsgeschichte, p. 7.
———. (2003c) Heredity old and new: French physicians and l'heredite naturelle in early 19th century. In J.H. Rheinberger and W. Muller S (eds): A Cultural History of Heredity II: 18th and 19th Centuries. Berlin: Max Planck Institut fur Wissenschaftsgeschichte, p. 17.
———. (2004) In the cradle of heredity; French physicians and L'Heredite Naturelle in the early 19th century. Journal of the History of Biology 37:39-72.
———. (2006) Storytelling, statistics and hereditary thought: the narrative support of early statistics. Studies in the History and Philosophy of Biology and Biomedical Sciences 37:41-58.
Lucas, P. (1847a) Traite Philosophique et Physiologique de l'Heredite Naturelle dans les Etats de Sante et de Maladie du Systeme Nerveux, Vol. 1. Paris: J.B. Bailliere.
———. (1847b) Traite Philosophique et Physiologique de l'Heredite Naturelle dans les Etats de Sante et de Maladie du Systeme Nerveux, Vol. 1, p. 472.

MacKinder, D. (1857) Deficiency of fingers transmitted through six generations. British Medical Journal 1:845-846.
"A many toed and fingered family." (1834) London Medical Gazette 14:65.
Marcet, A. (1817) An Essay on the Chemical History and Medical Treatment of Calculous Disorders. London: Longman.
Martin, P.J. (1818) Case of hereditary ichthyosis. Medico-Chirurgical Transactions 9:52-55.
Meryon, E. (1836a) The Physical and Intellectual Constitution of Man Considered. London: Smith, Elder and Co., p. 100.
———. (1836b) The Physical and Intellectual Constitution of Man Considered, p. 116.
———. (1851) On fatty degeneration of the voluntary muscles. Lancet 2:588-589.
———. (1852) On granular and fatty degeneration of the voluntary muscles. Medico-Chirurgical Transactions 35:73-85.
———. (1864) Practical and Pathological Researches on the Various Forms of Paralysis. London: Churchill.
Motulsky, A.G. (1959) Joseph Adams (1756-1818) A forgotten founder of medical genetics. Archives of Internal Medicine 104:490-496.
Muller-Wille, S. and H.J. Rheinberger. (2005) Introduction. In S. Muller-Wille and H.J. Rheinberger (eds): A Cultural History of Heredity III: 19th and Early 20th Centuries. Berlin: Max Planck Institut fur Wissenschaftsgeschichte, p. 5.
Newman, C. (1957) The Evolution of Medical Education in the Nineteenth Century. London: Oxford University Press, p. 92.
Newport, G. (1852) Notes on the impregnation of the ovum in the Amphibia. Proceedings of the Royal Society London 6:171-172.
———. (1854) Researches on the impregnation of the ovum in the Amphibia. Philosophical Transactions 144:229-244.
Nicholl, W. (1816) Account of a curious imperfection of vision. Medico-Chirurgical Transactions 6:477-481.
———. (1818) Account of a case of defective power to distinguish colors. Medico-Chirurgical Transactions 9:359-363.
Norris, W. (1820) Case of fungoid tumor. Edinburgh Medical and Surgical Journal 16:562-565.
Osborne, J. (1835) Account of a hemorrhagic diathesis existing in a family, and also a peculiar appearance of the iris belonging to a family. Dublin Journal of Medicine and Chemical Sciences 7:32-35.
Paget, J. (1853a) Lectures on Surgical Pathology, Vol. 2. London: Longman, pp. 244-245.
———. (1853b) Lectures on Surgical Pathology, Vol. 2, pp. 328-329.
———. (1853c) Lectures on Surgical Pathology, Vol. 2, pp. 538-539.
———. (1857) On the hereditary transmission of tendencies to cancer and other tumors. Medical Times and Gazette 15:191-193.
Pettigrew, A. (1833) Phenomenon of the skin. Lancet 2:146-147.
Pickells, A. (1852) Hemorrhagic diathesis exemplified in two brothers. Edinburgh Medical and Surgical Journal 77:1-10.
Prater, H. (1842) Suggestions for the prevention of hereditary diseases. Lancet 2:500-506, 546-552.
Saunders, J.C. (1811) A Treatise on Some Practical Points Relating to Diseases of the Eye. London: Longman, p. 134.

Scudamore, C. (1823) A Treatise on the Nature and Cure of Gout and Gravel, 4th ed. London: Longman, p. 55.
Seton, A. (1824) On the variation in the colours of peas from cross-segregation. Transactions of the Horticultural Society of London 5:236.
Sieveking, E.H. (1858) On Epilepsy. London: Churchill, p. 94.
Simpson, J. (1842) Antiquarian instances of leprosy and leper hospitals in Scotland and England. Part III. The etiological history of the disease. Edinburgh Medical and Surgical Journal 57:405-429.
Sorsby, A. (1934) Anophthalmos: An unpublished manuscript by James Briggs giving the first account of the familial occurrence of the condition. British Journal of Ophthalmology 18:469-474.
Stanley, E. (1853) Development of numerous exostoses in the same subject. Medical Times and Gazette 7:37.
Steinau, J.H. (1843a) A Pathological and Philosophical Essay on Hereditary Diseases. London: Simpkin, Marshall, pp. 4-6.
———. (1843b) A Pathological and Philosophical Essay on Hereditary Diseases, pp. 7-8.
———. (1843c) A Pathological and Philosophical Essay on Hereditary Diseases, p. 26.
———. (1843d) A Pathological and Philosophical Essay on Hereditary Diseases, pp. 9-11.
———. (1843e) A Pathological and Philosophical Essay on Hereditary Diseases, p. 37.
———. (1843f) A Pathological and Philosophical Essay on Hereditary Diseases, p. 44.
Streatfield, J.F. (1857a) Six cases of cataract in one family. Royal London Ophthalmic Hospital Report 1:104.
———. (1857-1859b) Coloboma irides. Royal London Ophthalmic Hospital Report 1:153-155.
———. (1857c) Seven cases of strabismus in one family. Royal London Ophthalmic Hospital Reports 1:260-262.
"Surgical lecture." (1824) Lancet 4:69.
Thomson, J. (1858) On the comparative influence of the male and female parent upon progeny. Edinburgh Medical Journal 4:501-504, 696-699.
Thurnan, J. (1831) Two cases in which the skin, hair and teeth were very imperfectly developed. Medico-Chirurgical Transactions 31:71-82.
Usher, C.H. (1911-1912) A pedigree of colour-blindness. Transactions of the Ophthalmologic Society of the United Kingdom 32:352-362.
Walker, A. (1839a) Intermarriage. New York: Langley.
———. (1839b) Intermarriage, p. 1.
———. (1839c) Intermarriage, p. 131.
———. (1839d) Intermarriage, pp. 131-132.
———. (1839e) Intermarriage, p. 137.
———. (1839f) Intermarriage, p. 372.
———. (1839g) Intermarriage, p. 139.
———. (1839h) Intermarriage, p. 142.
———. (1839i) Intermarriage, p. 241.
———. (1839j) Intermarriage, pp. 180-181.
Waller, J.C. (2001) Ideas of heredity, reproduction and eugenics in Britain, 1800-1875. Studies in the History and Philosophy of Biology and Biomedical Sciences 32:459-465.

———. (2002a) The illusion of an explanation: The concept of hereditary disease. Journal of the History of Medicine 57:445.
———. (2002b) The illusion of an explanation: The concept of hereditary disease. Journal of the History of Medicine 57:410-411.
———. (2002c) The illusion of an explanation: The concept of hereditary disease. Journal of the History of Medicine 57:411.
———. (2002d) The illusion of an explanation: The concept of hereditary disease. Journal of the History of Medicine 57:423.
———. (2002e) The illusion of an explanation: The concept of hereditary disease. Journal of the History of Medicine 57:419-420.
———. (2002f) The illusion of an explanation: The concept of hereditary disease. Journal of the History of Medicine 57:433.
———. (2002g) The illusion of an explanation: The concept of hereditary disease. Journal of the History of Medicine 57:431.
Watson, T. (1844) Lectures on the Principles and Practice of Physick. Philadelphia: Lea and Blanchard.
———. (1848a) Lectures on the Principles and Practice of Physic, Vol. 1. London: Longman, pp. 109-110.
———. (1848b) Lectures on the Principles and Practice of Physic, Vol. 1, p. 335.
Whitehead, J. (1857a) On the Transmission from Parent to Offspring of Some Forms of Disease and of Morbid Taints and Tendencies, 2nd ed. London: Churchill, p. 28.
———. (1857b) On the Transmission from Parent to Offspring of Some Forms of Disease and of Morbid Taints and Tendencies, p. 24.
———. (1857c) On the Transmission from Parent to Offspring of Some Forms of Disease and of Morbid Taints and Tendencies, p. 7.
———. (1857d) On the Transmission from Parent to Offspring of Some Forms of Disease and of Morbid Taints and Tendencies, p. 24.
———. (1857e) On the Transmission from Parent to Offspring of Some Forms of Disease and of Morbid Taints and Tendencies, p. 29.
———. (1857f) On the Transmission from Parent to Offspring of Some Forms of Disease and of Morbid Taints and Tendencies, pp. 76-77.
Wilmot, S. (1841) A case of hemorrhagic diathesis. Dublin Journal of Medical Science 19:234-240.
Wilson, G. (1855) Researches on Colour Blindness. Edinburgh: Sutherland and Knox, pp. 14-18.
Wright, W. (1830) Causes and treatment of deafness. Lancet 2:464-466.
Yelloly, J. (1829) Remarks on the tendency to calculous disease. Philosophical Transactions 119:55-81.
Zirkle, C. (1946) The early history of the idea of the inheritance of acquired characters and of pangenesis. Transactions of the American Philosophical Society 35:117-118.

CHAPTER SEVEN

Barlow, N. (ed). (1959a) The Autobiography of Charles Darwin. New York: Harcourt, Brace and Company, pp. 29-30.
———. (1959b) The Autobiography of Charles Darwin, p. 47.
———. (1959c) The Autobiography of Charles Darwin, p. 48.
———. (1959d) The Autobiography of Charles Darwin, p. 46.

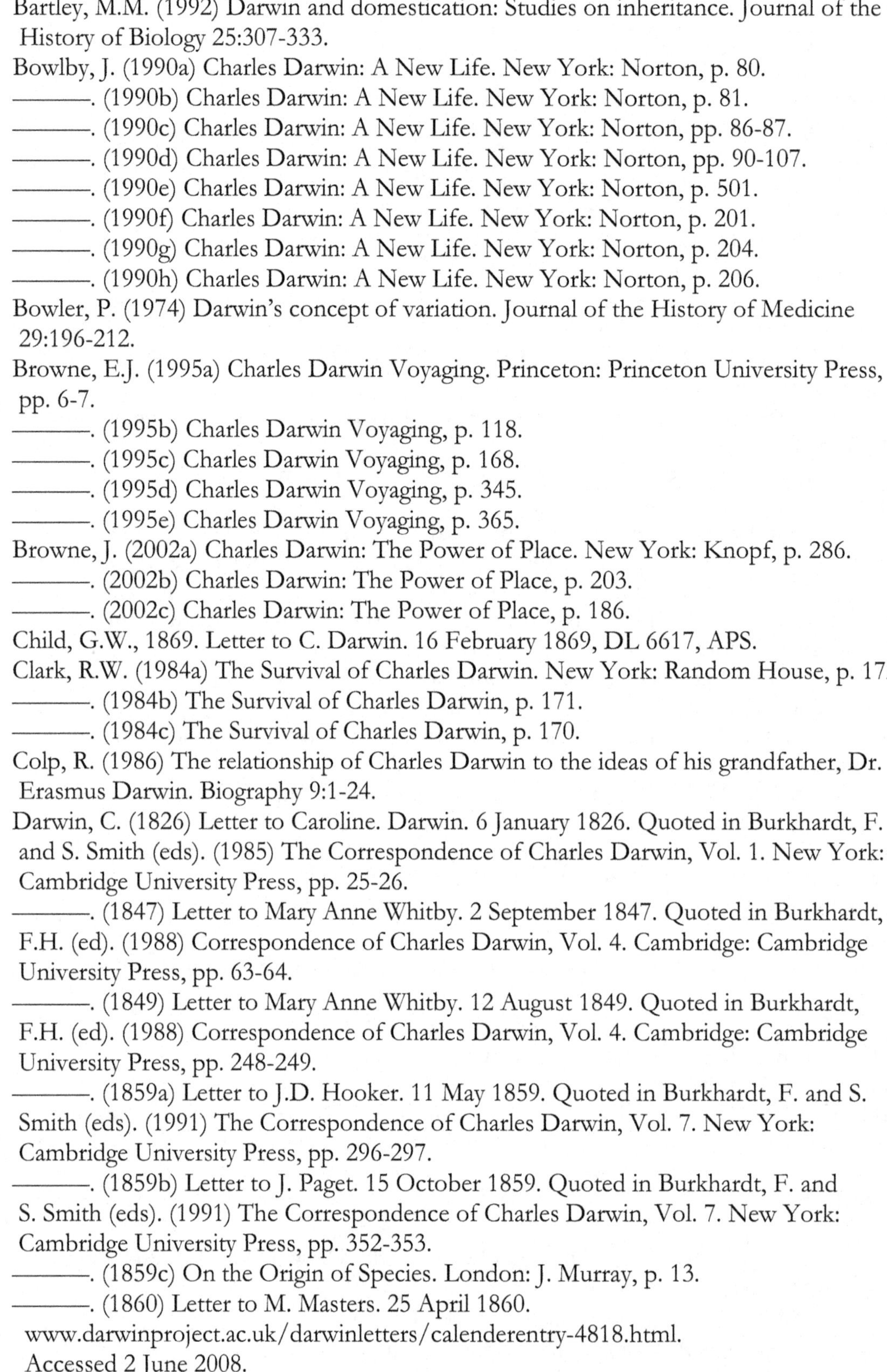

Bartley, M.M. (1992) Darwin and domestication: Studies on inheritance. Journal of the History of Biology 25:307-333.
Bowlby, J. (1990a) Charles Darwin: A New Life. New York: Norton, p. 80.
———. (1990b) Charles Darwin: A New Life. New York: Norton, p. 81.
———. (1990c) Charles Darwin: A New Life. New York: Norton, pp. 86-87.
———. (1990d) Charles Darwin: A New Life. New York: Norton, pp. 90-107.
———. (1990e) Charles Darwin: A New Life. New York: Norton, p. 501.
———. (1990f) Charles Darwin: A New Life. New York: Norton, p. 201.
———. (1990g) Charles Darwin: A New Life. New York: Norton, p. 204.
———. (1990h) Charles Darwin: A New Life. New York: Norton, p. 206.
Bowler, P. (1974) Darwin's concept of variation. Journal of the History of Medicine 29:196-212.
Browne, E.J. (1995a) Charles Darwin Voyaging. Princeton: Princeton University Press, pp. 6-7.
———. (1995b) Charles Darwin Voyaging, p. 118.
———. (1995c) Charles Darwin Voyaging, p. 168.
———. (1995d) Charles Darwin Voyaging, p. 345.
———. (1995e) Charles Darwin Voyaging, p. 365.
Browne, J. (2002a) Charles Darwin: The Power of Place. New York: Knopf, p. 286.
———. (2002b) Charles Darwin: The Power of Place, p. 203.
———. (2002c) Charles Darwin: The Power of Place, p. 186.
Child, G.W., 1869. Letter to C. Darwin. 16 February 1869, DL 6617, APS.
Clark, R.W. (1984a) The Survival of Charles Darwin. New York: Random House, p. 172.
———. (1984b) The Survival of Charles Darwin, p. 171.
———. (1984c) The Survival of Charles Darwin, p. 170.
Colp, R. (1986) The relationship of Charles Darwin to the ideas of his grandfather, Dr. Erasmus Darwin. Biography 9:1-24.
Darwin, C. (1826) Letter to Caroline. Darwin. 6 January 1826. Quoted in Burkhardt, F. and S. Smith (eds). (1985) The Correspondence of Charles Darwin, Vol. 1. New York: Cambridge University Press, pp. 25-26.
———. (1847) Letter to Mary Anne Whitby. 2 September 1847. Quoted in Burkhardt, F.H. (ed). (1988) Correspondence of Charles Darwin, Vol. 4. Cambridge: Cambridge University Press, pp. 63-64.
———. (1849) Letter to Mary Anne Whitby. 12 August 1849. Quoted in Burkhardt, F.H. (ed). (1988) Correspondence of Charles Darwin, Vol. 4. Cambridge: Cambridge University Press, pp. 248-249.
———. (1859a) Letter to J.D. Hooker. 11 May 1859. Quoted in Burkhardt, F. and S. Smith (eds). (1991) The Correspondence of Charles Darwin, Vol. 7. New York: Cambridge University Press, pp. 296-297.
———. (1859b) Letter to J. Paget. 15 October 1859. Quoted in Burkhardt, F. and S. Smith (eds). (1991) The Correspondence of Charles Darwin, Vol. 7. New York: Cambridge University Press, pp. 352-353.
———. (1859c) On the Origin of Species. London: J. Murray, p. 13.
———. (1860) Letter to M. Masters. 25 April 1860. www.darwinproject.ac.uk/darwinletters/calenderentry-4818.html. Accessed 2 June 2008.

———. (1863) Letter to H.B. Dobell. 21 April 1863. Quoted in Burkhardt F.H. (ed). (1999) Correspondence of Charles Darwin, Vol. 11. Cambridge: Cambridge University Press, pp. 345-346.

———. (1866). Letter to A. Wallace. 6 February 1866 DL 4989 APS.

———. (1868a). Letter to J.D. Hooker. 14 July 1868 DL 6276 APS.

———. (1868b) Letter to J.D. Hooker. 23 February 1868. Quoted in Darwin, F. (ed). (1887) The Life and Letters of Charles Darwin. New York: Appleton, pp. 259-261.

———. (1868c) The Variation of Animals and Plants under Domestication, Vol. 2. London: John Murray. Chapter 27.

———. (1868d) The Variation of Animals and Plants under Domestication, Vol. 2. Chapter 27, p. 429.

———. (1868e) The Variation of Animals and Plants under Domestication, Vol. 2. Chapter 27, p. 448.

———. (1868f) The Variation of Animals and Plants under Domestication, Vol. 2. Chapter 27, p. 432.

———. (1868g) The Variation of Animals and Plants under Domestication, Vol. 2. Chapter 27, p. 461.

———. (1868h) The Variation of Animals and Plants under Domestication, Vol. 2. Chapter 27, pp. 476-477.

———. (1868i) The Variation of Animals and Plants under Domestication, Vol. 2. Chapter 27, pp. 478-479.

———. (1868j) The Variation of Animals and Plants under Domestication, Vol. 2. Chapter 27, p. 451.

———. (1868k) The Variation of Animals and Plants under Domestication, Vol. 2. Chapter 27, pp. 445-446.

———. (1868l) The Variation of Animals and Plants under Domestication, Vol. 2. Chapter 27, p. 473.

———. (1873) Letter to A. De Candolle. 18 January 1873. Quoted in Darwin, F. (1903) More Letters of Charles Darwin. New York: Appleton, Vol. 1, p. 348

———. (1893a) The Variation of Animals and Plants under Domestication, 2nd ed., Vol. 2. London: Murray.

———. (1893b) The Variation of Animals and Plants under Domestication, 2nd ed., Vol. 2, pp. 373-374.

———. (1893c) The Variation of Animals and Plants under Domestication, 2nd ed., Vol. 2, p. 382.

———. (1963a) The Origin of Species, 1859 ed. New York: Washington Square Press, p. 7.

———. (1963b) The Origin of Species, 1859 ed., p. 140.

———. (1963c) The Origin of Species, 1859 ed., p. 348.

De Beer, G. (1964) Charles Darwin: Evolution by Natural Selection. Garden City: Doubleday.

Dobell, H.B. (1863a) Letter to C. Darwin. 20 April 1863. Quoted in Burkhardt, F.H. (ed). (1997) Correspondence of Charles Darwin, Vol. 11. Cambridge: Cambridge University Press, p. 331.

———. (1863b) Letter to C. Darwin. 12 May 1863. Quoted in Burkhardt, F.H. (ed). (1999) Correspondence of Charles Darwin, Vol. 11. Cambridge: Cambridge University Press, p. 406.
Geison, G.L. (1969) Darwin and heredity: The evolution of his hypothesis of pangenesis. Journal of the History of Medicine 24:406.
Katz-Sidlow, R.J. (1998) In the Darwin family tradition: Another look at Charles Darwin's ill health. Journal of the Royal Society of Medicine 91:485.
Keen, W.W., 1874. Letter to C. Darwin. 18 June 1874 DL 9500 APS.
King-Hele, D. (ed). (2003) Charles Darwin's The Life of Erasmus Darwin. Cambridge: Cambridge University Press.
Kohn, D. (1980a) Theories to work by: Rejected theories, reproduction and Darwin's path to natural selection. Studies in the History of Biology 1:86.
———. (1980b) Theories to work by: Rejected theories, reproduction and Darwin's path to natural selection. Studies in the History of Biology 1:80-83.
———. (1980c) Theories to work by: Rejected theories, reproduction and Darwin's path to natural selection. Studies in the History of Biology 1:127-128.
Lefevre, W. (2005) Inheritance of acquired characters: Heredity and evolution in late nineteenth-century Germany. In S. Muller-Wille and H.J. Rheinberger (eds): A Cultural History of Heredity III: 19th and Early 20th Centuries. Berlin: Max Planck Institut fur Wissenschaftsgeschichte, p. 55.
Lopez-Beltran, C. (2003) Heredity old and new: French physicians and l'heredite naturelle in early 19th century. In J.H. Rheinberger and W. Muller S (eds): A Cultural History of Heredity II: 18th and 19th Centuries. Berlin: Max Planck Institut fur Wissenschaftsgeschichte, p. 17.
Merrington, W.R. (1976) University College Hospital and its Medical School: A History. London: Heinemann.
"Obituary of William Sedgwick." (1905) British Medical Journal 2:1246.
Ogle, W., 1869. Letter to C. Darwin. 29 March 1869 DL 5470 APS.
Olby, R. (1963) Charles Darwin's manuscript of Pangenesis. British Journal of the History of Science 1:264.
Ospovat, D. (1981) The Development of Darwin's Theory. Cambridge: Cambridge University Press, pp. 41-42.
Paget, J. (1863) Letter to C. Darwin. 16 March 1863. Quoted in Burkhardt, F.H. (ed). (1997) Correspondence of Charles Darwin, Vol. 11. Cambridge: Cambridge University Press, p. 234.
Paget, S. (ed). (1903) Memoirs and Letters of Sir James Paget, 3rd ed. London: Longmans Green.
Platt, R. (1959) Darwin, Mendel and Galton. Medical History 3:87-99.
Richardson, E.W. (1916) A Veteran Naturalist, Being the Life and Work of W.B. Tegetmeier. London: Witherby.
Robinson, G. (1979) A Prelude to Genetics. Lawrence, Kansas: Coronado Press.
Rolleston, G. (1861) Letter to C. Darwin. 1 September 1861. Quoted in Burkhardt, F.H. (ed). (1994) Correspondence of Charles Darwin, Vol. 10. Cambridge: Cambridge University Press, p. 244-246.
Secord, J.A. (1985) Darwin and the breeders. In D. Kohn (ed): The Darwinian Heritage. Princeton: Princeton University Press, pp. 519-542.

Sedgwick, W. (1896) Notes on the influence of heredity in disease. British Medical Journal 1:458-462.
Tait, L. (1881). Letter to C. Darwin. 29 July 1881 DL 13257 APS.
Towers, B. (1968) The impact of Darwin's Origin of Species on medicine and biology. In F.N.L. Poynter (ed): Medicine and Science in the 1860s. Proceedings of the Sixth British Congress on the History of Medicine. London: Wellcome Institute of the History of Medicine, p. 53.
Van Dyck, W. (1882). Letter to C. Darwin. 25 January 1882 DL 13645 APS .
"Variation." (1999) Footnote 5. In F.H. Burkhardt (ed): Correspondence of Charles Darwin, Vol. 11. Cambridge: Cambridge University Press, p. 346.
Vorzimmer, P. (1963) Charles Darwin and blending inheritance. Isis 54:371-390.
Wade, W.S. (1873). Letter to C. Darwin. 11 September 1873 DL 9050 APS.
Webster, G. (1992) William Bateson and the science of form. In W. Bateson (ed): Materials for the Study of Variation. Baltimore: Johns Hopkins University Press, pp. xxix-lix.

Chapter Eight

Bernard, C. (1865) An Introduction to the Study of Experimental Medicine. New York: Macmillan, p. 146.
Bonner, T.N. (1995a) Becoming a Physician. Oxford: Oxford University Press, pp. 231-231.
———. (1995b) Becoming a Physician, pp. 259-264.
———. (1995c) Becoming a Physician, p. 245.
———. (1995d) Becoming a Physician, p. 275.
———. (1995e) Becoming a Physician, p. 300.
———. (1995f) Becoming a Physician, p. 282.
Booth, C.C. (1979) The development of clinical science in Britain. British Medical Journal 1:1469-1473.
Bradbury, J.B. (1880) Modern scientific medicine. Medical Times and Gazette 2:177-185.
Bristowe, J. (1887) A Treatise on the Theory and Practice of Medicine, 6th ed. London: H.C. Lea.
Brunton, T.L. (1897) The relationship of physiology, pharmacology, pathology and practical medicine. Nature 56:473-474.
Bynum, W.F. (1995) Science and the Practice of Medicine in the Nineteenth Century. Cambridge: Cambridge University Press, pp. 140-141.
Cowan, R.S. (1972a) Francis Galton's statistical ideas: the influence of eugenics. Isis 63:509-528.
———. (1972b) Galton's contribution to genetics. Journal of the History of Biology 5:389-412.
Cunningham, A, P. Williams (eds.): (1992) The Laboratory Revolution in Medicine. Cambridge: Cambridge University Press, pp. 146-147.
Darwin, C. (1868) The Variation of Animals and Plants under Domestication, Vol. 2. London: John Murray. Chapter 27.
———. (1871) Pangenesis. Nature 3:502-503.
"Editorial." (1863) Lancet 2:368-370.

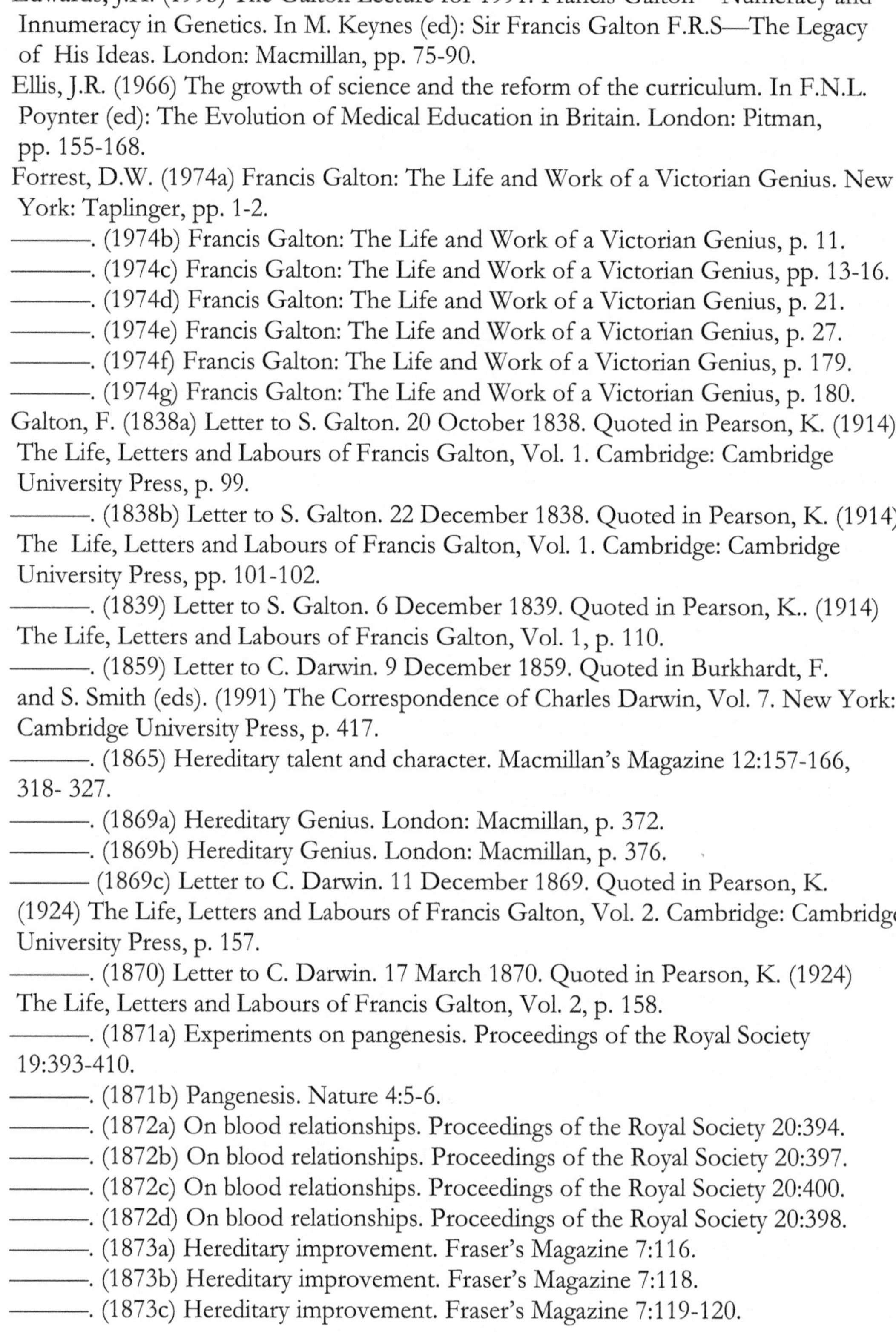

Edwards, J.H. (1993) The Galton Lecture for 1991: Francis Galton—Numeracy and Innumeracy in Genetics. In M. Keynes (ed): Sir Francis Galton F.R.S—The Legacy of His Ideas. London: Macmillan, pp. 75-90.
Ellis, J.R. (1966) The growth of science and the reform of the curriculum. In F.N.L. Poynter (ed): The Evolution of Medical Education in Britain. London: Pitman, pp. 155-168.
Forrest, D.W. (1974a) Francis Galton: The Life and Work of a Victorian Genius. New York: Taplinger, pp. 1-2.
———. (1974b) Francis Galton: The Life and Work of a Victorian Genius, p. 11.
———. (1974c) Francis Galton: The Life and Work of a Victorian Genius, pp. 13-16.
———. (1974d) Francis Galton: The Life and Work of a Victorian Genius, p. 21.
———. (1974e) Francis Galton: The Life and Work of a Victorian Genius, p. 27.
———. (1974f) Francis Galton: The Life and Work of a Victorian Genius, p. 179.
———. (1974g) Francis Galton: The Life and Work of a Victorian Genius, p. 180.
Galton, F. (1838a) Letter to S. Galton. 20 October 1838. Quoted in Pearson, K. (1914) The Life, Letters and Labours of Francis Galton, Vol. 1. Cambridge: Cambridge University Press, p. 99.
———. (1838b) Letter to S. Galton. 22 December 1838. Quoted in Pearson, K. (1914) The Life, Letters and Labours of Francis Galton, Vol. 1. Cambridge: Cambridge University Press, pp. 101-102.
———. (1839) Letter to S. Galton. 6 December 1839. Quoted in Pearson, K.. (1914) The Life, Letters and Labours of Francis Galton, Vol. 1, p. 110.
———. (1859) Letter to C. Darwin. 9 December 1859. Quoted in Burkhardt, F. and S. Smith (eds). (1991) The Correspondence of Charles Darwin, Vol. 7. New York: Cambridge University Press, p. 417.
———. (1865) Hereditary talent and character. Macmillan's Magazine 12:157-166, 318- 327.
———. (1869a) Hereditary Genius. London: Macmillan, p. 372.
———. (1869b) Hereditary Genius. London: Macmillan, p. 376.
——— (1869c) Letter to C. Darwin. 11 December 1869. Quoted in Pearson, K. (1924) The Life, Letters and Labours of Francis Galton, Vol. 2. Cambridge: Cambridge University Press, p. 157.
———. (1870) Letter to C. Darwin. 17 March 1870. Quoted in Pearson, K. (1924) The Life, Letters and Labours of Francis Galton, Vol. 2, p. 158.
———. (1871a) Experiments on pangenesis. Proceedings of the Royal Society 19:393-410.
———. (1871b) Pangenesis. Nature 4:5-6.
———. (1872a) On blood relationships. Proceedings of the Royal Society 20:394.
———. (1872b) On blood relationships. Proceedings of the Royal Society 20:397.
———. (1872c) On blood relationships. Proceedings of the Royal Society 20:400.
———. (1872d) On blood relationships. Proceedings of the Royal Society 20:398.
———. (1873a) Hereditary improvement. Fraser's Magazine 7:116.
———. (1873b) Hereditary improvement. Fraser's Magazine 7:118.
———. (1873c) Hereditary improvement. Fraser's Magazine 7:119-120.

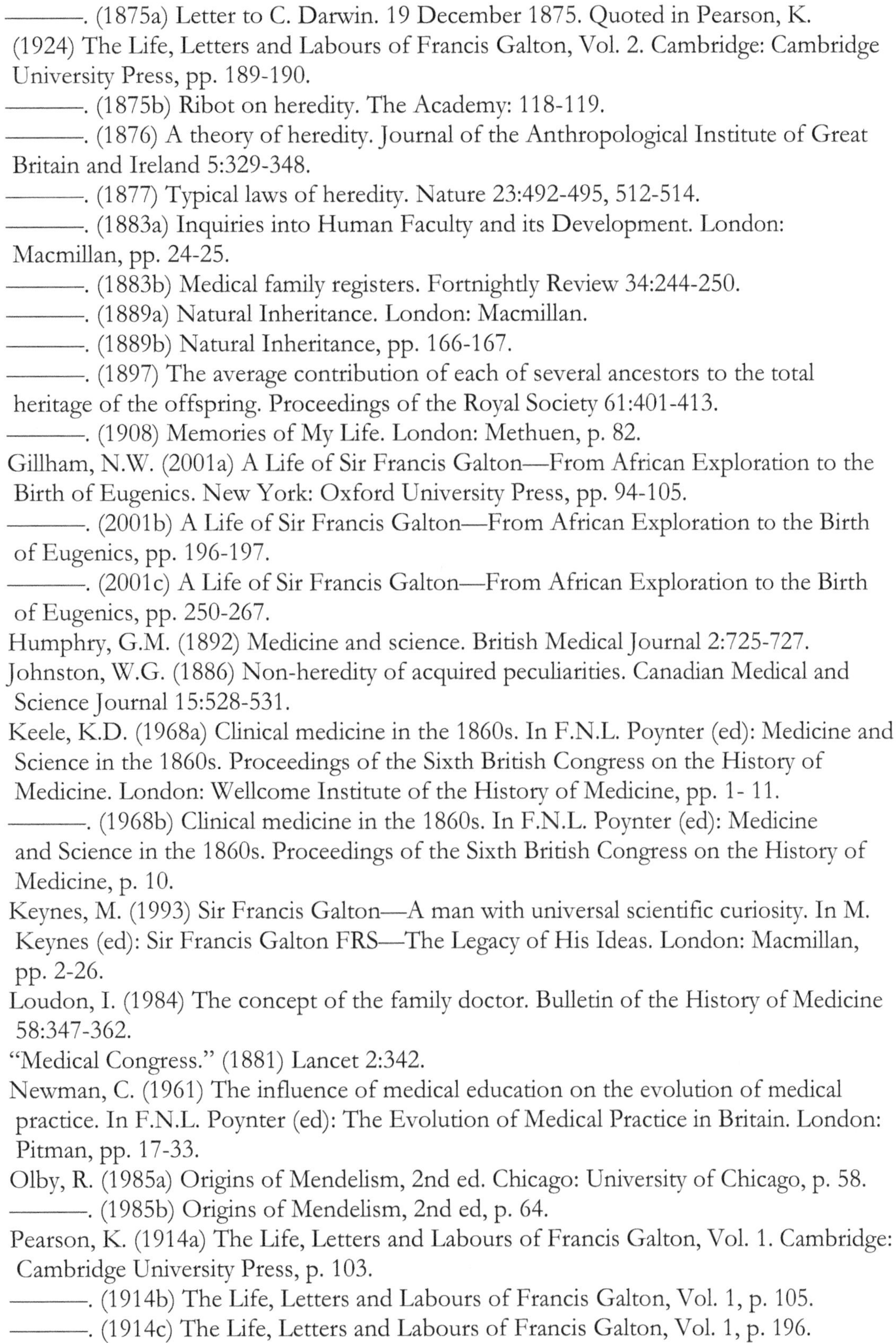

———. (1875a) Letter to C. Darwin. 19 December 1875. Quoted in Pearson, K. (1924) The Life, Letters and Labours of Francis Galton, Vol. 2. Cambridge: Cambridge University Press, pp. 189-190.

———. (1875b) Ribot on heredity. The Academy: 118-119.

———. (1876) A theory of heredity. Journal of the Anthropological Institute of Great Britain and Ireland 5:329-348.

———. (1877) Typical laws of heredity. Nature 23:492-495, 512-514.

———. (1883a) Inquiries into Human Faculty and its Development. London: Macmillan, pp. 24-25.

———. (1883b) Medical family registers. Fortnightly Review 34:244-250.

———. (1889a) Natural Inheritance. London: Macmillan.

———. (1889b) Natural Inheritance, pp. 166-167.

———. (1897) The average contribution of each of several ancestors to the total heritage of the offspring. Proceedings of the Royal Society 61:401-413.

———. (1908) Memories of My Life. London: Methuen, p. 82.

Gillham, N.W. (2001a) A Life of Sir Francis Galton—From African Exploration to the Birth of Eugenics. New York: Oxford University Press, pp. 94-105.

———. (2001b) A Life of Sir Francis Galton—From African Exploration to the Birth of Eugenics, pp. 196-197.

———. (2001c) A Life of Sir Francis Galton—From African Exploration to the Birth of Eugenics, pp. 250-267.

Humphry, G.M. (1892) Medicine and science. British Medical Journal 2:725-727.

Johnston, W.G. (1886) Non-heredity of acquired peculiarities. Canadian Medical and Science Journal 15:528-531.

Keele, K.D. (1968a) Clinical medicine in the 1860s. In F.N.L. Poynter (ed): Medicine and Science in the 1860s. Proceedings of the Sixth British Congress on the History of Medicine. London: Wellcome Institute of the History of Medicine, pp. 1- 11.

———. (1968b) Clinical medicine in the 1860s. In F.N.L. Poynter (ed): Medicine and Science in the 1860s. Proceedings of the Sixth British Congress on the History of Medicine, p. 10.

Keynes, M. (1993) Sir Francis Galton—A man with universal scientific curiosity. In M. Keynes (ed): Sir Francis Galton FRS—The Legacy of His Ideas. London: Macmillan, pp. 2-26.

Loudon, I. (1984) The concept of the family doctor. Bulletin of the History of Medicine 58:347-362.

"Medical Congress." (1881) Lancet 2:342.

Newman, C. (1961) The influence of medical education on the evolution of medical practice. In F.N.L. Poynter (ed): The Evolution of Medical Practice in Britain. London: Pitman, pp. 17-33.

Olby, R. (1985a) Origins of Mendelism, 2nd ed. Chicago: University of Chicago, p. 58.

———. (1985b) Origins of Mendelism, 2nd ed, p. 64.

Pearson, K. (1914a) The Life, Letters and Labours of Francis Galton, Vol. 1. Cambridge: Cambridge University Press, p. 103.

———. (1914b) The Life, Letters and Labours of Francis Galton, Vol. 1, p. 105.

———. (1914c) The Life, Letters and Labours of Francis Galton, Vol. 1, p. 196.

———. (1924a) The Life, Letters and Labours of Francis Galton, Vol. 2. Cambridge: Cambridge University Press, p. 177.
———. (1924b) The Life, Letters and Labours of Francis Galton, Vol. 2, p. 82.
———. (1924c) The Life, Letters and Labours of Francis Galton, Vol. 2, p. 118.
———. (1924d) The Life, Letters and Labours of Francis Galton, Vol. 2, p. 359.
Robinson, G. (1979a) A Prelude to Genetics. Lawrence, Kansas: Coronado Press, p. 33.
———. (1979b) A Prelude to Genetics, p. 41.
Romano, T.M. (1997) Gentlemanly versus scientific ideals: John Burdon Sanderson, medical education and the failure of the Oxford school of physiology. Bulletin of the History of Medicine 71:224-248.
Shortt, S.E.D. (1983) Physicians, science and status: Issues in the professionalization of Anglo-American medicine in the nineteenth century. Medical History 27:51-68.
Smith, J.M. (1993) Galton and evolutionary theory. In M. Keynes (ed): Sir Francis Galton FRS—The Legacy of His Ideas. London: Macmillan, pp. 158-169.
Waller, J.C. (2001) Ideas of heredity, reproduction and eugenics in Britain, 1800-1875. Studies in the History and Philosophy of Biology and Biomedical Sciences 32:479.
Youngson, A.J. (1979) The Scientific Revolution of Victorian Medicine. London: Helm, p. 16.

CHAPTER NINE

Aitken, W. (1888) On the progress of scientific pathology. British Medical Journal 2:348-359.
Anderson, W. (1886) Congenital malformation of hands and feet transmitted through four generations. British Medical Journal 1:1107-1108.
Barber, H. (1864) Case of a hereditary malformation. Medical Mirror 1:758-760.
Barbour, H. (1894) Some aspects of heredity. Edinburgh Medical Journal 40:602-609.
Blacher, L.I. (1982a) The Problem of the Inheritance of Acquired Characters. New Delhi: American Publishing Co., pp. 186-187.
———. (1982b) The Problem of the Inheritance of Acquired Characters, p. 87.
———. (1982c) The Problem of the Inheritance of Acquired Characters, pp. 89-90.
———. (1982d) The Problem of the Inheritance of Acquired Characters, p. 91.
———. (1982e) The Problem of the Inheritance of Acquired Characters, p. 98.
———. (1982f) The Problem of the Inheritance of Acquired Characters, p. 111.
Brown-Sequard, C.E. (1875) On the hereditary transmission of effects of certain injuries to the nervous system. Lancet 1:7-8.
Bryce, T.H. (1896) On recent views as to the part the nucleus plays in development. Glasgow Medical Journal 45:81-95.
Campbell, H. (1889) The Causation of Disease. London: Lewis, p. 40.
———. (1897) Should epileptics marry? Lancet 1:914.
Charles, R.H. (1893) Morphological peculiarities in the Panjabi and their bearing on the question of the transmission of acquired characters. Journal of Anatomy 28:271-280.
Clark, F. (1886) Heredity. St. Thomas's Hospital Report 14:21-30.
Cross, F.R. (1885) Cases of congenital malformation of the eye. British Medical Journal 2:1153.

Darwin, C. (1863) Letter to H.B. Dobell. 21 April 1863. Quoted in Burkhardt, F.H. (ed). (1999) Correspondence of Charles Darwin, Vol. 11. Cambridge: Cambridge University Press, p. 345-346.
Dobell, H.B. (1863) Letter to C. Darwin. 20 April 1863. Quoted in Burkhardt, F.H. (ed). (ed). (1997) Correspondence of Charles Darwin, Vol. 11. Cambridge: Cambridge University Press, p. 331.
Duckworth, D.D. (1889) A Treatise on Gout. London: Griffin, pp. 128-131.
Felkin, R.W. (1888) Heredity: Its influence on man in health and disease. Edinburgh Health Society Lectures 8:55-72.
Galton, F. (1875) Letter to C. Darwin. 3 November 1875. Quoted in Pearson, K. (1924) The Life, Letters and Labours of Francis Galton, Vol. 2. Cambridge: Cambridge University Press, p. 182.
Gaskoin, G. (1880) An epitome of fifty cases of ichthyosis. St. George's Hospital Report 10:588-606.
Granville, J.M. (1880) A note on intention in the determination of sex and the mental and physical inheritance of children. Lancet 2:650-652.
Gubbin, W.R. (1894) Heredity and disease. Medical Times and Hospital Gazette 22:2-4, 18-20, 37-38, 52-54.
Gunn, R.M. (1889) Congenital malformations of the eyeball. Ophthalmic Review 8:193-202, 225-234, 257-262.
Hamilton, D.J. (1900) On heredity in disease. Scottish Medical and Surgical Journal 6:289-320.
Harker, J. (1865) Malformation of the hands. Lancet 2:389.
Hutchinson, H. (1946) Jonathan Hutchinson. London: Heinemann.
Hutchinson, J. (1866) Report on cases of congenital amaurosis. Royal London Ophthalmic Hospital Reports 5:347-352.
———. (1875) Heredity. British and Foreign Medical and Chirurgical Review 56:53-71.
———. (1881a) Heredity. Medical Press and Gazette 1:523-524, 547-548.
———. (1881b) Heredity. Medical Press and Circular 2:1-2, 22-23, 44-47, 65-67.
———. (1889a) Notes on heredity. Archives of Surgery 1:242-244.
———. (1889b) The pedigree of disease. Wood's Medical and Surgical Monograph 1:5-114.
———. (1890a) On heredity in reference to disease. Archives of Surgery 1:289-306.
———. (1890b) On heredity in reference to disease. Archives of Surgery 2:42-53.
———. (1896) Lecture on the pedigree of disease. In T.C. Allbutt (ed): System of Medicine, Vol. 1. London: Macmillan, pp. 35-46.
Johnston, W.G. (1886) Non-heredity of acquired peculiarities. Canadian Medical and Science Journal 15:528-531.
"Jonathan Hutchinson." (1921) Dictionary of National Biography 1912-1921:279-280.
Lang, W. (1885) Congenital aniridia. Transactions of the Ophthalmological Society of the United Kingdom 5:207.
Lauder, W. (1886) Heredity in relation to disease. Manchester Health Lectures for the People 10:113-136.
Lee, R.J. (1888) Case of mental defect in a child due to maternal disturbance caused by a dream. Medical Press and Circular 46:505.
Leslie, G. (1881) On hereditary transmission of disease: Method of graphic representation. Edinburgh Medical Journal 27:795-799.
———. (1882) Heredity and disease. Edinburgh Medical Journal 27:641-642.

Liston, A. (1865) Monstrosity in a child following a fright to the mother in the third month of pregnancy. Medical Times and Gazette 2:333.
Lithgow, R.A.O. (1887) From generation to generation: a prelude to the study of heredity. Provincial Medical Journal 6:116-119, 157-160.
Lithgow, R. (1889a) Heredity. London: Balliere, p. 6.
———. (1889b) Heredity. London: Balliere, preface.
Lopez-Beltran, C. (2003) Heredity old and new: French physicians and l'heredite naturelle in early 19th century. In J.H. Rheinberger and W. Muller S (eds): A Cultural History of Heredity II: 18th and 19th Centuries. Berlin: Max Planck Institut fur Wissenschaftsgeschichte, p. 10.
Lucas, P. (1847) Traite Philosophique et Physiologique de l'Heredite Naturelle dans les Etats de Sante et de Maladie du Systeme Nerveux, Vol. 1. Paris: JB Bailliere.
Lucas, R.C. (1892) On a case of hereditary suppression of fingers. Lancet 2:462-464.
Manning, F.N. (1886) A contribution to the study of heredity. Journal and Proceedings of the Royal Society of New South Wales 19:197-204.
Marsh, F. (1889) Double polydactylism, double harelip, complete cleft palate, and double talipes varus. Lancet 2:739.
Maudlsey, H. (1862) Considerations with regard to hereditary influence. Journal of Mental Science 8:482-512.
Maudsley, M. (1863) Considerations with regard to hereditary influence. Journal of Mental Science 9:506-530.
McKendrick, J.G. (1888a) On the modern cell theory and the phenomena of fecundation. Proceedings of the Philosophical Society of Glasgow 19:111-113.
———. (1888b) On the modern cell theory and the phenomena of fecundation. Proceedings of the Philosophical Society of Glasgow 19:116.
Montagu, A. (1979a) The Elephant Man, 2nd ed. New York: Dutton, pp. 13-14.
———. (1979b) The Elephant Man, 2nd ed, pp. 14-16.
———. (1979c) The Elephant Man, 2nd ed, p. 18.
———. (1979d) The Elephant Man, 2nd ed, pp. 28-36.
———. (1979e) The Elephant Man, 2nd ed, p. 37.
Montgomery-Smith, W.T. (1888) A family history of digital deformities. Guy's Hospital Reports 30:115-116.
Morris, J.P. (1865) On the hereditary transmission through four generations of an abnormality. Anthropological Review 3:183.
Murray, J. (1860) Contribution to teratology. British and Foreign Medico-Chirurgical Review 26:502-509.
Newman, C. (1957) The Evolution of Medical Education in the Nineteenth Century. London: Oxford University Press.
Oliver, T. (1900) Physiology and pathology of inheritance. Lancet 2:1335-1341.
Parker, R.W. and H.B. Robinson (1887) Inherited congenital deformity of hands and feet. Lancet 1:729-730.
———. (1887) A case of inherited congenital malformation of the hands and feet. Transactions of the Clinical Society of London 20:181-189.
Phillips, J. (1887) Four cases of spurious hermaphroditism in one family. Transactions of the Obstetrical Society of London 28:158-168.
Pope, H.C. (1889) The beginnings of disease. Illustrated Medical News (London) 5:155-162.
Reid, G.A. (1900) Heredity in disease. Scottish Medical and Surgical Journal 6:510-533.

Ribot, T. (1875) Heredity. New York: Appleton.
Savage, G.H. (1897) Heredity and neurosis. Brain 20:1-21.
Sedgwick, W. (1861) On sexual limitation in hereditary disease. British and Foreign Medico-Chirurgical Review 27:477-489.
———. (1863a) On the influence of sex in hereditary disease. British and Foreign Medical and Chirurgical Review 31:445-478.
———. (1863b) On the influence of sex in hereditary disease. British and Foreign Medical and Chirurgical Review 32:159-197.
Smith, D. (1882) Retinitis pigmentosa. Ophthalmic Review 1:30-32.
Snell, S. (1887) Congenital defects of the eye and ear. Practitioner 38:261-266.
Strahan, S.A.K. (1892a) Marriage and Disease: A Study of Heredity and the More Important Family Degenerations. London: Kegan, Paul, Trench, Tribner, p. 1.
———. (1892b) Marriage and Disease: A Study of Heredity and the More Important Family Degenerations, p. 4.
———. (1892c) Marriage and Disease: A Study of Heredity and the More Important Family Degenerations, p. 67.
———. (1892d) Marriage and Disease: A Study of Heredity and the More Important Family Degenerations, pp. 301-302.
Struthers, J. (1863) On the variation in the numbers of fingers and toes and the number of phalanges in man. Edinburgh New Philosophical Journal 18:83-111.
Stubbe, H. (1972) History of Genetics. Cambridge: MIT Press, pp. 247-251.
Sym, W.G. (1890) Albinism. Transactions of the Ophthalmologic Society of the United Kingdom 11:218-219.
Talbot, E.S. (1894) Etiology of Osseous Deformities. Chicago: W.T. Keenan.
Thomson, J.A. (1888) The history and theory of heredity. Proceedings of the Royal Society of Edinburgh 16:91-116.
Treves, F. (1884) Report of societies. British Medical Journal 2:1140.
———. (1885a) A case of congenital deformity. Transactions of the Pathological Society of London 36:494-498.
———. (1885b) Reports of societies. British Medical Journal 1:595.
Turner, W. (1889) Heredity. Report of the British Association for the Advancement of Science:756-771.
Whitfield, H. (1862) The hereditary transmission of mental and physical impressions. British Medical Journal 1:601-602.

Chapter Ten

Abbott, F.C. (1892) Congenital dislocation of radius. Lancet 1:800.
Anderson, J.W. (1893) Friedreich's ataxia. Glasgow Medical Journal 40:168-174.
Anderson, T. (1863) Hereditary deaf mutism. Medical Times and Gazette 2:247-248.
Anderson, T.M. (1883) On a unique case of tricorexis nodosa. Lancet 2:140-141.
———. (1887) A Treatise on Diseases of the Skin. London: Griffin, p. 55.
———. (1889) Note on a rare form of skin disease: xeroderma pigmentosum. British Medical Journal 1:1284-1285.
———. (1892) Xeroderma pigmentosum. Glasgow Medical Journal 37:150-151.
Anderson, W. (1886) Congenital malformation of hands and feet transmitted through four generations. British Medical Journal 1:1107-1108.

Annandale, T. (1866) The Malformations, Diseases and Injuries of the Fingers and Toes. Philadelphia: Lippincott, p. 36.
Anstie, F.E. (1880) Alcoholism. In J.R. Reynolds (ed): A System of Medicine, Vol. 1. Philadelphia: Lea's, pp. 670-690.
Atherton, A.B. (1894) Case of inherited fragility of bones. Dominion Medical Monthly 2:1-3.
Atwood, W.T. (1897) Two cases of congenital hereditary night blindness. Royal London Ophthalmic Hospital Reports 14:260-263.
Babington, B.G. (1865) Hereditary epistaxis. Lancet 2:362-363.
Barber, H. (1864) Case of a hereditary malformation. Medical Mirror 1:758-760.
Batten, R.D. (1896) A family suffering from hereditary optic atrophy. Transactions of the Ophthalmological Society of the United Kingdom 16:125-130.
Beecher, H.K. (1960) Disease and the Advancement of Basic Science. Cambridge: Harvard University Press, p. 12.
Bell, B. (1868) An account of three cases of congenital cataract in one family. Edinburgh Medical Journal 13:1063-1067.
Bennett, A.H. (1879) Analysis of 100 cases of epilepsy. British Medical Journal 1:379, 419, 846.
Benson, A.H. (1893) Nephritis of obscure origin in several children of one family. Lancet 1:588.
Berry, G.A. (1888) Note on a marked instance of heredity in a form of cataract. Ophthalmic Review 7:1-6.
Bickerton, M.T. (1886) Colour blindness. Liverpool Medico-Chirurgical Journal 6:369-378.
Bickerton, T.H. (1886) Remarks on colour blindness. Lancet 2:392-394.
Boon, A.P. (1892) Albinism. Leeward Islands Medical Journal 2:135.
Bramwell, B. (1895) Diseases of the Spinal Cord, 3rd ed. Edinburgh: Clay, pp. 229-230.
Brigstocke, C.A. (1872) Cases of hemophilia. British Medical Journal 2:122.
Brock, E.H. (1893) Three cases of Friedreich's disease. Lancet 1:139.
Brooke, H.G. (1893) Epithelioma adenoides cystica. British Journal of Dermatology 4:269-286.
Browne, A. (1888) Optic atrophy in three brothers. Transactions of the Ophthalmological Society of the United Kingdom 8:235-239.
Browne, E. (1888) Optic atrophy in three brothers. British Medical Journal 1:1338.
Brunton, T.L. (1880) Diabetes mellitus. In J.R. Reynolds (ed): A System of Medicine, Vol. 3. Philadelphia: Henry C. Lea's Son, pp. 585-612.
Burton-Fanning, F.W. (1895) Hereditary congenital nystagmus. Lancet 2:1497.
Buzzard, T. (1887) Two cases of Thomsen's disease. Lancet 1:972-974.
Campbell, D.A. (1888) Causative influence of heredity in progressive muscular atrophy. Maritime Medical News 1:77-79.
Campbell, H.J. (1887) Diabetes mellitus. Guy's Hospital Reports 29:181-232.
Cant, W.J. (1886) A family of four children affected with retinitis pigmentosa. Ophthalmic Review 5:245-246.
Carpenter, G. (1899) Clavicle deformity. Lancet 1:13.
Carter, R.B. (1890) Colour vision and colour blindness. Nature 42:55-59.
Chapman, P.M. (1884) Thomsen's disease. Brain 6:131-136.

Church, W.M. (1874) Hereditary character of some forms of xanthelasma palpebrorum. St. Bart's Hospital Reports 10:65-70.
Clarke, J.M. (1889) An account of three cases of Friedreich's disease, or hereditary ataxia. Lancet 1:570-571.
———. (1894) A case of Friedreich's ataxia. British Medical Journal 2:1294-1297.
———. (1897) On Huntington's chorea. Brain 20:22-34.
Clay, R.H. (1889) Three cases of diabetes insipidus in one family. Lancet 1:1188-1189.
Clemesha, J.C. (1897) Thomsen's disease: A family history. Lancet 2:1039-1040.
Clubbe, W.H. (1872) Hereditariness of stone. Lancet 1:204.
Coley, F.C. (1894) A pseudohypertrophic family. British Medical Journal 1:399-400.
Cook, A. and B. Sweeten (1890) A case of Thomsen's disease. British Medical Journal 1:73.
Cotes, C. (1890) Exostoses. Lancet 2:924.
Cotes, C.E. (1891) A case of hereditary multiple exostoses. Transactions of the Clinical Society of London 24:228-229.
Couch, J. (1895) A family history of herniae. Lancet 2:1043.
Crocker, H.R. (1883) Three cases of xeroderma pigmentosum. Proceedings of the Royal Medical and Chirurgical Society of London 1:234-235.
———. (1884) Three cases of xeroderma pigmentosum. Medical Times and Gazette 1:433-434.
———. (1887) Diseases of the Skin. London: Lewis, p. 354.
———. (1893) Hereditary alopecia neurotica. British Journal of Dermatology 5:176-177.
Davidson, D. (1886) Congenital blindness from optic atrophy and pigmentary retinitis. British Medical Journal 1:72.
Davy, J. (1861) On the present state of knowledge in regard to colour blindness. Transactions of the Royal Society of Edinburgh 37:441-480.
Dobell, H. (1862) A contribution to the natural history of hereditary transmission. Lancet 2:619-620.
———. (1863) A contribution to the natural history of hereditary transmission. Medico-Chirurgical Transactions 46:25-28.
Doyne, R. (1899) Peculiar condition of choroiditis occurring in several members of the same family. Transactions of the Ophthalmological Society of the United Kingdom 19:71.
Drake-Brockman, H.E. (1892) Remarkable case of polydactylism. British Medical Journal 2:1167-1168.
Dreschfeld, A. (1890) Thomsen's disease. British Medical Journal 1:429.
Dreschfeld, J. (1876) A family predisposed to locomotor ataxy. Liverpool and Manchester Medical and Surgical Report 4:93-98.
Drysdale, A. (1885) On migraine. Medical Press and Circular 39:488-494.
Durham, A.E. (1868) A case of the hemorrhagic diathesis. Guy's Hospital Reports 13:489-493.
Eccles, M. (1896) Exostoses. Lancet 2:1682.
Echeverri, M.G. (1880) Marriage and hereditariness of epileptics. Journal of Mental Science 26:346-369.
Eve, F.S. (1889) Haemophilia. Lancet 2:1002-1003.

Fagge, C.H. (1868) Skin and its appendages. Transactions of the Pathological Society of London 19:434.
Finlayson, J. (1882) Hemorrhagic diathesis in three generations. Glasgow Medical Journal 18:1-7.
Forbes, T. (1897) Cystic disease of the kidneys and liver. St. Bart's Hospital Reports 33:181-227.
Fotherby, H.A. (1886) The history of a family in which a similar hereditary deformity appeared in five generations. British Medical Journal 1:975-976.
Freeman, W.T. (1900) Eczema and the allied disorders. Lancet 2:398-401.
Frew, W. (1887) Case of diabetes mellitus in a girl of nine years with hereditary history. Glasgow Medical Journal 27:272-274.
Fulton, J. (1881) On pseudohypertrophic paralysis. Canada Lancet 13:225-228.
Gairdner, W.J. (1880) Angina pectoris and allied states. In J.R. Reynolds (ed): A System of Medicine, Vol. 2. Philadelphia: Henry C. Lea's Son, pp. 665-706.
Galton, F. (1886) Family likeness in eye colour. Proceedings of the Royal Society 40:402-416.
Gee, S. (1877) A contribution to the history of polydipsia. St. Bart's Hospital Reports 13:79-80.
———. (1884) Nervous disorders affecting a whole family. St. Bart's Hospital Reports 20:12-14.
———. (1889) Hereditary infantile spastic paraplegia. St. Bart's Hospital Reports 25:81-83.
Given, J.C. (1896) Diabetes and neurotic inheritance. Lancet 1:1425.
Goodhart, J.H. and G. Carpenter (1888) Cases of hereditary ataxia. Transactions of the Clinical Society of London 21:268-276.
Goodlee, A. (1884) Cases. Medical Times and Gazette 1:180-181.
Goodridge, H.F.A. (1882) Two cases of pseudohypertrophic muscular paralysis. Brain 5:268-271.
Gowers, W.R. (1879a) Pseudohypertrophic Muscular Paralysis. London: Churchill, p. 23.
———. (1879b) Pseudohypertrophic Muscular Paralysis, p. 24.
———. (1879c) Clinical lecture on pseudohypertrophic muscular paralysis. Lancet 2:737-750.
———. (1880) Epilepsy. Medical Times and Gazette 1:227-229.
———. (1881) A family affected with locomotor ataxy. Transactions of the Clinical Society of London 14:1-5.
———. (1885) Epilepsy. New York: Wood, pp. 6-10.
———. (1893a) A Manual of Diseases of the Nervous System, 2nd ed., Vol. 2. London: Churchill, p. 837.
———. (1893b) A Manual of Diseases of the Nervous System, 2nd ed., Vol. 2, p. 506.
———. (1893c) A Manual of Diseases of the Nervous System, 2nd ed., Vol. 1, p. 461.
Graham, J. (1886) A case of hemophilia. Australasian Medical Gazette 6:245-247.
Greenish, R.W. (1880) A case of hereditary tendency to fragilitus ossium. British Medical Journal 1:966-967.
Griffiths, J. (1892) Enchondroma following on hereditary multiple exostoses. Transactions of the Pathological Society of London 43:154-156.
Gunn, D. (1898) Family cataracts. Ophthalmic Review 17:141-142.

Gunn, R.M. (1882) Peculiar appearance of the retina in the vicinity of the optic disc in several members of one family. Transactions of the Ophthalmologic Society of the United Kingdom 3:110-113.
Habershon, S.A. (1888) Hereditary optic atrophy. Transactions of the Ophthalmological Society of the United Kingdom 8:190-234.
Harbinson, A. (1880) Sclerosis of the nervous centres mostly cerebral. Medical Press and Circular 80:123-125.
Harker, J. (1865) Malformation of the hands. Lancet 2:389.
Hawkins, F. (1894) Three cases of pseudohypertrophic paralysis in members of one family. Transactions of the Clinical Society of London 27:267-268.
Heath, C. (1868) Two cases of hereditary hemorrhagic diathesis. British Medical Journal 1:25.
"The hemorrhagic diathesis." (1884) British Medical Journal 1:686.
Herringham, W. (1888) Muscular atrophy of the peroneal type affecting many members of a family. Brain 11:230-236.
Higgens, C. (1881) Three cases of simple atrophy of the optic nerves, occurring in members of the same family. Lancet 2:869.
Hinshelwood, M. (1889) An isolated case of Friedreich's disease. Lancet 2:645.
Hodge, G. (1897) Three cases of Friedreich's ataxia. British Medical Journal 1:1405-1406.
Hope, J. (1887) A case of hemophilia. Australasian Medical Gazette 7:7.
Hulme, E. (1862) Malposition and cataractous state of the lenses. Lancet 2:618.
Hunter, W.B. (1889) Notes on three cases of xeroderma pigmentosum. British Medical Journal 2:69-70.
Huntington, G. (1872) On chorea. Medical and Surgical Reporter 26:317-321.
———. (1910) Recollections of Huntington's chorea as I saw it at East Hampton, Long Island during my boyhood. Journal of Nervous and Mental Diseases 39:255-257.
Hutchinson, J. (1866) Report on cases of congenital amaurosis. Royal London Ophthalmic Hospital Reports 5:347-352.
———. (1869) Notes on miscellaneous cases. Royal London Ophthalmic Hospital Reports 6:277-283.
———. (1876) Symmetrical central choroido-retinal disease occurring in senile persons. Royal London Ophthalmic Hospital Reports 8:231-244.
———. (1880) Multiple exostoses. Lancet 2:732.
———. (1882) On retinitis pigmentosa and allied disorders, as illustrating the laws of heredity. Ophthalmic Review 1:2-7, 26-30.
———. (1886) Congenital absence of hair and mammary glands. Medico-Chirurgical Transactions 51:473-477.
———. (1890a) The future of dermatology. British Medical Journal 2:440-442.
———. (1890b) On heredity in reference to disease. Archives of Surgery 2:42-53.
———. (1892a) Congenital defect in sight of three children. Archives of Surgery 4:271-272.
———. (1892b) Congenital defects and inherited proclivities. Archives of Surgery 4:305-308.
Jamieson, W.A. (1880) On cleft palate and incisor teeth: An instance of heredity. Edinburgh Medical Journal 26:117-120.
Jeaffreson, C.S. (1886) Cataract. Lancet 1:386-388.

Jones, R. (1896) The discovery of a bullet lost in the wrist by means of the Roentgen rays. Lancet 1:476-477.

Kingdon, E.C. (1894) Symmetrical changes of the macula lutea in an infant. Transactions of the Ophthalmological Society of the United Kingdom 14:129.

Kingdon, E. (1892) A rare fatal disease of infancy with symmetrical changes of the macula latea. Transactions of the Ophthalmological Society of the United Kingdom 12:126-137.

Kingdon, E. and J.S.R. Russell (1897) Infantile cerebral degeneration with symmetrical changes in the macula. Medico-Chirurgical Transactions 80:87-118.

Lang, W. (1885) Congenital aniridia. Transactions of the Ophthalmological Society of the United Kingdom 5:207.

———. (1888) Concommitant convergent strabismus. Royal London Ophthalmic Hospital Reports 12:133-148.

"The late Mr. Matthew Arnold." (1888) British Medical Journal 1:866.

Lawford, J.B. (1888) Congenital hereditary defect of ocular movements. Transactions of the Ophthalmological Society of the United Kingdom 8:262-274.

———. (1889a) Amblyopia and nystagmus. St. Bart's Hospital Reports 17:163-165.

———. (1889b) Atrophy of optic nerves. St. Bart's Hospital Reports 17:157-166.

Laycock, T. (1866) Nyctalopia with partial deafness in five children of the same family. Medical Times and Gazette 1:412.

Legg, J.W. (1871) Four cases of hemophilia. St. Bart's Hospital Reports 7:23-31.

———. (1872a) A Treatise on Hemophilia. London: HK Lewis.

———. (1872b) A Treatise on Hemophilia, p. 126.

———. (1876) Case of hemophilia. Lancet 2:856.

———. (1881) Report on hemophilia with a note on the hereditary descent of colour blindness. St. Bart's Hospital Reports 17:303-320.

Lindsay, J. (1893) Three cases of doubtful sex in one family. Glasgow Medical Journal 39:161-165.

Lingard, A. (1884) The hereditary transmission of hypospadius and its transmission by indirect atavism. Lancet 1:703.

Little, F. (1896) Three cases of pseudohypertrophic paralysis in one family. Transactions of the Clinical Society of London 29:238-239.

Liveing, E. (1873) Megrim, Sick Headaches. London: Churchill.

Lloyd Owen, D.C. (1882) An illustration of hereditary nystagmus. Ophthalmic Review 1:239-242.

Love, J.K. (1896a) Deaf Mutism. Glasgow: MacLehose, p. 88.

———. (1896b) Deaf Mutism, p. 99.

———. (1896c) Deaf Mutism, p. 128.

Lucas, R.C. (1881) On a remarkable incidence of hereditary tendency to the production of supernumerary digits. Guy's Hospital Reports 25:417-419.

———. (1888) On the congenital absence of an upper lateral incisor tooth as a forerunner of harelip and cleft palate. Transactions of the Clinical Society of London 21:64-66.

MacLehose, N.M. (1897) Hereditary congenital nystagmus associated with head movements. Ophthalmic Review 16:207-211.

MacLeod, M.D. (1882) On chorea. Journal of Mental Science 27:194-200.

Macphail, D. (1882) Pseudohypertrophic paralysis in four brothers. Glasgow Medical Journal 18:1-7.
Mason, F. (1877) On Hare Lip and Cleft Palate. London: Churchill, p. 18.
Maudsley, H. (1870) Relations between body and mind. Lancet 1:609-612.
M'caw, J. (1886) Hemophilia. Dublin Journal of Medical Science 81:507-510.
McIlraith, C.H. (1892) Notes on some cases of diabetes insipidus with marked family and hereditary tendencies. Lancet 2:767-768.
Menzies, W.F. (1892) Cases of hereditary chorea. Journal of Mental Science 38:560-568.
———. (1893) Cases of hereditary chorea. Journal of Mental Science 39:50-62.
Meryon, E. (1866a) On granular degeneration of the voluntary muscles. Lancet 1:258-260.
———. (1866b) On granular degeneration of the voluntary muscles. Medico-Chirurgical Transactions 49:45-51.
——— (1870) Cases of granular degeneration of the voluntary muscles. British Medical Journal 2:32-33.
M'gillivray, A. (1895) Hereditary congenital nystagmus associated with head movements. Ophthalmic Review 14:252-262.
M'Hardy, M.M. (1879) Cataract. St. George's Hospital Reports 9:479-485.
Miles, P. (1883) Two cases of heredity. Ophthalmic Review 2:48-49.
Mitchell, A. (1863) Interesting cases of deaf mutism. Medical Times and Gazette 2:164.
Montgomery-Smith, W.T. (1888) A family history of digital deformities. Guy's Hospital Reports 30:115-116.
Moore, M. (1880) Report of the history of a family, three members of which are subject to pseudohypertrophic muscular paralysis. Lancet 1:949-950.
Moreton, A. (1886) Hemophilia. Lancet 1:692-693.
Morgan, G. (1896) Skiagram of a case of polydactylism. Lancet 2:1599.
Morgan, J.H. (1890) Hereditary type of white hair in the forehead. British Medical Journal 2:85.
Morris, J.P. (1865) On the hereditary transmission through four generations of an abnormality. Anthropological Review 3:183.
Morton, A.S. (1892) Two cases of hereditary night blindness. Transactions of the Ophthalmologic Society of the United Kingdom 13:147-149.
———. (1893) Two cases of hereditary stationary night blindness. Transactions of the Ophthalmological Society of the United Kingdom 13:147-150.
Morton, J. (1894) A case of Friedreich's disease. Indian Medical Record 6:11.
Morton, S. (1879) Congenital displacement of both lenses occurring in seven members of one family. Royal London Ophthalmic Hospital Reports 9:435-439.
Muir, J.S. (1884) Note of a curious instance of abnormal development of adventitious fingers and toes, as illustrating the influence of heredity in five generations. Glasgow Medical Journal 21:420-423.
Murray, J. (1860) Contribution to teratology. British and Foreign Medico-Chirurgical Review 26:502-509.
"The narrowness of specialization." (1870) Lancet 1:1027.
Nettleship, E. (1880) Congenital day-blindness with colour blindness. St. Bart's Hospital Reports 10:37-48.

———. (1886) On some forms of congenital and infantile amblyopia. Royal London Ophthalmic Hospital Reports 11:353-399.
Newell, F.W. (1980) The Ophthalmological Society of the United Kingdom—Its first hundred years. American Journal of Ophthalmology 89:605-607.
Newman, D. (1897) Cases of cystic disease of the kidney. Glasgow Medical Journal 47:324-328.
Nicholson, F. (1889) Pseudohypertrophic muscular paralysis occurring in four brothers. Lancet 1:1081-1082.
Nolan, M.J. (1895) Three cases of Friedreich's ataxia. Dublin Journal of Medical Science 99:369-382.
Ogilvie, F.M. (1896) Optic atrophy in three brothers. Transactions of the Ophthalmological Society of the United Kingdom 16:111-124.
Ogle, J.A. (1872) On hereditary transmission of structural peculiarities. British and Foreign Medico-Chirurgical Review 44:510-521.
Oliver, C. (1892) Symmetrically placed opacities of the cornea occurring in mother and son. Ophthalmic Review 11:349-351.
Oliver, J. (1886) The study of epilepsy. Medical Press and Circular 43:350-352.
Oliver, T. (1886) Clinical notes on hemophilia. Lancet 2:526-529.
———. (1900) Physiology and pathology of inheritance. Lancet 2:1335-1341.
Ormerod, J.A. (1885a) Muscular atrophy after measles in three members of a family. Brain 7:334-342.
———. (1885b) On the so-called hereditary ataxia, first described by Friedreich. Brain 7:105-131.
———. (1887) Some of the observations on Friedreich's ataxia. Brain 10:461-473.
Ormerod, M. (1888) Friedreich's disease. Lancet 1:422.
Osler, W. (1885) Hemophilia. In W. Pepper (ed): System of Medicine, Vol. 3. Philadelphia: Lea Brothers, pp. 931-939.
———. (1896) Lectures on angina pectoris and related disorders. New York Medical Journal 64:250.
Page, H. (1874) Transmission through three generations of microphthalmos, iridemia, and nystagmus. Lancet 2:193-194.
Page, H.W. (1887) A case of haemophilia. Lancet 1:1028.
Pavy, F.W. (1885) Heredity and glycosuria. British Medical Journal 2:1049-1052.
Pendred, V. (1898) Hereditary keratosis palmae et plantaris. British Medical Journal 1:1132-1133.
Phillips, L.C.P. (1895) A case of xeroderma pigmentosum. St. Bart's Hospital Reports 31:221-223.
Pirie, G.E. (1892) A case of pseudohypertrophic muscular paralysis in an early stage. British Medical Journal 1:384.
Pole, W. (1893) On the present state of knowledge and opinion in regard to colour blindness. Transactions of the Royal Society of Edinburgh 37:441-480.
Poore, G. (1873) Hereditary exostoses. Lancet 2:771.
Powell, R.D. (1880) Aneurism of the thoracic aorta. In J.R. Reynolds (ed): A System of Medicine, Vol. 2. Philadelphia: Henry C. Lea's Son, pp. 838-858.
Power, D'A. (1882) Case of hereditary locomotor ataxy. St. Bart's Hospital Reports 18:305-308.

Price, W. (1863) On an extreme case of exostoses. Lancet 1:631-632.
Pritchard, O. (1883) Hereditary predisposition to fracture. Lancet 2:394.
Pye-Smith, P. (1883) Dislocation of radial head. Lancet 2:993.
Radmore, M. (1884) Remarkable history of hemophilia. Lancet 1:294.
Rayleigh, Lord. (1892) Report of the Committee on Colour Vision. Proceedings of the Royal Society 51:281-396.
Reid, T. (1887) Xeroderma pigmentosum. Glasgow Medical Journal 28:301-302.
Reynolds, J.R. (1880) Epilepsy. In J.R. Reynolds (ed): A System of Medicine, Vol. 1. Philadelphia: Lea's, pp. 762-783.
Roberts, C. (1882) Colour blindness as a racial character. Lancet 1:124.
Roberts, F.T. (1880) Tumors and new growths of the kidney. In J.R. Reynolds (ed): A System of Medicine, Vol. 3. Philadelphia: Henry C. Lea's Son, pp. 718-736.
Robertson, A. (1891) Hydrophthalmos. Transactions of the Ophthalmological Society of the United Kingdom 11:239-240.
Robinson, T. (1893) A case of multiple pedunculated exostoses. British Medical Journal 2:11.
Rook, A. (1979) Dermatology in Britain in the late nineteenth century. British Journal of Dermatology 100:3-11.
Rose, W. (1891) On Hare Lip and Cleft Palate. London: Lewis, p. 24.
Russell, J. (1869) Two cases of Ducchene's paralysis with muscular degeneration. Medical Times and Gazette 1:571-572.
Russell, J.W. (1894) Two cases of hereditary chorea occurring in twins. Birmingham Medical Review 35:31.
Russell, W. (1889) The influence of hereditary predisposition in epilepsy. Glasgow Medical Journal 31:434-435.
Salter, H.H. (1860) On asthma. London: Churchill.
Sandler, E.A. (1898) Hemophilia. Birmingham Medical Review 44:45.
Sankey, H.R. (1878) Two cases of microcephalic idiotcy in one family. Brain 1:391-399.
Schurr, P.W. (1985) Outline of the history of the Section of Neurology of the Royal Society of Medicine. Journal of the Royal Society of Medicine 78:146-148.
Sedgwick, W. (1861a) On sexual limitation in hereditary disease. British and Foreign Medico-Chirurgical Review 27:477-489.
———. (1861b) On sexual limitation in hereditary disease. British and Foreign Medico-Chirurgical Review 28:198-214.
———. (1862) Hereditary amaurosis. Medical Times and Gazette 1:309.
———. (1863a) On the influence of sex in hereditary disease. British and Foreign Medical and Chirurgical Review 31:445-478.
———. (1863b) On the influence of sex in hereditary disease. British and Foreign Medical and Chirurgical Review 32:159-197.
———. (1882) Atavism. British Medical Journal 2:922.
Shaw, J.E. (1897) Case of hemophilia with joint lesions. Bristol Medico-Chirurgical Journal 15:240-245.
Shuttleworth, G.E. (1886) The relation of marriages of consanguinity to mental unsoundness. British Medical Journal 2:581.
Simi, A. (1867) Retinitis pigmentosa occurring in three brothers. Ophthalmic Review 3:278-279.

Simpson, J.C. (1894) Report of five cases of pseudohypertrophic paralysis occurring in one family. Medical Press and Circular 57:57-59.
Skelton, H. (1887) Three cases of haemophilia in the same family. Lancet 1:874.
Smith, J. (1884) Two cases of hemophilia. Bristol Medico-Chirurgical Journal 2:264-269.
Smith, P. (1894) On an instance of hereditary glaucoma. Ophthalmic Review 13:215-226.
Smith, R. (1888) On recent developments in germ theory. Bristol Medico-Chirurgical Journal 6:225-264.
Smith, W.G. (1892) Recent advances in the etiology of diseases of the skin. Dublin Journal of Medical Science 93:1-13.
Smith, W.R. and J.S. Norwell (1894) Hereditary malformation of hands and feet. British Medical Journal 2:8-10.
Snell, S. (1886) Nyctalopia (retinitis pigmentosa) occurring in several members of one family. Ophthalmic Review 5:72-74.
Solomon, J.V. (1885) Clinical lecture on congenital cataract. Lancet 2:375-376.
Spokes, S. (1890) Enamel hypoplasia. Transactions of the Odontological Society of Great Britain 22:229-232.
Sproule, J. (1863) Hereditary nature of hare lip. British Medical Journal 1:412.
Spurway, J. (1896) Hereditary tendency to fracture. British Medical Journal 2:844.
Stawell, A.R. (1895) Two cases of Friedreich's disease. Australian Medical Journal 17:452-460.
Steven, J.L. (1889) Cases of trichorexis nodosa with a hereditary history. Glasgow Medical Journal 31:459.
Stewart, J. (1899) Clinical observations in chorea. Edinburgh Medical Journal 5:262-263.
Story, J.A. (1885) Hereditary amaurosis. Transactions of the Academy of Medicine of Ireland 3:23-28.
Story, J.B. (1885) Hereditary amaurosis. Ophthalmic Review 4:33-38.
Strahan, S.A.K. (1892) Marriage and Disease: A Study of Heredity and the More Important Family Degenerations. London: Kegan, Paul, Trench, Tribner, p. 307.
Streatfield, J.F. (1882) Observations on some congenital diseases of the eye. Lancet 1:303-305.
Struthers, J. (1863) On the variation in the numbers of fingers and toes and the number of phalanges in man. Edinburgh New Philosophical Journal 18:83-111.
———. (1873) On hereditary supracondylar process in man. Lancet 1:231-232.
Suckling, C. (1887a) Hereditary optic atrophy. Lancet 2:1271.
———. (1887b) The leg type of progressive muscular atrophy. British Medical Journal 1:66.
———. (1889a) Hereditary ataxia. British Medical Journal 1:1119.
———. (1889b) Hereditary chorea. Birmingham Medical Review 26:162.
———. (1889c) Hereditary chorea. British Medical Journal 2:1039.
Swanzy, H.R. (1873) Cases of congenital hemeralopia. Irish Hospital Gazette 1:84-86.
———. (1897) An address on some of the congenital anomalies of the eye. British Medical Journal 2:1249-1252.
Sym, W.G. (1890a) Albinism. Transactions of the Ophthalmologic Society of the United Kingdom 11:218-219.
———. (1890b) A case of hereditary amaurosis. Edinburgh Medical Journal 36:1131-1136.

Symonds, H. (1898) Two cases of night blindness. British Medical Journal 1:212.
Tay, W. (1884) A third instance in the same family of symmetrical changes of the yellow spot of each eye of an infant. Transactions of the Ophthalmological Society of the United Kingdom 4:158-159.
———. (1892a) A fourth instance of symmetrical changes in the yellow spot region of an infant. Transactions of the Ophthalmological Society of the United Kingdom 12:125-126.
——— .(1892b) Symmetrical retinal disease in infants. British Medical Journal 1:1022.
Taylor, J. (1891) Hereditary optic atrophy. British Medical Journal 2:1313.
———. (1894a) Three cases of pseudohypertrophic paralysis. Transactions of the Clinical Society of London 27:266-267.
———. (1894b) Two cases of Friedreich's ataxia. Practitioner 53:335-342.
Taylor, S.J. (1892) Hereditary optic atrophy. Transactions of the Ophthalmological Society of the United Kingdom 12:146-156.
Teevan, A. (1863) Stone in the bladder, hereditary and congenital. Lancet 1:386.
Thompson, J.A. (1889) Notes on a case of hereditary tendency to cataract in early childhood. Transactions of the Ophthalmologic Society of the United Kingdom 10:141-145.
———. (1890) Note on a case of hereditary tendency to cataract in early childhood. Transactions of the Ophthalmological Society of the United Kingdom 10:141-145.
Thompson, T. (1889) Hereditary tendency to cataract. Lancet 2:1282.
Thomson, J.D. (1892) Congenital malformation of hands and feet. British Medical Journal 1:1188-1190.
Tooth, H.H. (1886) Peroneal type of progressive muscular atrophy. London: Lewis.
Tooth, H. (1889) On hereditary progressive muscular atrophy. St. Bart's Hospital Reports 25:141-149.
Tressiden, W.E. (1893) Three cases of hereditary ataxy. Lancet 2:304.
Treves, F. (1886) A case of hemophilia. Lancet 2:533-534.
Tubby, A.H. (1894) A case of "lobster claw deformity" of the feet and partial suppresion of the fingers with remarkable hereditary history. Lancet 1:396-397.
Turner, W. (1883) Note on a hereditary deformity of the hand. Journal of Anatomy 18:463-464.
———. (1889) Heredity. Report of the British Association for the Advancement of Science:756-771.
Walker, J.W. (1872) On hemophilia. British Medical Journal 1:605-606.
Warden, C. (1887) Deaf mutism and consanguineous marriages. British Medical Journal 2:455-456.
West, J. (1884) Chorea in adult males. British Medical Journal 1:14-15.
White, W.H. (1889) On Thomsen's disease. Guy's Hospital Reports 46:329-360.
Whitlaw, W. (1885) Two cases of pseudohypertrophic paralysis. Medical Times and Gazette 1:273-275.
Whyte, J.M. (1898) Four cases of Friedreich's ataxia. Brain 21:72-136.
Wightman, J.P. (1894) Notes and family history of cases of hemophilia. Lancet 1:535-536.
Wilson, C. (1890) Some cases of hereditary enlargement of the spleen. Transactions of the Clinical Society of London 23:162-172.

Wilson, C. and D. Stanley (1892) A sequel to some cases of hereditary enlargement of the spleen. Transactions of the Clinical Society of London 26:163-171.
Wilson, E. (1869) On ekzema. Journal of Cutaneous Medicine 3:105-117.
Wilson, G. (1896) Hereditary polydactylism. Journal of Anatomy 30:437-449.
Winter, W.H.T. (1880) Some clinical observations on two cases of hemophilia. Dublin Journal of Medical Science 70:202-208.
Wolfe, J.R. (1879) Colour sight and colour blindness. Medical Times and Gazette 1:372-374; 419-421.
Wood, T.O. (1896) Three cases of hereditary congenital nystagmus. Transactions of the Medical Society of London 19:412-413.
Wordsworth, J. (1878) Congenital displacement of both lenses in six males in one family. Medical Press and Circular 25:110-111.
Young, D. (1898) Hereditary digital abnormality. British Medical Journal 2:715.
Young, J. (1889) On a case of hemophilia. Lancet 2:951.

Chapter Eleven

Ackerknecht, E.H. (1982) Diathesis: The word and the concept in medical history. Bulletin of the History of Medicine 56:317-325.
Adams, J. (1814) A Treatise on the Supposed Hereditary Properties of Diseases. London: Callow, p. 38.
Alborn, T. (2001a) Insurance against germ theory: Commerce and conservatism in late-Victorian medicine. Bulletin of the History of Medicine 75:406-445.
———. (2001b) Insurance against germ theory: Commerce and conservatism in late-Victorian medicine. Bulletin of the History of Medicine 75:414.
———. (2001c) Insurance against germ theory: Commerce and conservatism in late-Victorian medicine. Bulletin of the History of Medicine 75:417.
———. (2001d) Insurance against germ theory: Commerce and conservatism in late-Victorian medicine. Bulletin of the History of Medicine 75:433.
Andrew, J. (1884) The etiology of phthisis. Lancet 1:693-698, 785-788, 833-838.
Barling, G. (1891) Tubercule. Medical Press and Circular 51:423-426.
Barrett, J.W. and P. Webster (1891) A case of multiple adenomata. Australian Medical Journal 13:425-426.
———. (1892) Multiple sudariparous adenomata. British Medical Journal 1:272-273.
Barwell, R. (1894) The improbability of a parasitic origin of malignant disease. Lancet 2:180-182, 430-431, 678-679, 1024-1025.
Beecher, H.K. (1960) Disease and the Advancement of Basic Science. Cambridge: Harvard, p. 12.
Bennett, J.H. (1880) Phthisis pulmonalis. In J.R. Reynolds (ed): A System of Medicine, Vol. 2. Philadelphia: Henry C. Lea's Son, pp. 107-144.
Blake, T.W. (1891) Cancer and phthisis. British Medical Journal 2:846.
"Book review." (1846) British and Foreign Medico-Chirurgical Review 22:124-155.
Brand, A.T. (1903) The exogenesis of cancer. Quarterly Medical Journal 11:177-196.
Buchanan, J.R.M. (1900) The etiology of cancer with special reference to the parasitic theory. Liverpool Medico-Chirurgical Journal 20:149-161.
Budd, R. (1887) Is cancer contagious? Lancet 2:1091.
Butlin, H.T. (1895) Is cancer hereditary? British Medical Journal 1:1006.

Cameron, H.C. (1886) The etiological and clinical aspects of carcinoma. Glasgow Medical Journal 35:354-368.
Coats, J. (1889) On the nature of constitutional susceptibility to disease. British Medical Journal 2:409-414.
Darwin, C. (1893) The Variation of Animals and Plants under Domestication, 2nd ed., Vol. 2. London: Murray.
Davies, C.A. (1900) Consanguinity as a factor in the etiology of tuberculosis. British Medical Journal 2:904-906.
Dean, G. (1891) Dr. Russell's characteristic microorganisms of cancer. Lancet 1:768.
Dunn, H.P. (1886) Theory of cancerous inheritance. Lancet 1:148-150.
Elsner, F.W. (1886) Etiology of tuberculosis. Australasian Medical Gazette 6:12-15, 36-38.
Fee, E. and D. Porter. (1992) Public health, preventive medicine and professionalization: England and America in the nineteenth century. In A. Wear (ed): Medicine in Society. Cambridge: Cambridge University Press, pp. 249-275.
Fox, W. (1880) Diseases of the stomach. In J.R. Reynolds (ed): A System of Medicine, Vol. 3. Philadelphia: Henry C. Lea's Son, pp. 17-131.
Galloway, J. (1893) The abstract of the Morton Lectures on the parasitism of protozoa in carcinoma. Lancet 1:231-234.
Galton, F. (1889) Natural Inheritance. London: Macmillan.
Garrod, A.B. (1880a) Rheumatism. In J.R. Reynolds (ed): A System of Medicine, Vol. 1. Philadelphia: Lea's, pp. 558-575.
———. (1880b) Gout. In J.R. Reynolds (ed): A System of Medicine, Vol. 1, pp. 512-550.
Garrod, A.E. and E.H. Cooke (1888) On an attempt to determine the frequency of rheumatic family histories amongst non-rheumatic patients. Lancet 2:110.
Green, T.H. (1883) A lecture on the tubercule bacillus and phthisis. British Medical Journal 1:193-194.
Greenhow, A. (1862) Phthisis. Medical Times and Gazette 1:362.
Hamilton, D.J. (1900) On heredity in disease. Scottish Medical and Surgical Journal 6:289-320.
Hansen, G. (1875) On the etiology of leprosy. British and Foreign Medico-Chirurgical Review 55:459-489.
Hardman, W. (1894) The heredity of cancer. British Medical Journal 1:1358.
Hartshorne, H. (1880) Scrofula. In J.R. Reynolds (ed): A System of Medicine, Vol. 1. Philadelphia: Lea's, pp. 497-511.
Haviland, A. (1895) Cancer causes. Lancet 1:1049-1050.
Howlett, E.H. (1893) A family history of cancer. Quarterly Medical Journal 2:313-319.
Hutchinson, J. (1891) Sebaceous tumors of the scalp. Archives of Surgery 3:336-337.
———. (1896a) Illustrations of the laws of heredity. Archives of Surgery 7:128-132.
———. (1896b) Relation of the study of dermatology to general medicine. Lancet 2:440-441.
James, A. (1888) Pulmonary Phthisis. Edinburgh: Pentland, pp. 90-92.
Kanthrack, A. (1891) A characteristic organism of cancer. British Medical Journal 1:579-580.
Lauder, W. (1886) Heredity in relation to disease. Manchester Health Lectures for the People 10:113-136.
Lithgow, R.A.O. (1887) From generation to generation: a prelude to the study of heredity. Provincial Medical Journal 6:116-119, 157-160.

———. (1887) Heredity. London: Bailliere, p. 73.
Love, J.K. (1896) Deaf Mutism. Glasgow: MacLehose, p. 128.
Mahomed, F.A. and F. Galton (1882) An inquiry into the physiognamy of phthisis by the method of "composite portraiture." Guy's Hospital Reports 25:1-18.
Marsh, H. (1886) Diseases of the Joints. London: Cassel, pp. 97-98.
Marshall, J. (1889) Cancer and cancerous diseases. Lancet 2:1045-1048.
McAldowie, A. (1879) On the modification of cancer by hereditary transmission. British Medical Journal 1:44.
Monsaurat, K.W. (1900) The parasite of cancer. Liverpool Medico-Chirurgical Journal 20:318-324.
Oliver, T. (1900) Physiology and pathology of inheritance. Lancet 2:1335-1341.
Osler, W. (1892a) The Principles and Practice of Medicine. New York: Appleton, p. 270.
———. (1892b) The Principles and Practice of Medicine. New York: Appleton, p. 28.
———. (1892c) The Principles and Practice of Medicine. New York: Appleton, p. 287.
———. (1892d) The Principles and Practice of Medicine. New York: Appleton, p. 256.
———. (1892e) The Principles and Practice of Medicine. New York: Appleton, pp. 251-259.
———. (1892f) The Principles and Practice of Medicine. New York: Appleton, p. 185.
Parsons, J.I. (1900) The parasitic theory of cancer. British Gynacological Journal 16:56-67.
Pasteur, W. (1897) An epidemic of infantile paralysis occurring in children of the same family. Transactions of the Clinical Society of London 30:143-150.
Pollock, J.E. (1883a) Modern theories and treatments of phthisis. Medical Times and Gazette 1:605-607.
———. (1883b) Tuberculosis. Lancet 1:717-721.
Power, J.H. (1898) The history of a cancerous family. British Medical Journal 2:154.
Robertson, R. (1882) Family history in relation to contagion in phthisis pulmonalis. British Medical Journal 2:624-626.
Ruffer, M.A. and H.G. Plimmer (1893) Further researches on parasitic protozoans found in cancerous tumors. Journal of Pathology and Bacteriology 2:3-25.
Russell, A. (1900a) A contribution to the etiology of cancer. Birmingham Medical Review 47:257-275.
———. (1900b) A contribution to the etiology of cancer. Birmingham Medical Review 47:334-353.
———. (1900c) A contribution to the etiology of cancer. Birmingham Medical Review 48:12-24.
Russell, W. (1890) An address on a characteristic organism of cancer. British Medical Journal 2:1356-1360.
Sedgwick, W. (1863a) On the influence of sex in hereditary disease. British and Foreign Medical and Chirurgical Review 32:159-197.
———. (1863b) On the influence of sex in hereditary disease. British and Foreign Medical and Chirurgical Review 31:445-478.
Silcock, A.Q. (1891) Hereditary melanotic sarcoma of the choroid. Transactions of the Pathological Society of London 43:140-141.
Simon, J. (1892) Some points of science and practice concerning cancer. St. Thomas's Hospital Reports 20:221-236.

Simpson, J. (1842) Antiquarian instances of leprosy and leper hospitals in Scotland and England. Part III. The etiological history of the disease. Edinburgh Medical and Surgical Journal 57:405-429.
Smith, G.B. (1900) The infectivity of malignant growths. Edinburgh Medical Journal 7:1-14.
Snow, H. (1880) The etiology of cancer. Lancet 2:1012.
Snow, H.L. (1883) Clinical Notes on Cancer. London: Churchill, pp. 18-23.
Snow, H. (1885) Is cancer hereditary? British Medical Journal 2:690-692.
———. (1891) The Proclivity of Women to Certain Cancerous Diseases. London: Churchill, p. 27.
———. (1893a) A Treatise, Practical and Theoretical, on Cancer. London: Churchill.
———. (1893b) The so-called "parasitic protozoa" of mammary carcinoma. Lancet 2:1182-1183.
———. (1893c) The nature of cancer. Lancet 2:235-237.
———. (1898) Twenty Two Years Experience in Treating Cancerous and other Tumors. London: Bailliere, pp. 15-16.
Squire, A.B. (1880) Elephantiasis graecorum. In J.R. Reynolds (ed): A System of Medicine, Vol. 3. Philadelphia: Lea's Son, pp. 947-950.
Squire, J.E. (1894) The influence of heredity in phthisis. British Medical Journal 2:1364-1365.
———. (1895) The influence of heredity in phthisis. Medico-Chirurgical Transactions 78:67-87.
———. (1897) Heredity in phthisis. American Journal of Medical Science 114:537-542.
Steven, J.L. (1892) The pathological and clinical aspects of tuberculosis as an infectious disease. Glasgow Medical Journal 37:15-41.
Strahan, S.A.K. (1892a) Marriage and Disease: A Study of Heredity and the More Important Family Degenerations. London: Kegan, Paul, Trench, Tribner, p. 199.
———. (1892b) Marriage and Disease: A Study of Heredity, p. 182.
Taylor, G.G.S. and F.H. Barendt (1893) Three cases of adenoma sebaceum in one family. British Journal of Dermatology 5:360-363.
Thin, G. (1892) On the origin and spread of leprosy at Parcent in Spain. Lancet 1:134-136.
Thomas, W.R. (1888) On the etiology and curability of phthisis. British Medical Journal 1:239-240.
Vellemin, J.A. (1862) Du Tubercule au Point de Vue de son Siege, de son Evolution, et de sa Nature. Paris: J.B. Bailliere.
Waller, J.C. (2002a) The illusion of an explanation: The concept of hereditary disease. Journal of the History of Medicine 57:410-448.
———. (2002b) The illusion of an explanation: The concept of hereditary disease. Journal of the History of Medicine 57:419-420.
———. (2002c) The illusion of an explanation: The concept of hereditary disease. Journal of the History of Medicine 57:423.
———. (2002d) The illusion of an explanation: The concept of hereditary disease. Journal of the History of Medicine 57:432.
———. (2002e) The illusion of an explanation: The concept of hereditary disease. Journal of the History of Medicine 57:443.

Weindling, P. (1992) From infectious to chronic diseases: changing patterns of sickness in the nineteenth and twentieth centuries. In A. Wear (ed): Medicine in Society. Cambridge: Cambridge University Press, pp. 303-316.
Williams, C.J.B. and C.T. Williams. (1887) Pulmonary Consumption. London: Longmans, pp. 56-77.
Williams, G.R. (1891) Remarks on the pathogeny of cancer, with special reference to the microbe theory. Lancet 2:606-607.
Williams, W.R. (1884) The family history of cancer patients. British Medical Journal 1:1039-1040.
———. (1886) The family history of cancer patients. Lancet 1:146-147.
———. (1887) Cancer and phthisis as correlated diseases. Lancet 1:977.
———. (1895) Is cancer hereditary? British Medical Journal 1:1007.
Wilson, P.K. (2003) Erasmus Darwin on hereditary disease: Conceptualizing heredity in Enlightenment English medical writings. In J.H. Rheinberger and W. Muller S (eds): A Cultural History of Heredity II: 18th and 19th Centuries. Berlin: Max Planck Institut fur Wissenschaftsgeschichte, p. 120.
Woodhead, G.S. (1892) The bearing of recent biological researches on the practice of medicine and surgery. Lancet 1:77.
Woods, R. and J. Woodward. (1961) Mortality, poverty, and the environment. In F.N.L. Poynter (ed): The Evolution of Medical Practice in Britain. London: Pitman, pp. 20-29.
Woodward, J. (1961) Medicine and the city in the nineteenth-century experience. In F.N.L. Poynter (ed): The Evolution of Medical Practice in Britain, pp. 67-68.
Worboys, M. (2000a) Spreading Germs: Disease Theories and Medical Practice in Britain, 1865-1900. Cambridge: Cambridge University Press, p. 176.
———. (2000b) Spreading Germs: Disease Theories and Medical Practice in Britain, 1865-1900, p. 42.
———. (2000c) Spreading Germs: Disease Theories and Medical Practice in Britain, 1865-1900, pp. 197-198.
———. (2000d) Spreading Germs: Disease Theories and Medical Practice in Britain, 1865-1900, p. 198.
———. (2000e) Spreading Germs: Disease Theories and Medical Practice in Britain, 1865-1900, pp. 205-206.
———. (2000f) Spreading Germs: Disease Theories and Medical Practice in Britain, 1865-1900, p. 206.
———. (2000g) Spreading Germs: Disease Theories and Medical Practice in Britain, 1865-1900, pp. 206-207.
———. (2000h) Spreading Germs: Disease Theories and Medical Practice in Britain, 1865-1900, p. 31.

Chapter Twelve

"A censor of scientific method" (1915) British Medical Journal 1:16-17.
Adami, J.G. (1901a) An address on theories of inheritance. British Medical Journal 1:1317-1323.
———. (1901b) On theories of inheritance. Montreal Medical Journal 30:425-449.
———. (1901c) On theories of inheritance with special reference to the inheritance of acquired conditions in man. New York Medical Journal 73:925-936.
———. (1906) The dominance of the nucleus. Montreal Medical Journal 35:581-596.

———. (1907) The dominance of the nucleus. Canadian Journal of Medicine and Surgery 21:143-162.

Adami, M. (1930) J. George Adami—A Memoir. London: Constable and Co.

Adler, J.E. and J. McIntosh (1909-1910) Histological examination of a case of albinism. Biometrika 7:237-243.

"An investigation into the etiology of cancer" (1900) British Medical Journal 2:932.

Barrington, A. and K. Pearson. (1909a) A First Study of the Inheritance of Vision and the Relative Influence of Heredity and Environment on Sight, Memoir V. London: Dulau, p. 4.

———. (1909b) A First Study of the Inheritance of Vision, p. 60.

———. (1909c) A First Study of the Inheritance of Vision, p. 61.

Bateson, B. (1928a) William Bateson, F.R.S. Naturalist: His Essays and Addresses. Cambridge: Cambridge University Press, p. 62.

———. (1928b) William Bateson, F.R.S. Naturalist, p. 126.

Bateson, W. (1894a) Materials for the Study of Variation. Baltimore: Johns Hopkins University Press, p. 568.

———. (1894b) Materials for the Study of Variation, p. 514.

———. (1899) Hybridisation and cross-breeding as a method of scientific investigation. Journal of the Royal Horticultural Society 24:59-66.

———. (1902a) The facts of heredity in light of Mendel's discovery. Report to the Evolution Committee of the Royal Society 1:125-160.

———. (1902b) Letter to K. Pearson. 13 May 1902 (P 631/4).

———. (1902c) Mendel's Principles of Heredity: A Defence. Cambridge: Cambridge University Press, p. 125.

———. (1902d) Mendel's Principles of Heredity: A Defence, pp. 76-80.

———. (1902e) The facts of heredity in light of Mendel's discovery. Report to the Evolution Committee of the Royal Society 1:131.

———. (1902f) The facts of heredity in light of Mendel's discovery. Report to the Evolution Committee of the Royal Society 1:133.

———. (1904) Heredity and variation. British Medical Journal 2:448-449.

———. (1905-1906a) Albinism in Sicily. Biometrika 4:231-232.

———. (1905b) Letter to E. Nettleship. 15 July 1905 (P 329).

———. (1906a) An address on Mendelian heredity and its application to man. Brain 29:157-175.

———. (1906b) An address on Mendelian heredity and its application to man. British Medical Journal 2:61-67.

———. (1906c) Letter to E. Nettleship. 13 April 1906 (P 329).

———. (1906d) Letter to E. Nettleship. 1 February 1906 (P 329).

———. (1906e) Letter to E. Nettleship. 13 October 1906 (P 329).

———. (1907a) Facts limiting the theory of heredity. Science 26:649-660.

———. 1907b. Letter to E. Nettleship. 7 January 1907 (P 329).

———. (1908-1909a) Heredity. Proceedings of the Royal Society of Medicine 2:22-30.

———. (1908b) Letter to E. Nettleship. 31 March 1908 (P 329).

———. (1909a) Mendel's Principles of Heredity. Cambridge: Cambridge University Press.

———. (1909b) Mendel's Principles of Heredity, p. 195.

———. (1911a) Hereditary nystagmus. Lancet 1:1278.

———. (1911b) Hereditary transmission. Lancet 1:1682.

———. (1913) Address on heredity. Lancet 2:451-454.

———. (1914a) Heredity. Cincinnati Lancet Clinic 112:312-317.

———. (1914b) Presidential address. Australian Medical Journal 1:179, 197.

———. (ed). (1915a) Report of the Eighty-Fourth Meeting of the British Association for the Advancement of Science. London: Murray.

———. (ed). (1915b) Report of the Eighty-Fourth Meeting of the British Association for the Advancement of Science, p. 26.

———. (ed). (1915c) Report of the Eighty-Fourth Meeting of the British Association for the Advancement of Science, pp. 3-7.

———. 1925. Notes for lecture to University College Medical Society 17 November 1925 (C G8C-18).

Batten, F.E., 1908. Letter to W. Bateson. 27 November 1908 (B 2763).

Beard, J. (1904) Heredity in its biological and psychiatrical aspects. British Medical Journal 2:963-965.

Bearn, A.G. (1993a) Archibald Garrod and the Individuality of Man. Oxford: Clarendon.

———. (1993b) Archibald Garrod and the Individuality of Man, p. 42.

Bevan-Lewis, W. (1909) On the biological factor in heredity. Journal of Mental Science 55:591-630.

Bluhm, A. (1912) Problems in Eugenics. London: Eugenics Education Society.

Bond, C.J. (1905) The correlation of sex and disease. British Medical Journal 2:1094.

Bramwell, B. (1902) The causation and prevention of phthisis. Lancet 2:6-10, 61-64, 132-136, 200-204, 274-280.

Brownlee, J. (1910-1911) The inheritance of complex growth forms, such as stature, on Mendel's theory. Proceedings of the Royal Society of Edinburgh 31:251-256.

Bulloch, W., (1909) Letter to K. Pearson. 14 June 1909 (P 205/6).

———. (1911-1915) Letters to K. Pearson. 1911-1915 (P 647/5).

———. (1913) Letter to K. Pearson. 4 April 1913 (P 647/5).

Burton-Fanning, F.W. (1902) The etiology of pulmonary tuberculosis. Practitioner 68:317-326.

Catarinich, J. (1914) Huntington's chorea. Australian Medical Journal 3:1509-1510.

Chambers, D.W. (1991) Does distance tyrannize science? In R.W. Home (ed): International Science and National Scientific Identity. London: Kluwer, pp. 19-29.

Church, W.S. (1909) Influence of Heredity on Disease. London: Longmans, Green.

Clarke, E. (1903) Hereditary nystagmus. Ophthalmoscope 1:86.

———. (1910) Letter to W. Bateson. ?9 February 1910 (B 2709).

Clippingdale, S.D. (1918) Hereditary abnormality. Lancet 2:802.

Cock, A.G. (1973) William Bateson, Mendelism, and Biometry. Journal of the History of Biology 6:1-36.

Cock, A.G. and D.R. Forsdyke (2008a) Treasure Your Exceptions—The Science and Life of William Bateson. New York: Springer, p. 140.

———. (2008b) Treasure Your Exceptions—The Science and Life of William Bateson, p. 242.

———. (2008c) Treasure Your Exceptions—The Science and Life of William Bateson, pp. 230-231.

———. (2008d) Treasure Your Exceptions—The Science and Life of William Bateson, pp. 336-338.

Cockayne, E.A. (1914-1915) A piebald family. Biometrika 10:197-200.

Coleman, W. (1970) William Bateson. In C.C. Gillispie (ed): Dictionary of Scientific Biography, Vol. 1. New York: Scribners, pp. 505-506.

Cowan, R.S. (1972) Galton's contribution to genetics. Journal of the History of Biology 5:389-412.

Cragg, E. and H. Drinkwater (1916-1917) Hereditary absence of phalanges through five generations. Journal of Genetics 6:81-89.

Darbshire, A.D. (1902) Note on the results of crossing Japanese waltzing mice and European albino mice. Biometrika 2:101-104.

———. (1907) Mendelism. Nature 76:73-74.
Darden, L. (1977) William Bateson and the promise of Mendelism. Journal of the History of Biology 10:87-106.
Davenport, C.B. (1910) Letter to K. Pearson. 5 February 1910. Quoted in Kim, K.-M. (1994) Explaining Scientific Consensus—The Case of Mendelian Genetics. New York: Guilford, p. 132.
Drinkwater, H. (1907a) Letter to W. Bateson. 29 May 1907 (B 2781).
———. (1907b) Letter to W. Bateson. 26 June 1907 (B 2783).
———. (1907c) Letter to W. Bateson. 13 December 1907 (B 2784).
———. (1907d) Letter to W. Bateson. 2 June 1907 (B 2782).
———. (1907e) Proof of seminar presented at Royal Society of Edinburgh 1907 (P 381).
———. (1908a) An account of a brachydactylous family. Liverpool Medico-Chirurgical Journal 28:408-414.
———. (1908b) Letter to W. Bateson. 7 October 1908 (B 2758).
———. (1908c) Recent theories and experiments in heredity. British Medical Journal 2:1538-1541.
———. (1909) Mendelian heredity in asthma. British Medical Journal 1:88.
———. (1910) A Lecture on Mendelism. London: J.M. Dent.
———. (1911) Letter to K. Pearson. 8 March 191 (P 309).
———. (1912-1913) Account of family showing minor brachydactyly. Journal of Genetics 2:21-40.
———. (1913-1914a) Minor brachydactyly No. 2. Journal of Genetics 3:217-220.
———. (1913b) Study of a brachydactylous family. Report of the Fourth International Congress on Genetics p. 549.
———. (1914-1915) A second brachydactylous family. Journal of Genetics 4:323-340.
———. (1916a) Hereditary abnormal segmentation of the index and middle fingers. Journal of Anatomy 50:177-186.
———. (1916b) Letter to W. Bateson. 18 April 1916 (B 2804).
———. (1917a) The inheritance of normal and pathologic traits in man. Practitioner 98:257-278.
———. (1917b) Phalangeal anarthrosis (synostosis, ankylosis) transmitted through fourteen generations. Proceedings of the Royal Society of Medicine 10:60-68 Pathology.
Dunn, L.C. (1991) A Short History of Genetics. Ames, Iowa: Iowa State University Press.
Eccles, W.A. (1912) Letter to K. Pearson. January 1912 (P 892/5).
Eisenhart, C. (1970) Karl Pearson. In C.C. Gillispie (ed): Dictionary of Scientific Biography, Vol. 10. New York: Scribners, pp. 447-469.
Elderton, E.M. (1909) Relative strength of nurture and nature. Eugenics Laboratory Lecture Series 3:33.
———. (1910) A First Study of the Influence of Parental Alcoholism on the Physique and Ability of the Offspring, Eugenics Laboratory Memoir X. London: Dulau.
Farabee, W.C. (1905) Inheritance of digital malformations in man. Peabody Museum of American Archaeology and Ethnology Papers 3:67-80.
Farmer, J.B., J.E.S. Moore, and C.E. Walker (1906) On the cytology of malignant growths. Proceedings of the Royal Society 77B:336-353.
Farrall, L. (1975) Controversy and conflict in science: A case study—The English biometric school and Mendel's laws. Social Studies in Science 5:269-301.
Farrall, L.A. (1985a) The Origins and Growth of the English Eugenics Movement 1865-1925. New York: Garland Publishing Co.
———. (1985b) The Origins and Growth of the English Eugenics Movemet, p. 176-177.

———. (1985c) The Origins and Growth of the English Eugenics Movement, p. 134.
———. (1985d) The Origins and Growth of the English Eugenics Movement, pp. 150-151.
Fildes, P. (1909) Hemophilia. London Hospital Gazette 16:48-51.
Firth, R.H. (1909) Some modern views regarding heredity and variation. Journal of the Royal Army Medical Corps 13:633-646.
Froggatt, P. and N.C. Nevin (1971) The 'law of ancestral heredity' and the Mendelian-Ancestrian controversy in England, 1889-1906. Journal of Medical Genetics 8:1-36.
Galton, F. (1889) Natural Inheritance. London: Macmillan.
Garrod, A.E. (1902a) The incidence of alkaptonuria. Lancet 2:1616-1620.
———. (1902b) Letter to W. Bateson. 11 January 1902. Quoted in Bearn, A.G. (1993) Archibald Garrod and the Individuality of Man. Oxford: Clarendon, pp. 59-61.
———. (1902c) Letter to W. Bateson. 20 March 1902. Quoted in ———. (1993) Archibald Garrod and the Individuality of Man, .p. 61.
———. (1902d) Letter to W. Bateson. 22 March 1902 (B G7h-4).
———. (1902e) Letter to W. Bateson. 8 June 1902 (B G7h-05).
———. (1903a) Letter to W. Bateson. 5 June 1903. Quoted in Bearn, A.G. (1993) Archibald Garrod and the Individuality of Man. Oxford: Clarendon, p. 64.
———. (1903b) Uber chemische Individualitat und die chemische Missbildungen. Pflugers Archiv fur die Gesamte Physiologie 97:410-418.
———. (1908) Inborn errors of metabolism. Lancet 2:1-7, 73-79, 142-148, 214-220.
Gask, G.E. (1918) Letter to W. Bateson. 20 January 1918 (B 2552).
Gillham, N.W. (2001a) A Life of Sir Francis Galton—From African Exploration to the Birth of Eugenics. New York: Oxford University Press.
———. (2001b) A Life of Sir Francis Galton, p. 339.
———. (2001c) A Life of Sir Francis Galton, p. 347.
———. (2001d) A Life of Sir Francis Galton, p. 349.
———. (2001e) A Life of Sir Francis Galton, p. 352.
Gossage, A. (1907a) Letter to W. Bateson. 16 November 1907 (B 2745).
———. (1907b) Letter to W. Bateson. 9 May 1907 (B 2741).
———. (1908-1909a) Discussion. Proceedings of the Royal Society of Medicine 2:86-89.
———. (1908b) The inheritance of certain human abnormalities. Quarterly Journal of Medicine 1:331-344.
———. (1908c) Letter to W. Bateson. 24 November 1908 (B 2748).
———. (1908d) Letter to W. Bateson. 25 June 1908 (B 2747).
———. (1908e) Letter to W. Bateson. 6 June 1908 (B 2744).
———. (1909) Letter to W. Bateson. 3 October 1909 (B 2764).
———. (1910a) Letter to W. Bateson. 11 April 1910 (B 2766).
———. (1910b) Letter to W. Bateson. 20 November 1910 (B 2767).
———. (1910c) Letter to W. Bateson. 10 January 1910 (B 2765).
Gossage, A.M. and E.R. Carling (1910-1911) Multiple cartilaginous exostoses. Proceedings of the Royal Society of Medicine 4:1-22 Medicine.
Gowers, W. (1908-1909a) Heredity. Proceedings of the Royal Society of Medicine 2:15-22.
———. (1908b) Heredity in diseases of the nervous system. British Medical Journal 2:1541-1543.
———. (1908c) Heredity in diseases of the nervous system. Lancet 2:1506-1508.
Greenwood, M. (1908) Discussion. Proceedings of the Royal Society of Medicine 1:162-164.
———. (1940) Karl Pearson. Dictionary of National Biography 1931-1940:681-684.
Hall, G.A.M. (1928) Hereditary brachydactyly and intraphalangeal ankylosis. Annals of Eugenics 3:265-268.

Harman, N.B. (1908-1909) Discussion. Proceedings of the Royal Society of Medicine 2:135.
Herringham, C.J. (1903) Letter to W. Bateson. 19 December 1903 (C G50-2).
———. (1906) Letter to W. Bateson. 14 January 1906 (C G50-12).
Herringham, W.P. (1902) Letter to W. Bateson. 6 July 1902 (C G5n-13).
———. (1904) Letter to E. Nettleship. 28 November 1904 (P 330).
Higgit, R., 1998. Personal communication. 5 January 1998, from The Manuscript and Rare Book Division of the Library at the University College London.
Hillier, W.T. and I. Tritsch (1904) Heredity in cancer. Archives of Middlesex Hospital 2:104-126.
Hutchinson, J. (1905) Letter to K. Pearson. 4 February 1905 (P 205/20).
Jones, J.S. (1993) The Galton Laboratory—University College London. In M. Keynes (ed): Sir Francis Galton FRS—The Legacy of His Ideas. London: Macmillan, pp. 190-194.
Jordan, H.E. (1912) The place of eugenics in the medical curriculum. In Problems in Eugenics. London: Eugenics Education Society, pp. 396-398.
Kevles, D.J. (1980) Genetics in the US and Great Britain 1890-1930: A review with speculations. Isis 71:441-455.
———. (1985a) In the Name of Eugenics. New York: Knopf.
———. (1985b) In the Name of Eugenics, p. 337.
———. (1985c) In the Name of Eugenics, p. 57.
———. (1985d) In the Name of Eugenics, p. 104.
Kim, K.-M. (1994a) Explaining Scientific Consensus—The Case of Mendelian Genetics. New York: Guilford, p. 30.
———. (1994b) Explaining Scientific Consensus—The Case of Mendelian Genetics, pp. 58-62.
———. (1994c) Explaining Scientific Consensus—The Case of Mendelian Genetics, pp. 58-62.
———. (1994d) Explaining Scientific Consensus—The Case of Mendelian Genetics, p. 65.
———. (1994e) Explaining Scientific Consensus—The Case of Mendelian Genetics, p. 78.
———. (1994f) Explaining Scientific Consensus—The Case of Mendelian Genetics, p. xviii.
———. (1994f) Explaining Scientific Consensus—The Case of Mendelian Genetics, pp. 81-82.
Knight, D. (1991) Tyrannies of distance in British science. In R.W. Home (ed): International Science and National Scientific Identity. London: Kluwer, p. 40.
Lawford, J.B. (1922) Memoir of Edward Nettleship. Treasury of Human Inheritance 2(I):ix-xv.
Lewis, T. (1906) Letter to K. Pearson. 1906 (P 185).
———. (1908-1909) Addendum to Memoir: Split hand and split foot deformities. Biometrika 6:117-118.
Lewis, T. and D. Embleton (1908-1909) Split hand and split foot deformities. Biometrika 6:26-58.
Lucas, R.C. (1904) The hereditary bias and early environment in their relation to the diseases and defects of children. Lancet 2:278-283.
MacLeod, R. (1988) From imperial to national science. In R. MacLeod (ed): The Commonwealth of Science. Melbourne: Oxford University Press, p. 57.
Macpherson, J. (1904) Letter to K. Pearson. 21 January 1904 (P 757/1).
———. 1908. Letter to K. Pearson. 23 May 1908 (P 757/1).

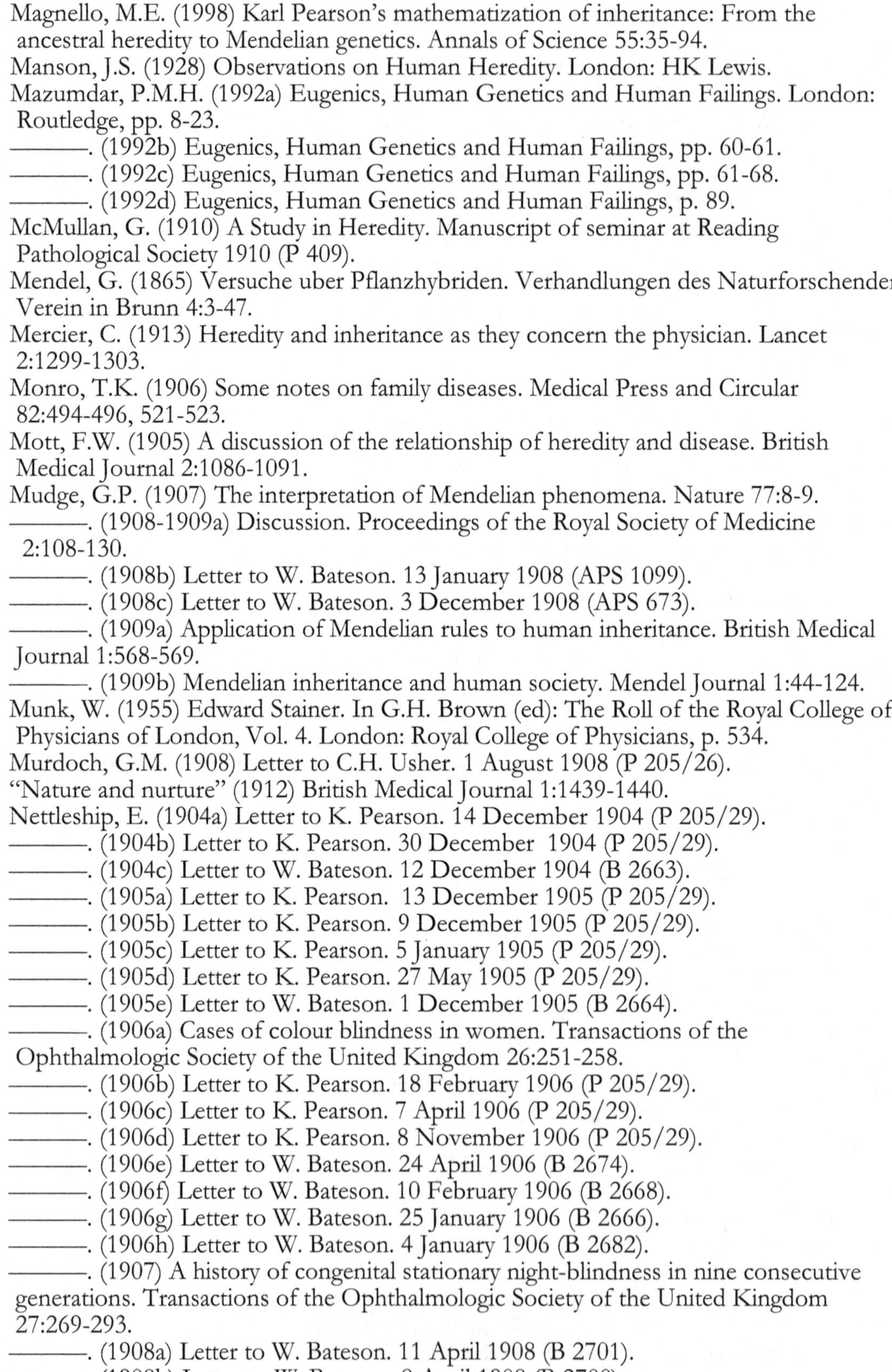

Magnello, M.E. (1998) Karl Pearson's mathematization of inheritance: From the ancestral heredity to Mendelian genetics. Annals of Science 55:35-94.

Manson, J.S. (1928) Observations on Human Heredity. London: HK Lewis.

Mazumdar, P.M.H. (1992a) Eugenics, Human Genetics and Human Failings. London: Routledge, pp. 8-23.

———. (1992b) Eugenics, Human Genetics and Human Failings, pp. 60-61.

———. (1992c) Eugenics, Human Genetics and Human Failings, pp. 61-68.

———. (1992d) Eugenics, Human Genetics and Human Failings, p. 89.

McMullan, G. (1910) A Study in Heredity. Manuscript of seminar at Reading Pathological Society 1910 (P 409).

Mendel, G. (1865) Versuche uber Pflanzhybriden. Verhandlungen des Naturforschender Verein in Brunn 4:3-47.

Mercier, C. (1913) Heredity and inheritance as they concern the physician. Lancet 2:1299-1303.

Monro, T.K. (1906) Some notes on family diseases. Medical Press and Circular 82:494-496, 521-523.

Mott, F.W. (1905) A discussion of the relationship of heredity and disease. British Medical Journal 2:1086-1091.

Mudge, G.P. (1907) The interpretation of Mendelian phenomena. Nature 77:8-9.

———. (1908-1909a) Discussion. Proceedings of the Royal Society of Medicine 2:108-130.

———. (1908b) Letter to W. Bateson. 13 January 1908 (APS 1099).

———. (1908c) Letter to W. Bateson. 3 December 1908 (APS 673).

———. (1909a) Application of Mendelian rules to human inheritance. British Medical Journal 1:568-569.

———. (1909b) Mendelian inheritance and human society. Mendel Journal 1:44-124.

Munk, W. (1955) Edward Stainer. In G.H. Brown (ed): The Roll of the Royal College of Physicians of London, Vol. 4. London: Royal College of Physicians, p. 534.

Murdoch, G.M. (1908) Letter to C.H. Usher. 1 August 1908 (P 205/26).

"Nature and nurture" (1912) British Medical Journal 1:1439-1440.

Nettleship, E. (1904a) Letter to K. Pearson. 14 December 1904 (P 205/29).

———. (1904b) Letter to K. Pearson. 30 December 1904 (P 205/29).

———. (1904c) Letter to W. Bateson. 12 December 1904 (B 2663).

———. (1905a) Letter to K. Pearson. 13 December 1905 (P 205/29).

———. (1905b) Letter to K. Pearson. 9 December 1905 (P 205/29).

———. (1905c) Letter to K. Pearson. 5 January 1905 (P 205/29).

———. (1905d) Letter to K. Pearson. 27 May 1905 (P 205/29).

———. (1905e) Letter to W. Bateson. 1 December 1905 (B 2664).

———. (1906a) Cases of colour blindness in women. Transactions of the Ophthalmologic Society of the United Kingdom 26:251-258.

———. (1906b) Letter to K. Pearson. 18 February 1906 (P 205/29).

———. (1906c) Letter to K. Pearson. 7 April 1906 (P 205/29).

———. (1906d) Letter to K. Pearson. 8 November 1906 (P 205/29).

———. (1906e) Letter to W. Bateson. 24 April 1906 (B 2674).

———. (1906f) Letter to W. Bateson. 10 February 1906 (B 2668).

———. (1906g) Letter to W. Bateson. 25 January 1906 (B 2666).

———. (1906h) Letter to W. Bateson. 4 January 1906 (B 2682).

———. (1907) A history of congenital stationary night-blindness in nine consecutive generations. Transactions of the Ophthalmologic Society of the United Kingdom 27:269-293.

———. (1908a) Letter to W. Bateson. 11 April 1908 (B 2701).

———. (1908b) Letter to W. Bateson. 8 April 1908 (B 2700).

———. (1909) On some hereditary diseases of the eye. The Bowman Lecture. Transactions of the Ophthalmologic Society of the United Kingdom 29:i-cxcviii.
———. (1911) On some cases of hereditary nystagmus. Transactions of the Ophthalmologic Society of the United Kingdom 31:159-202.
———. (1912a) Letter to W. Bateson. 5 June 1912 (B 2726).
———. (1912b) A pedigree of congenital night blindness with myopia. Transactions of the Ophthalmologic Society of the United Kingdom 32:21-45.
———. (1912c) Some unusual pedigrees of colour blindness. Transactions of the Ophthalmologic Society of the United Kingdom 32:309-336.
Nettleship, E. and A.H. Thompson (1912-1913) A pedigree of Leber's disease. Proceedings of the Royal Society of Medicine 6:8-16 Ophthalmology.
Norton, B.J. (1975) Biology and philosophy: The methodological foundations of biometry. Journal of the History of Biology 8:85-93.
Olby, R. (1987) William Bateson's introduction of Mendelism to England: A reassessment. British Journal for the History of Science 30:399-420.
Oliver, C. (1892) Symmetrically placed opacities of the cornea occurring in mother and son. Ophthalmic Review 11:349-351.
Oliver, T. (1900) Physiology and pathology of inheritance. Lancet 2:1335-1341.
Ormerod, J.A. (1908a) The Harveian Oration for 1908: On Heredity in Relation to Disease. London: Adland.
———. (1908b) Heredity in relation to disease. Lancet 2:1199-1203.
Pearson, E.S. (1936) Karl Pearson: An appreciation of some aspects of his life and work. Biometrika 28:204.
———. (1938a) Karl Pearson. Cambridge: Cambridge University Press.
———. (1938b) Karl Pearson, p. 56.
Pearson, K. (1897) Letter to F. Galton. 12 February 1897. Quoted in Pearson, K. (ed). (1930) The Life, Letters and Labours of Francis Galton, Vol. 3A. Cambridge: Cambridge University Press, pp. 127-128.
———. (1898) Mathematical contributions to the study of evolution. On the law of ancestral heredity. Proceedings of the Royal Society 62:386-412.
———. (1900) Mathematical contribution to the theory of evolution Part III. On the inheritance of eye colour in man. Philosophical Transactions 195A:1-21.
———. (1902-1903a) The law of ancestral heredity. Biometrika 2:211-228.
———. (1902b) Letter to W. Bateson. 9 January 1902 (P 631/4).
———. (1903a) Letter to W. Bateson. 26 May 1903 (P 907/2).
———. (1903b) Mathematical contribution to the study of evolution XII. On a generalised theory of alternative evolution with special reference to Mendel's laws. Proceedings of the Royal Society 72:505-509.
———. (1904a) Notes from Weldon lectures (P 263/3).
———. (1904b) Letter to C.C. Hurst. Quoted in Kim, K.-M. (1994) Explaining Scientific Consensus—The Case of Mendelian Genetics. New York: Guilford, p. 86.
———. (1904c) Letter to E. Nettleship. 5 December 1904 (P 205/42).
———. (1904d) Letter to E. Nettleship. 23 November 1904 (P 205/42).
———. (1904e) Mathematical contribution to the theory of evolution. XII. On a generalized theory of alternative inheritance with special reference to Mendel's laws. Philosophical Transactions 203A:53-86.
———. (1904f) A Mendelian's view on the law of ancestral heredity. Biometrika 3:109-112.
———. (1904g) Report on certain cancer statistics. Archives of Middlesex Hospital 2:127-137.
———. (1905a) Letter to C.H. Usher. 2 January 1905 (P 205/46).
———. (1905b) Letter to E. Nettleship. 30 October 1905 (P 205/42).

———. (1905c) Letter to E. Nettleship. (P 205/43).
———. (1906a) Letter to E. Nettleship. 25 September 1906 (P 205/43).
———. (1906b) Mendel's Law: Lecture notes (P 159/2).
———. (1906c) On the Inheritance of the Physical, Moral and Intellectual Characters in Man. Notes for Manchester University lecture 16 November 1906 (P 64).
———. (1907) Letter to E. Nettleship. 17 November 1907 (P 205/43).
———. (1908-1909a) Discussion. Proceedings of the Royal Society of Medicine 2:54-60.
———. (1908b) Letter to E. Nettleship. 13 December 1908 (P 205/44).
———. (1908c) Letter to E. Nettleship. 28 October 1908 (P 205/44).
———. (1908-1909d) Note on inheritance in man. Biometrika 6:327-328.
———. (1908e) On inheritance of the deformity known as split hand or lobster claw. Biometrika 6:69-79.
———.(1909a) Introduction. Treasury of Human Inheritance 1(I):i.
———. (1909b) Letter to E. Nettleship. 20 March 1909 (P 205/45).
———. (1909c) On the ancestral gametic correlation of a Mendelian population mating at random. Proceedings of the Royal Society 81B:225-229.
———. (1912) Darwinism, medical progress and eugenics. West London Medical Journal 17:165-193.
———. (1913) Letter to C.H. Usher. 25 February 1913 (P 205/46).
Pearson, K., E. Nettleship, and C.H. Usher. (1911-1913) A Monograph on Albinism in Man. London: Dulau.
Pockley, E. (1915) Leber's disease. Australian Medical Journal 1:189-190.
Porter, T.M. (2004a) Karl Pearson: The Scientific Life in a Statistical Age. Princeton: Princeton University Press.
———. (2004b) Karl Pearson: The Scientific Life in a Statistical Age, p. 246.
———. (2004c) Karl Pearson: The Scientific Life in a Statistical Age, pp. 238-241.
———. (2004d) Karl Pearson: The Scientific Life in a Statistical age, p. 3.
———. (2004e) Karl Pearson: The Scientific Life in a Statistical Age, p. 267.
———. (2004f) Karl Pearson: The Scientific Life in a Statistical Age, p. 258.
———. (2004g) Karl Pearson: The Scientific Life in a Statistical Age, p. 11.
———. (2004h) Karl Pearson: The Scientific Life in a Statistical Age, p. 280.
———. (2004i) Karl Pearson: The Scientific Life in a Statistical Age, pp. 69-73.
———. (2004j) Karl Pearson: The Scientific Life in a Statistical Age, pp. 271-272.
———. (2004k) Karl Pearson: The Scientific Life in a Statistical Age, p. 257.
Provine, W.B. (1971a) The Origins of Theoretical Population Genetics. Chicago: University of Chicago, p. 31.
———. (1971b) The Origins of Theoretical Population Genetics, pp. 32-33.
———. (1971c) The Origins of Theoretical Population Genetics, p. 62.
———. (1971d) The Origins of Theoretical Population Genetics, p. 58.
———. (1971e) The Origins of Theoretical Population Genetics, pp. 63-64.
———. (1971f) The Origins of Theoretical Population Genetics, pp. 73-80.
———. (1971g) The Origins of Theoretical Population Genetics, pp. 85-86.
———. (1971h) The Origins of Theoretical Population Genetics, p. 86.
———. (1971i) The Origins of Theoretical Population Genetics, p. 87.
———. (1971j) The Origins of Theoretical Population Genetics, pp. 86-90.
———. (1971k) The Origins of Theoretical Population Genetics, p. 88.
Punnett, R.C. (1907-1908) Mendelism in relation to disease. Proceedings of the Royal Society of Medicine 1:135-165 Epidemiology.
———. (1908) Discussion. Proceedings of the Royal Society of Medicine 1:167-168.
———. (1912) Genetics and eugenics. Problems in Eugenics. Papers Communicated to the First International Eugenics Congress, p. 137.

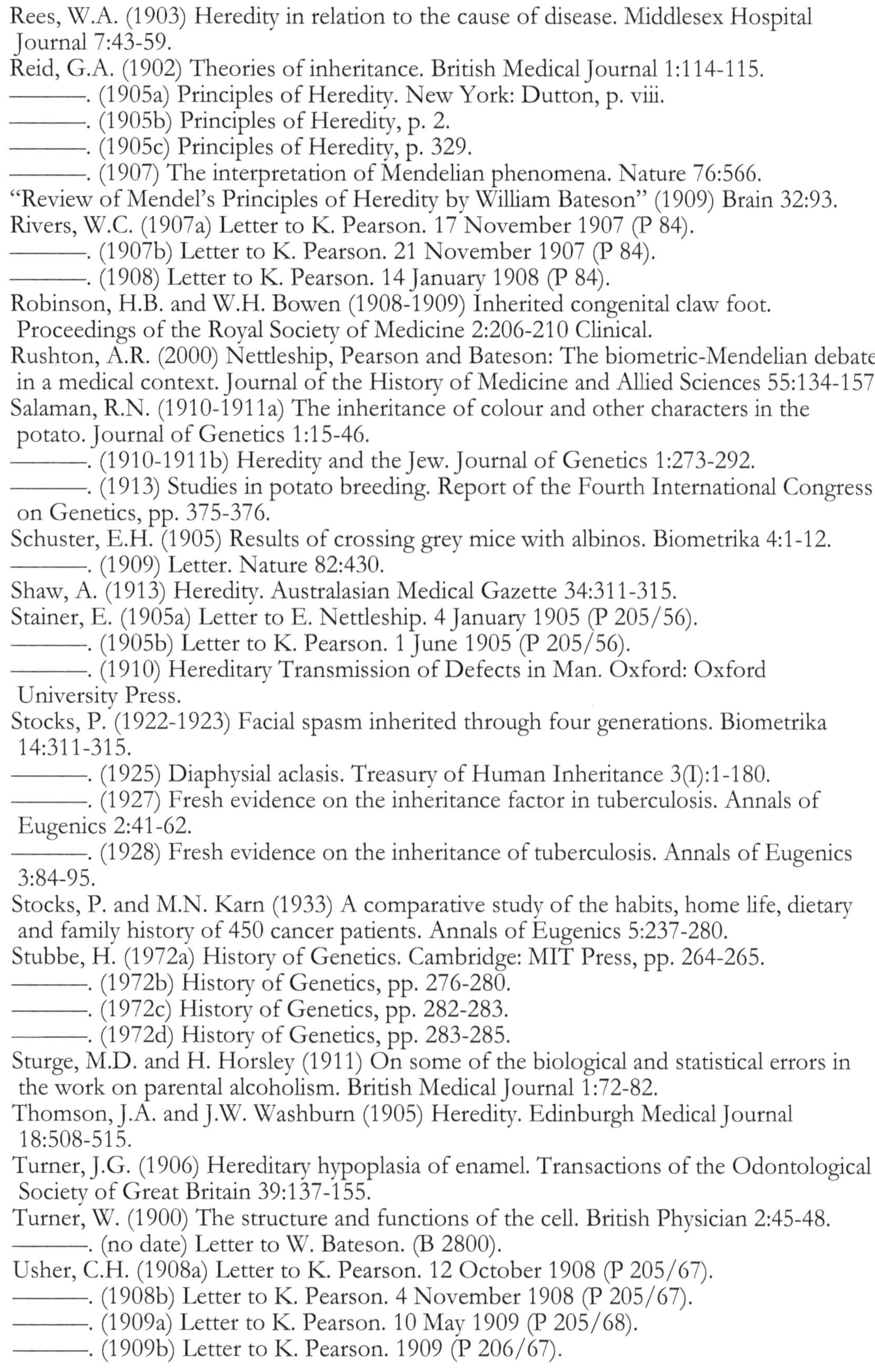

Rees, W.A. (1903) Heredity in relation to the cause of disease. Middlesex Hospital Journal 7:43-59.

Reid, G.A. (1902) Theories of inheritance. British Medical Journal 1:114-115.

———. (1905a) Principles of Heredity. New York: Dutton, p. viii.

———. (1905b) Principles of Heredity, p. 2.

———. (1905c) Principles of Heredity, p. 329.

———. (1907) The interpretation of Mendelian phenomena. Nature 76:566.

"Review of Mendel's Principles of Heredity by William Bateson" (1909) Brain 32:93.

Rivers, W.C. (1907a) Letter to K. Pearson. 17 November 1907 (P 84).

———. (1907b) Letter to K. Pearson. 21 November 1907 (P 84).

———. (1908) Letter to K. Pearson. 14 January 1908 (P 84).

Robinson, H.B. and W.H. Bowen (1908-1909) Inherited congenital claw foot. Proceedings of the Royal Society of Medicine 2:206-210 Clinical.

Rushton, A.R. (2000) Nettleship, Pearson and Bateson: The biometric-Mendelian debate in a medical context. Journal of the History of Medicine and Allied Sciences 55:134-157.

Salaman, R.N. (1910-1911a) The inheritance of colour and other characters in the potato. Journal of Genetics 1:15-46.

———. (1910-1911b) Heredity and the Jew. Journal of Genetics 1:273-292.

———. (1913) Studies in potato breeding. Report of the Fourth International Congress on Genetics, pp. 375-376.

Schuster, E.H. (1905) Results of crossing grey mice with albinos. Biometrika 4:1-12.

———. (1909) Letter. Nature 82:430.

Shaw, A. (1913) Heredity. Australasian Medical Gazette 34:311-315.

Stainer, E. (1905a) Letter to E. Nettleship. 4 January 1905 (P 205/56).

———. (1905b) Letter to K. Pearson. 1 June 1905 (P 205/56).

———. (1910) Hereditary Transmission of Defects in Man. Oxford: Oxford University Press.

Stocks, P. (1922-1923) Facial spasm inherited through four generations. Biometrika 14:311-315.

———. (1925) Diaphysial aclasis. Treasury of Human Inheritance 3(I):1-180.

———. (1927) Fresh evidence on the inheritance factor in tuberculosis. Annals of Eugenics 2:41-62.

———. (1928) Fresh evidence on the inheritance of tuberculosis. Annals of Eugenics 3:84-95.

Stocks, P. and M.N. Karn (1933) A comparative study of the habits, home life, dietary and family history of 450 cancer patients. Annals of Eugenics 5:237-280.

Stubbe, H. (1972a) History of Genetics. Cambridge: MIT Press, pp. 264-265.

———. (1972b) History of Genetics, pp. 276-280.

———. (1972c) History of Genetics, pp. 282-283.

———. (1972d) History of Genetics, pp. 283-285.

Sturge, M.D. and H. Horsley (1911) On some of the biological and statistical errors in the work on parental alcoholism. British Medical Journal 1:72-82.

Thomson, J.A. and J.W. Washburn (1905) Heredity. Edinburgh Medical Journal 18:508-515.

Turner, J.G. (1906) Hereditary hypoplasia of enamel. Transactions of the Odontological Society of Great Britain 39:137-155.

Turner, W. (1900) The structure and functions of the cell. British Physician 2:45-48.

———. (no date) Letter to W. Bateson. (B 2800).

Usher, C.H. (1908a) Letter to K. Pearson. 12 October 1908 (P 205/67).

———. (1908b) Letter to K. Pearson. 4 November 1908 (P 205/67).

———. (1909a) Letter to K. Pearson. 10 May 1909 (P 205/68).

———. (1909b) Letter to K. Pearson. 1909 (P 206/67).

———. (1909c) Letter to K. Pearson. 21 March 1909 (P 205/68).
Vernon, H.M. (1908) Discussion. Proceedings of the Royal Society of Medicine 1:161-162.
Vine, B. (2002) The Blood Doctor. New York: Shaye Areheart, p. 3.
"Vision in relation to heredity and environment" (1909) Nature 81:49.
Von Tschermak-Seysenegg, E. (1951) The rediscovery of Gregor Mendel's work. Journal of Heredity 42:163-171.
Walker, C.E. (1904) The nature and etiology of cancer. Lancet 2:467-468.
Weldon, W. (1893) On certain correlated variations in *Carcinus moenas*. Proceedings of the Royal Society 54:318-329.
Weldon, W.F. (1901-1902) Mendel's laws of inheritance in peas. Biometrika 1:228-254.
———. (1904) Albinism in Sicily and Mendel's laws. Biometrika 3:107-109.
———. (1905a) Current theories of the hereditary process. Lancet 1:42, 180, 307, 512, 584, 657, 732, 810.
———. (1905b) Theories of hereditary processes. British Medical Journal 1:441-442, 505-506.
Williams, R., 1997. Personal communication from the Search Service, Royal Society of Medicine Library, London. 10 December 1997.
Woods, F.A. (1902-1903) Mendel's laws and some records of rabbit breeding. Biometrika 2:299-306.
Yearsley, M. (1913a) Letter to W. Bateson. 15 September 1913 (B 3126).
———. (1913b) Letter to W. Bateson. 17 September 1913 (B 3127).
———. (1914-1915) The problem of deafness and its prevention. Eugenics Review 6:116-129.
Yule, G.U. (1902) Mendel's laws and their probable relations to intra-racial heredity. New Phytologist 1:183-207.
———. (1995) Karl Pearson. Dictionary of National Biography CD-ROM. Oxford: Oxford University Press.
Zirkle, C. (1964) Some oddities in the delayed discovery of Mendelism. Journal of Heredity 55:65-72.

Chapter Thirteen

"A case of hemophilia with anomalous family history" (1909) Guy's Hospital Gazette 23:68.
Adair-Dighton, C.A. (1912) Four generations of blue sclerotics. Ophthalmoscope 10:188-189.
Adami, J. (1917) Adaptation to disease. British Medical Journal 1:872-873.
Adams, P.H. (1909) 1. A family with congenital displacement of lenses. 2. A family with congenital opacities of lenses. Transactions of the Ophthalmologic Society of the United Kingdom 29:274-278.
Adie, W.J. (1925-1926a) A family with progressive familial cerebral (so-called cerebro-macular) degeneration. Proceedings of the Royal Society of Medicine 19:1-2 Children.
———. (1925-1926b) Von Recklinghausen's disease in three generations. Proceedings of the Royal Society of Medicine 19:11 Neurology.
Adler, J.E. and J. McIntosh (1909-1910) Histological examination of a case of albinism. Biometrika 7:237-243.
Aitkin, J. (1909) Congenital, hereditary and family hematuria. Lancet 2:444-446.
Alexander, J. (1922) Fragilitas ossium. British Medical Journal 1:677.
Ali Khan, W. (1926) Pedigree of lamellar cataract. British Journal of Ophthalmology 10:387-389.

Alport, A.C. (1927) Hereditary familial and congenital hemorrhagic nephritis. British Medical Journal 1:504-506.

Anderson, W. (1886) Congenital malformation of hands and feet transmitted through four generations. British Medical Journal 1:1107-1108.

Apert, E. (1914) The laws of Naudin-Mendel. An interpretation of the statistics of Pearson et al. on albinism in man. Journal of Heredity 5:492-495.

Atkinson, E.M. (1921-1922) A case of hereditary polydactylism. British Journal of Surgery 9:298-301.

Back, F. (1926) Huntington's chorea. British Medical Journal 2:60-61.

Baildon, F.J. (1912) Amaurotic family idiocy. Liverpool Medico-Chirurgical Journal 32:308-313.

Ballantyne, A.J. (1908) Multiple telangiectases. Glasgow Medical Journal 70:256-259.

Bangson, J.S. (1926) Several generations of achondroplasia. Journal of Heredity 17:393-395.

Barnes, S. (1924) Case of progressive lenticular degeneration and hepatic cirrhosis. Brain 47:239-240.

Barnes, S. and E.W. Hurst (1925) Hepatolenticular degeneration. Brain 48:279-334.

Barr, J. (1922) Mendelism. Medical Press and Circular 113:171-175.

Bateson, W. (1909) Mendel's Principles of Heredity. Cambridge: Cambridge University Press.

———. (1911) Hereditary nystagmus. Lancet 1:1278.

———. (1913) Address on heredity. Lancet 2:451-454.

Batten, F.E. (1902a) A familial type of paralysis allied to the myopathies and Friedreich's disease. Transactions of the Clinical Society of London 35:205-206.

———. (1902-1903b) Three cases of progressive spinal muscle atrophy. Transactions of the Clinical Society of London 36:226-228.

———. (1903) Cerebral degeneration with symmetrical changes in the maculae of two members of one family. Transactions of the Ophthalmologic Society of the United Kingdom 23:386-390.

———. (1910-1911) Progressive spinal muscular atrophy. Proceedings of the Royal Society of Medicine 4:53-84 Neurology.

———. (1911) Progressive spinal muscular atrophy of infants and young children. Brain 33:433-463.

———. (1914) Family cerebral degeneration with macular change. Quarterly Journal of Medicine 7:444-454.

Batten, F.E. and G. Holmes (1912-1913) Progressive spinal muscular atrophy of infants. Brain 35:38-49.

Batten, F.E. and M.A. Jukes (1914-1915) Amaurotic family idiocy. Proceedings of the Royal Society of Medicine 8:89 Children.

Batten, F.E. and M.S. Mayou (1914-1915) Family cerebral degeneration with macular changes. Proceedings of the Royal Society of Medicine 8:70-80 Ophthalmology.

Batten, R. (1909) Two cases of hereditary optic atrophy in a family. Transactions of the Ophthalmologic Society of the United Kingdom 29:144-150.

Battle, W.H. and S.G. Shattock (1907-1908) A remarkable case of diffuse cancellous osteoma. Proceedings of the Royal Society of Medicine 1:83-94 Pathology.

Beaumont, M.W. (1900) Family tendency to ophthalmoplegia externa. Transactions of the Ophthalmologic Society of the United Kingdom 20:258-264.

Berrisford, P.B. (1916) Statistical notes on glioma retinae. Royal London Ophthalmic Hospital Report 20:296-331.

Bickerton, E. (1904) Hereditary optic atrophy in two brothers. Transactions of the Ophthalmologic Society of the United Kingdom 24:178-180.

Birt, A. (1908) A case of Thomsen's disease by a sufferer. Montreal Medical Journal 37:771-784.
Blegvad, O. and H. Haxthausen (1921) Blue sclerotics and brittle bones with macular atrophy of the skin and zonular cataract. British Medical Journal 2:1071-1072.
Bond, C.J. (1912-1913) On heterochromia irides in man and animals from the genetic point of view. Journal of Genetics 2:99-128.
Bosanquet, W.C. (1908) Diabetes mellitus in two brothers. Lancet 1:14-15.
Bowen, W.H. (1908-1909) Case of spontaneous occurrence of congenital deaf-mutism. Proceedings of the Royal Society of Medicine 2:81-83 Otology.
Bradburne, A. (1912) Hereditary ophthalmoplegia in five generations. Transactions of the Ophthalmologic Society of the United Kingdom 32:142-153.
———. (1916) Retinitis pigmentosa in five sisters. Ophthalmic Review 35:65-70.
Brain, W.R. (1925) The mode of inheritance of hereditary ataxia. Quarterly Journal of Medicine 18:351-358.
———. (1926) The inheritance of epilepsy. Quarterly Journal of Medicine 19:299-310.
———. (1927) Heredity in simple goitre. Quarterly Journal of Medicine 20:303-319.
Bramwell, B. (1903) Case of hereditary ichthyosis of the palms and soles. Clinical Studies 1:77-80.
———. (1904) Hereditary optic atrophy. Clinical Studies 2:44-55.
———. (1907a) Angioneurotic edema. Clinical Studies 5:374-387.
———. (1907-1908b) Diabetes mellitus. Clinical Studies 6:263-266.
———. (1907c) Hemophilia. Clinical Studies 5:368-370.
———. (1907d) Hereditary webbing of second and third toes of the left foot. Clinical Studies 5:373-374.
Branch, C.W. (1905) An epileptic family. British Medical Journal 1:1330.
Bride, T.M. (1923) Case of glioma of the retina. Transactions of the Ophthalmologic Society of the United Kingdom 43:653-654.
Bronson, E. (1917) On fragilitis ossium and its association with blue sclerotics and otosclerosis. Edinburgh Medical Journal 18:248-281.
———. (1918) Osteogenesis imperfecta. Proceedings of the Royal Society of Medicine 12:15-17 Children.
Brush, S.G. (2002) How theories became knowledge: Morgan's chromosome theory of heredity in America and Britain. Journal of the History of Biology 35:471-535.
Bryant, J.H. (1905a) Two cases of the peroneal type of family amyotrophy. Brain 28:355-356.
Bryant, J. (1905b) Two cases of the peroneal type of family amyotrophy. Transactions of the Clinical Society of London 38:195-199.
Buchanan, L. (1923) Blue sclerotics. Transactions of the Ophthalmologic Society of the United Kingdom 43:352-354.
Bulloch, W. (1909a) Angioneurotic edema. Treasury of Human Inheritance 1(IXa):38-49.
———. (1909b) Chronic hereditary trophedema. Treasury of Human Inheritance 1(VIIIa):32-38.
Bulloch, W. and P. Fildes (1911) Hemophilia. Treasury of Human Inheritance 1(XIVa)):169-347.
Bulmer, E. (1929) Hereditary angioneurotic edema. British Medical Journal 1:766.
Bunch, J.L. (1913) Hereditary Dupuytren's contracture. British Journal of Dermatology 25:279-283.
Burroughs, A.E. (1924) Two cases of Leber's disease. Transactions of the Ophthalmologic Society of the United Kingdom 44:339-403.
Burrows, H. (1911) Blue sclerotics and brittle bones. British Medical Journal 2:16.
Butler, T.H. (1908) An albino family. Ophthalmoscope 6:589.

Buzzard, A. (1916-1917) Case of Huntington's chorea. Proceedings of the Royal Society of Medicine 10:48 Neurology.
Buzzard, E.F. (1907) Case of Huntington's chorea. Proceedings of the Royal Society of Medicine 1:12 Neurology.
Cairns, H.W.B. (1925) Heredity in polycystic disease of the kidneys. Quarterly Journal of Medicine 18:359-392.
Cameron, C. (1920) The family history in a case of angioneurotic edema. Lancet 2:849-850.
Cammidge, P.J. (1928) Diabetes mellitus and heredity. British Medical Journal 2:738-740.
Campbell, M.H. and E.C. Ware (1926) Heredity in acholuric jaundice. Quarterly Journal of Medicine 19:333-355.
Cane, C.B. (1909) Epidermolysis bullosa. British Medical Journal 1:1114-1116.
Carlyll, H.B. and F.W. Mott (1910-1911) Seven cases of amaurotic idiocy. Proceedings of the Royal Society of Medicine 4:147-148 Pathology.
Castle, W.F.R. (1922-1923) Case of epidermolysis bullosa. Proceedings of the Royal Society of Medicine 16:53-54 Dermatology.
———. (1924-1925) Epidermolysis bullosa. Proceedings of the Royal Society of Medicine 18:25-26 Dermatology.
Catarinich, J. (1914) Huntington's chorea. Australian Medical Journal 3:1509-510.
Chase, L.A. (1927) Hereditary diabetes insipidus. Canadian Medical Association Journal 17:212-14.
Clark, W.E. (1916) A case of hereditary syndactyly. Lancet 2:434.
Clarkson, R.D. (1927) The causes of mental deficiency. Edinburgh Medical Journal 34:61-75.
Clegg, J.G. (1915) Remarks on dystrophies of the cornea and glaucoma. Transactions of the Ophthalmologic Society of the United Kingdom 35:245-253.
Clouston, H.R. (1929) A hereditary ectodermal dystrophy. Canadian Medical Association Journal 21:18-31.
Cock, A.G. (1983) William Bateson's recognition and eventual acceptance of the chromosome theory. Annals of Science 40:19-59.
———. (1989) Bateson's two Toronto addresses: 1. Chromosomal skepticism. Journal of Heredity 80:91-95.
Cockayne, E.A. (1914) Hereditary blue sclerotics and brittle bones. Ophthalmoscope 12:271-272.
Cockayne, E.A. (1913-1914) Case of hereditary blue sclerotics and brittle bones. Proceedings of the Royal Society of Medicine 7:101-102 Children.
———. (1914-1915) A piebald family. Biometrika 10:197-200.
———. (1926) Case of brittle bones and blue sclerotics. Proceedings of the Royal Society of Medicine 19:51 Children.
———. (1927) Heredity in relation to cancer. Cancer Review 2:337-347.
Cockayne, E.A. and J. Attlee (1914-1915) Amaurotic family idiocy in an English child. Proceedings of the Royal Society of Medicine 8:65-66 Ophthalmology.
Collier, A.J. (1908-1909) Two cases of peroneal atrophy. Proceedings of the Royal Society of Medicine 2:31-32 Neurology.
Collier, J. (1903) Two cases of peroneal atrophy. Brain 26:149.
Collins, E.T. (1905) Two children in the same family with congenital opacity of the cornea. Transactions of the Ophthalmologic Society of the United Kingdom 25:49-50.
Cooper, H. (1910) A series of cases of congenital ophthalmoplegia externa. British Medical Journal 1:917.
Cowen, S.O. (1922) Familial hemolytic splenomegaly. Australian Medical Journal 2:545-561.

Cox, R. (1915) A case of multiple exostoses with hereditary history. Lancet 2:701.
Cragg, E. and H. Drinkwater (1916-1917) Hereditary absence of phalanges through five generations. Journal of Genetics 6:81-89.
Crew, F.A.E. (1925) Sex determination. Nature 115:574-577.
———. (1926) The mechanism of inheritance. British Medical Journal 2:285-289.
———. (1927a) Organic Inheritance in Man. London: Oliver and Boyd, pp. 139-144.
———. (1927b) Organic Inheritance in Man, p. 2.
———. (1927c) Organic Inheritance in Man, p. 21.
———. (1928) Genetical aspects of natural immunity and disease resistance. Edinburgh Medical Journal 35:301-321.
Critchley, M. (1940) Samuel A.K. Wilson. Dictionary of National Biography 1931-1940:914-915.
Crivelli, L. (1920) Hereditary polydactylism. Australian Medical Journal 2:223.
Cunningham, J.F. (1909) A case of aniridia with a family history of the condition in four generations. Transactions of the Ophthalmologic Society of the United Kingdom 29:131-133.
Cuthbert, C.F. (1923) Heredity in alcaptonuria. Lancet 1:593-594.
Davenport, R.C. (1927) Choroidal sarcoma. British Journal of Ophthalmology 11:445-447.
Dawnay, A.H.P. (1905) Corneal opacities in members of the same family. Transactions of the Ophthalmologic Society of the United Kingdom 25:62.
Deachell, G.E. (1905) A case of dementia due to Huntington's chorea. Lancet 2:1252-1253.
Doncaster, E.L. (1910) Heredity and disease. British Medical Journal 1:308-312.
Doncaster, L. (1913-1914) Chromosomes, heredity and sex. Quarterly Journal of Microscopical Science 59:487-521.
———. (1920a) Genetic studies of *Drosophila*. Nature 105:405-406.
———. (1920b) An Introduction to the Study of Cytology. Cambridge: Cambridge University Press.
Doyne, R.W. and S. Stephenson (1905) Upon five cases of family degeneration of the cornea. Ophthalmoscope 3:213-221.
Dreschfeld, J.A. (1905) Thomsen's disease. Lancet 1:1136.
Drinkwater, H. (1907) An account of a brachydactylous family. Proceedings of the Royal Society of Edinburgh 28:35-37.
———. (1908) An account of a brachydactylous family. Liverpool Medico-Chirurgical Journal 28:408-414.
———. (1909) Mendelian heredity in asthma. British Medical Journal 1:88.
———. (1912-1913) Account of family showing minor brachydactyly. Journal of Genetics 2:21-40.
———. (1913-1914a) Minor brachydactyly No. 2. Journal of Genetics 3:217-220.
———. (1913b) Study of a brachydactylous family. Report of the Fourth International Congress on Genetics, p. 549.
———. (1914-1915) A second brachydactylous family. Journal of Genetics 4:323-340.
———. (1916) Hereditary abnormal segmentation of the index and middle fingers. Journal of Anatomy 50:177-186.
———. (1917) Phalangeal anarthrosis (synostosis, ankylosis) transmitted through fourteen generations. Proceedings of the Royal Society of Medicine 10:60-68 Pathology.
Drury, F. (1910) A case of xeroderma pigmentosum. Indian Medical Gazette 45:344-345.
Dukes, C. (1926) Single tumours of the large intestine and their relation to cancer. Proceedings of the Royal Society of Medicine 19:8-12 Proctology.

Dyke, S.C. and C.H. Budge (1922-1923) On the inheritance of specific isoagglutinable substances of human red cells. Proceedings of the Royal Society of Medicine 16:35-43 Pathology.
Eager, R. (1910) Notes on four cases of Huntington's chorea. Journal of Mental Science 56:506-509.
East, C.F.T. (1926) Familial telangiectasia. Lancet 1:332-334.
Eccles, W.A. (1918) The transmission of acquired deformities or war injuries, marriage and progeny. Medical Press and Circular 106:321-322.
Evans, J.W. (1908) Observations on a case of Huntington's chorea. Lancet 2:940.
Felling, A. and E. Ward (1920) A familial form of acoustic tumor. British Medical Journal 1:496-497.
Ferguson, J. (1903-1904) An epilepsy symposium. Canada Lancet 37:815-816.
Finlay, T. and A.M. Drennan (1916) Clinical observations on a case of hemophilia. Edinburgh Medical Journal 16:425-443.
Fisher, J.H. (1905) Coraliform cataract. Transactions of the Ophthalmologic Society of the United Kingdom 25:90-91.
Fitzwilliams, D.C.L. (1910) Hereditary cranio-cleido-dysostosis. Lancet 2:1466-1475.
Foggie, W.E. (1928) Hereditary hemorrhagic telangiectasia. Edinburgh Medical Journal 35:281-290.
Folker, H.H. (1909) Nodular opacity of the cornea in three generations. Transactions of the Ophthalmologic Society of the United Kingdom 29:42-52.
———. (1917) Fragilitas ossium. British Medical Journal 1:739.
Francis, A.E. (1902) Case of multiple exostoses. Lancet 1:1765.
Freeman, J. (1920) Toxic idiopathies. Proceedings of the Royal Society of Medicine 13:129-148.
Fuller, C.J. (1928-1929) Familial polycystic disease of the kidneys. Quarterly Journal of Medicine 22:567-574.
Galloway, R.M. (1912) Notes on the pigmentation of the human iris. Biometrika 8:267-299.
Garrod, A. (1928) The lessons of rare maladies. Lancet 1:1055-1060.
Garrod, A.E. and W.H. Hurtley (1912-1923) Congenital familial steatorrhea. Quarterly Journal of Medicine 6:242-258.
Gates, R.R. (1915) On the nature of mutation. Journal of Heredity 6:99-108.
———. (1925) Mutation. Nature 115:499-500.
———. (1926a) Aspects of physical and mental inheritance. Nature 118:663-665.
———. (1926b) Mendelian heredity and racial differences. Journal of the Royal Anthropological Institute 55:468-482.
———. (1927) Inter-racial inheritance in man. Verhandlungen der V. International Kongress for Vererbungswissenschaft 1:759-760.
———. (1929a) Blood groups in Canadian Indians and Eskimos. American Journal of Physical Anthropology 12:475-485.
———. (1929b) Heredity in Man. London: Constable.
Gilmore, E.R.W. (1927) Hereditary deformity of the fingers. British Medical Journal 2:935-936.
Goring, C. (1909) On the inheritance of the diathesis for phthisis and insanity. London: Dulau.
Gossage, A.M. (1908) The inheritance of certain human abnormalities. Quarterly Journal of Medicine 1:331-344.
Gossage, A.M. and E.R. Carling (1910-1911) Multiple cartilaginous exostoses. Proceedings of the Royal Society of Medicine 4:1-22 Medicine.
Gowers, W. (1908-1909a) Heredity. Proceedings of the Royal Society of Medicine 2:15-22.

———. (1908b) Heredity in diseases of the nervous system. British Medical Journal 2:1541-1543.

Graham, S. and J.S. Blacklock (1927) Gaucher's disease. Archive of Disease in Childhood 2:267-284.

Greene, S.H. (1907) Supernumerary digits and a history of heredity. Lancet 2:859-860.

Greenfield, J.G. and G. Holmes (1925) The histology of juvenile amaurotic idiocy. Brain 48:183-217.

Greenfield, J.G., F.J. Poynton, and F.M.R. Walshe (1923-1924) On progressive lenticular degeneration. Quarterly Journal of Medicine 17:385-403.

Griffith, A.H. (1917a) Hereditary glioma of the retina. British Journal of Ophthalmology 1:529-532.

———. (1917b) Hereditary glioma of the retina. Transactions of the Ophthalmologic Society of the United Kingdom 37:242-247.

———. (1917c) Hereditary retinal glioma. British Medical Journal 1:850.

Griffith, T. (1902) Remarks on a case of hereditary "localized" edema. British Medical Journal 1:1470-1471.

Gunn, A.R. (1907) Albinism in man. British Medical Journal 1:718-719.

———. (1912) Complete congenital dislocation of the lens—a family history. Ophthalmoscope 10:193-195.

Guthrie, L.G. (1902) Idiopathic or congenital heredity and family hematuria. Lancet 1:1243-1246.

Guthrie, L. (1910-1911) Two cases of muscular atrophy of the peroneal type. Proceedings of the Royal Society of Medicine 4:126-128 Clinical.

Hadfield, G. (1923) On hepatolenticular degeneration. Brain 46:147-178.

Halley, G. (1903) Heredity ichthyosis of the palms and soles. Scottish Medical and Surgical Journal 12:329-333.

Halliday, J. and A. Whiting (1909) The peroneal type of muscle atrophy. British Medical Journal 2:1114-1118.

Hamilton, A.S. (1911) Report of a case of hereditary muscular atrophy of the Charcot-Marie-Tooth type associated with cataract. Review of Neurology and Psychiatry 9:645-661.

Hancock, W.I. (1905) Nodular opacities of the cornea in mother and child. Transactions of the Ophthalmologic Society of the United Kingdom 25:64-66.

———. (1908) Hereditary optic atrophy. Royal London Ophthalmic Hospital Reports 17:167-177.

Harman, B. (1910) Congenital cataract. Treasury of Human Inheritance 1(XIIIa):126-160.

Harman, N.B. (1908) A study in heredity—six generations of piebalds. Medical Press and Circular 86:448.

———. (1909a) Congenital cataract—a pedigree of five generations. Transactions of the Ophthalmologic Society of the United Kingdom 29:101-108.

———. (1909b) Nine pedigrees of cataract. Transactions of the Ophthalmologic Society of the United Kingdom 29:296-306.

———. (1909c) A study in heredity—six generations of piebalds. Transactions of the Ophthalmologic Society of the United Kingdom 29:25-33.

———. (1910) Ten pedigrees of congenital and infantile cataract. Transactions of the Ophthalmologic Society of the United Kingdom 30:251-274.

———. (1914-1915a) Case of high myopia in an infant: hereditary and congenital. Proceedings of the Royal Society of Medicine 8:3 Ophthalmology.

———. (1914b) Congenital defect and inheritance. West London Medical Journal 19:93-110.

Harris, W. (1904) Case of familial tremor. Brain 27:288.

Hart, B. (1910) Phases of Evolution and Heredity. London: Rebman.
Hart, D.B. (1913) On the pressure experienced by the fetus in utero during pregnancy with special reference to achondroplasia. Edinburgh Medical Journal 10:496-501.
Haward, W. (1902) A case of fragilitas ossium. Transactions of the Clinical Society of London 35:38-42.
Hawkes, C.S. (1900) Hereditary optic atrophy. Australasian Medical Gazette 19:228-229.
Hawkins, H.P. and L.S. Dudgeon (1908-1909) Congenital family cholaemia. Quarterly Journal of Medicine 2:165-177.
Hay, P.J. and P.E. Naish (1923) Familial cerebro-retinal degeneration. Transactions of the Ophthalmologic Society of the United Kingdom 43:654-656.
Head, H. and E. Gardner (1904) Tremor in a case of family spastic paralysis. Brain 27:282-284.
Heaton, G. (1903) Two cases of fragilitis ossium. Midland Medical Journal 2:36-37.
Hertz, A.F. (1912) Case of hereditary intention tremor. Guy's Hospital Reports 66:133-134.
Hillier, W.T. and I. Tritsch (1904) Heredity in cancer. Archives of Middlesex Hospital 2:104-126.
Hine, M.L. (1923) Two cases of early familial maculo-cerebral degeneration. Proceedings of the Royal Society of Medicine 16:18-19 Ophthalmology.
Hine, M. (1928) An atypical case of retinitis pigmentosa. Transactions of the Ophthalmologic Society of the United Kingdom 48:160-166.
Hogg, C.A. (1902) Two cases of Huntington's chorea. Australasian Medical Gazette 21:400-404.
Hogg, G.H. (1928) Hereditary optic atrophy. Medical Journal of Australia 1:372-374.
Holland, H.T. (1924) Hereditary glaucoma affecting three generations. Indian Medical Gazette 59:408.
Holmes, G. (1907) An attempt to classify cerebellar disease. Brain 30:545-567.
Holmes, G. and L. Paton (1925) Cerebro-macular degeneration. Transactions of the Ophthalmologic Society of the United Kingdom 45:447-470.
Hope, W.B. and H. French (1908a) Persistent hereditary edema of the legs. Guy's Hospital Reports 62:5-31.
———. (1908b) Persistent hereditary edema of the legs with acute exacerbations (Milroy's disease). Quarterly Journal of Medicine 1:312-330.
Houghton, C.W. (1925) A case of familial osteochondromata. Guy's Hospital Gazette 39:583-586.
Hudson, A. (1903) Note on a case of congenital night blindness. Ophthalmoscope 1:89-90.
"Human blood relationships" (1922) Nature 110:738-739.
Hume, W.E. (1914) A case of amaurotic family idiocy. Review of Neurology and Psychiatry 12:281-287.
Humphreys, H. (1928) Human heredity. Birmingham Medical Review 3:322-336.
Hunter, C. (1916-1917) A rare disease in two brothers. Proceedings of the Royal Society of Medicine 10:104-115 Children.
Hunter, D. (1928) Achondroplasia in the third generation. Proceedings of the Royal Society of Medicine 21:1321-1324.
Hunter, D. and W. Evans (1929) Gaucher's disease. Proceedings of the Royal Society of Medicine 23:224.
Hunter, O.G. (1909) A case of polydactylism. Australasian Medical Gazette 28:545.
Hunter, W.K. (1900) Case of pseudohypertrophic paralysis. Glasgow Medical Journal 54:375-377.
Hurst, A. (1923) Hereditary familial congenital hemorrhagic nephritis. Guy's Hospital Reports 73:368-370.

Hurst, A.F. (1925) The pathogenesis of subacute combined degeneration of the spinal cord with special reference to its connection with Addison's anemia, achlorhydria and intestinal infection. Brain 48:217-232.
Hurst, C.C. (1907) On the inheritance of eye colour in man. Proceedings of the Royal Society 80B:85-96.
Hutchinson, R. (1910-1911) Case of splenomegaly. Proceedings of the Royal Society of Medicine 4:129-132 Clinical.
Jacob, F.H. and A. Fulton (1905) Keratosis palmaris et plantaris in five generations. British Medical Journal 2:125.
James, R.R. (1927) A pedigree of a family showing hereditary glaucoma. British Journal of Ophthalmology 11:438-443.
Jenkins, J.A. (1912a) Letter to W. Bateson. 26 December 1912 (B 3160).
———. 1912b. Letter to W. Bateson. 30 December 1912 (B 3161).
———. (1913-1914) Mendelian sex-factors in man. Journal of Genetics 3:121-122.
Jollye, F.W. (1902) Case of heredity of Huntington's chorea. British Medical Journal 2:1641-1642.
Jones, E. (1907) Hereditary spastic paraplegia. Review of Neurology and Psychiatry 5:98-106.
Jones, H. (1917) Huntington's chorea. Australian Medical Journal 1:376-377.
Jones, R. (1905) Huntington's chorea and dementia. Lancet 2:1831-1832.
Juler, H. (1902) Aniridia. Ophthalmic Review 21:22-23.
Kelly, A.B. (1906) Multiple telangiectases of the skin. Glasgow Medical Journal 65:411-422.
———. (1907-1908) Multiple telangiectases. Proceedings of the Royal Society of Medicine 1:45 Laryngology.
Kendall, G. and A.F. Hertz (1912) Hereditary familial congenital hemorrhagic nephritis. Guy's Hospital Reports 66:137-141.
Keyser, C.R. (1906) Achondroplasia. Lancet 1:1598-1602.
Kidd, F. (1910-1911) Case for diagnosis: imperfect osteogenesis. Proceedings of the Royal Society of Medicine 4:106-110 Clinical.
Krabbe, K.H. (1916) A new familial form of diffuse brain sclerosis. Brain 39:74-114.
———. (1920) Congenital familial spinal muscle atrophy. Brain 43:166-191.
Lane, J.K. (1901) Three cases of congenital ptosis. Glasgow Medical Journal 55:189-190.
Lane, M.H. (1912-1913) Hair and its heredity. Eugenics Review 4:257-283.
Langmead, F. (1909-1910) A case of hereditary multiple telangiectasis. Proceedings of the Royal Society of Medicine 3:109-110 Clinical.
Lawford, J.B. (1908) Examples of hereditary primary glaucoma. Royal London Ophthalmic Hospital Reports 17:57-68.
———. (1914) Notes on heredity of primary glaucoma. Royal London Ophthalmic Hospital Report 19:42-44.
Learmonth, J.R. (1920) The inheritance of specific iso-agglutinins in human blood. Journal of Genetics 10:141-148.
Ledbetter, T.A. (1925) A case of amaurotic family idiocy in an infant of non-Semitic parentage. Canadian Medical Association Journal 15:367-369.
Leslie, G. (1881) On hereditary transmission of disease: Method of graphic representation. Edinburgh Medical Journal 27:795-799.
Letchworth, T.W. (1928) Four cases of glioma retinae in one family. British Medical Journal 2:656.
Levy, A. (1907) Partial albinism with a curious heredity. Transactions of the Ophthalmologic Society of the United Kingdom 27:220-221.
Levy, A.H. (1922-1923) Case of amaurotic family idiocy. Proceedings of the Royal Society of Medicine 16:17-18 Opthalmology.

Lewis, T. (1909a) Hereditary split foot. Treasury of Human Inheritance 1(IIa):6-10.
———. (1909b) Polydactylism. Treasury of Human Inheritance 1(IIIa):10-14.
Lewis, T. and D. Embleton (1908-1909) Split hand and split foot deformities. Biometrika 6:26-58.
Lipscomb, W. (1915) A study in heredity. Australian Medical Journal 1:260-261.
Litchfield, W.F. (1917) A clinical and anatomical report of Friedreich's disease. Australian Medical Journal 1:135-140.
Lock, R.H. (1909) Recent Progress in the Study of Variation, Heredity and Evolution. London: Murray.
Lockhart-Mummery, P. (1925) Cancer and heredity. Lancet 1:427-429.
Loudon, J. (1925) Preliminary report on the Glover micro-organism as the specific cause of carcinoma. Canada Lancet and Practitioner 64:13-29.
Loudon, J. and J.M. McCormack (1925) Evidence in favor of the microbic origin of carcinoma. Canadian Journal of Medicine and Surgery 58:154-168.
Love, J. (1920) Hereditary deafness. Journal of Laryngology 35:263-268.
Love, J.K. (1921) Deafness and Mendelism. Maternity and Child Welfare 5:65-69.
MacGregor, R. (1926) A case of amaurotic family idiocy. Canadian Medical Association Journal 16:1362-1363.
MacKay, H. and A.M. Davidson (1929) Congenital ectodermal defect. British Journal of Dermatology 41:1-5.
Mackay, H. and F.D. McKenty (1927) Hereditary hemorrhagic telangiectasia. Canadian Medical Association Journal 17:65-67.
Macklin, M.T. (1926) Hereditary abnormalities of the eye I. Introduction: The laws of heredity and their exemplification in the inheritance of eye colour. Canadian Medical Association Journal 16:1340-1342.
———. (1927a) Hereditary abnormalities of the eye II. Inheritable defects involving the eyelids and their mode of transmission. Canadian Medical Association Journal 17:55-60.
———. (1927b) Hereditary abnormalities of the eye III(1). Anomalies of the entire eyeball. Canadian Medical Association Journal 17:327-331.
———. (1927c) Hereditary abnormalities of the eye III(2). Anomalies of the entire eyeball. Canadian Medical Association Journal 17:421-423.
———. (1927d) Hereditary abnormalities of the eye IV. Inheritable diseases affecting the conjunctiva. Canadian Medical Association Journal 17:697-702.
———. (1927e) Hereditary abnormalities of the eye V. Inheritable defects of the iris and lens. Canadian Medical Association Journal 17:937-942.
———. (1927f) Hereditary abnormalities of the eye VI (1). Inheritable defects involving the retina. Canadian Medical Association Journal 17:1191-1197.
———. (1927g) Hereditary abnormalities of the eye VI (2). Inheritable defects involving the retina. Canadian Medical Association Journal 17:1336-1342.
———. (1927h) Hereditary abnormalities of the eye VII. Inheritable defects involving eye muscles, refraction, etc. Canadian Medical Association Journal 17:1493-1498.
Macnab, A. (1907) Congenital opacity of the cornea in three members of one family. Ophthalmic Review 26:253.
Macnicol, M. (1910) A hemophiliac pedigree. Indian Medical Gazette 45:215-216.
Mandel, L. (1922-1923) Case of Tay-Sachs disease. Proceedings of the Royal Society of Medicine 16:55-56 Children.
Manson, J.S. (1911) Letter to W. Bateson. 12 May 1911 (B 2774).
———. (1915-1916) Hereditary syndactylism and polydactylism. Journal of Genetics 5:51-63.
———. (1928) Observations on Human Heredity. London: HK Lewis, pp. 76-77.

Marshall, L. (1902-1903) Digital abnormality. Reports of the Society for the Study of Diseases in Children 3:222-226.
Marshall, R. (1929) Notes on a family with brachydactyly. Archive of Disease in Childhood 4:385-388.
Mathew, P. (1908) A case of hereditary brachydactyly. British Medical Journal 2:969.
Mayou, M.S. (1904) Cerebral degeneration with symmetrical changes in the maculae. Transactions of the Ophthalmologic Society of the United Kingdom 24:142-145.
McDonagh, J.E.R. (1926) The etiology of cancer. Medical Press and Circular 121:111-114, 131-133.
McIntosh, G.A. (1907) A case of Huntington's chorea. Maritime Medical News 19:352-355.
Mehler, B. (2000) "Madge Thurlow Macklin." ISAR Biography. Notable American Women http://www.ferris.edu/isar/bios/macklin.htm. Accessed 20 June 2006.
Mekie, E.C. (1927) Hereditary hemorrhagic telangiectasis. British Medical Journal 1:423.
Mill, G. (1906) Huntington's chorea and heredity. British Medical Journal 2:1215.
Miller, R. and H. Perkins (1920) Congenital steatorrhea. Quarterly Journal of Medicine 14:1-9.
Moody, A.R. (1910) Friedreich's ataxia. Lancet 1:164-165.
Morgan, T.H. (1922a) Croonian Lecture—On the Mechanisms of Heredity. Proceedings of the Royal Society 94B:162-197.
———. (1922b) The mechanism of heredity. Nature 109:241-244, 275-278, 312-313.
Morgan, T.H., A.H. Sturtevant, H.J. Muller, C.B. Bridges (1915) The Mechanism of Mendelian Heredity. New York: Holt.
Moriet, A. (1921) Hereditary optic atrophy as a possible menace to the community. Australian Medical Journal 2:499-502.
Morley, E.B. (1914) Epidermolysis bullosa hereditaria. British Journal of Dermatology 26:35-42.
Morris, J.N. (1908) Hereditary cerebellar ataxia. Intercolonial Medical Journal of Australasia 13:185.
Mott, F.W. (1905) A discussion of the relationship of heredity and disease. British Medical Journal 2:1086-1091.
———. (1910) Hereditary aspects of nervous and mental diseases. British Medical Journal 2:1013-1020.
———. (1911-1912a) Hereditary transmission of disease. Medical Chronicle (Manchester) 55:63-92.
———. (1911-1912b) The inborn factor in nervous and mental disease. Proceedings of the Royal Society of Medicine 5:1-30 Neurology.
———. (1912) The inborn factor of nervous and mental disease. Brain 34:74-101.
———. (1913a) Inborn potentiality of the child. Science Progress in the Twentieth Century 8:307-321.
———. (1913b) The neuropathic inheritance. Journal of Mental Science 59:222-263.
———. (1925) Heredity in relation to mental disease. British Medical Journal 2:727-731.
Moxon, F. (1913-1914) Congenital diffuse non-inflammatory corneal opacity in two sisters. Proceedings of the Royal Society of Medicine 7:67-70 Ophthalmology.
———. (1914) Congenital diffuse non-inflammatory corneal opacity in two sisters. British Journal of Children's Diseases 11:257-259.
Muir, J. (1906) Eight generations of hemophilia in South Africa. South African Medical Record 4:300-302.
———. (1928) Heredity in hemophilia in South Africa. Journal of the Medical Association of South Africa 2:599-606.
Ness, B.R. (1908) Muscular dystrophy. Glasgow Medical Journal 70:35-41.

Nettleship, E. (1905) On heredity in the various forms of cataract. Royal London Ophthalmic Hospital Reports 16:179-246.
———. (1906a) Cases of colour blindness in women. Transactions of the Ophthalmologic Society of the United Kingdom 26:251-258.
———. (1906b) Some hereditary diseases of the eye. Ophthalmoscope 4:493-505, 549-556.
———. (1907a) A history of congenital stationary night-blindness in nine consecutive generations. Transactions of the Ophthalmologic Society of the United Kingdom 27:269-293.
———. (1907b) A history of night blindness in nine consecutive generations. Ophthalmic Review 26:250-251.
———. (1907-1908c) On retinitis pigmentosa and allied diseases. Royal London Ophthalmic Hospital Reports 17:1-56, 151-166, 333-426.
———. (1908a) A colour blind family. Transactions of the Ophthalmological Society of the United Kingdom 28:248-251.
———. (1908b) Lamellar cataract. Transactions of the Ophthalmologic Society of the United Kingdom 28:226-247.
———. (1908c) Senile cataract in husband and wife. Transactions of the Ophthalmologic Society of the United Kingdom 28:220-226.
———. (1909) On some Hereditary Diseases of the Eye: The Bowman Lecture. Transactions of the Ophthalmologic Society of the United Kingdom 29:i-cxcviii.
———. (1911a) Case of hereditary cataract, and a new pedigree of hereditary night blindness. Ophthalmic Review 30:377.
———. (1911b) On some cases of hereditary nystagmus. Transactions of the Ophthalmologic Society of the United Kingdom 31:159-202.
———. (1912a) A pedigree of congenital night blindness with myopia. Transactions of the Ophthalmologic Society of the United Kingdom 32:21-45.
———. (1912b) A pedigree of presenile or juvenile cataract. Transactions of the Ophthalmologic Society of the United Kingdom 32:337-352.
———. (1912c) Some unusual pedigrees of colour blindness. Transactions of the Ophthalmologic Society of the United Kingdom 32:309-336.
———. (1914) A pedigree of colour blindness including two colour blind females. Royal London Ophthalmic Hospital Reports 19:319-327.
Nettleship, E. and F.M. Ogilvie (1906) A peculiar form of hereditary congenital cataract. Transactions of the Ophthalmologic Society of the United Kingdom 26:191-207.
Nettleship, E. and A.H. Thompson (1912-1913) A pedigree of Leber's disease. Proceedings of the Royal Society of Medicine 6:8-16 Ophthalmology.
Newsholme, H.P. (1910) A pedigree showing biparental inheritance of webbed toes. Lancet 2:1690-1691.
Newton, R.E. (1902) Glioma of retina. Australasian Medical Gazette 21:236-237.
Nicol, W. (1915) A pedigree of hereditary nystagmus. Ophthalmoscope 13:224-231.
Ogilvie, G. (1907-1908) Hereditary spastic paralysis. Proceedings of the Royal Society of Medicine 1:91-92 Neuroology.
Oliver, G.H. (1913) Thirteen cases of hereditary transmission of retinitis pigmentosa in two generations. Ophthalmoscope 11:407-408.
Oliver, J. (1912-1913) Chorea. Eugenics Review 4:39.
Ord, A.G. (1925) A case of hereditary deforming dyschondroplasia. Lancet 2:178-179.
Osler, W. (1908) On hereditary multiple telangiectasae with recurring hemorrhages. Quarterly Journal of Medicine 1:53-58.
———. (1910) Female hemophiliacs and de novo cases of hemophilia. Lancet 1:1226.
Owens, S.A. (1905) Glioma retinae. Royal London Ophthalmologic Hospital Report 16:323-369.

Palmer, F.S. (1906) Friedreich's ataxia. Brain 29:406-407.
Parker, R.W. and M.B. Robinson (1887) A case of inherited congenital malformation of the hands and feet. Transactions of the Clinical Society of London 20:181-189.
Parkinson, J.P. (1912) Pseudohypertrophic muscular paralysis. Clinical Journal 40:317-318.
Parsons, P.H. (1906) Case of Recklinghausen's disease. Medical Press and Circular 81:68-69.
Paterson, D. (1921-1922) Familial cerebral degeneration. Proceedings of the Royal Society of Medicine 15:46 Children.
———. (1926) Case of familial microcephaly. Proceedings of the Royal Society of Medicine 19:60 Children.
Paterson, D. and E.A. Carmichael (1924) A form of familial cerebral degeneration chiefly affecting the lenticular nucleus. Brain 47:207-231.
Paton, L. (1907) Congenital nystagmus with incomplete albinism. Transactions of the Ophthalmological Society of the United Kingdom 27:219-220.
Paul, S.N. (1918) Hereditary angiomata (telangiectases) with epistaxis. British Journal of Dermatology 30:27-32.
Peacocke, G. (1905) Hodgkin's disease occurring in twins. Dublin Journal of Medical Science 120:85-89.
Pearson, K. (1904) Report on certain cancer statistics. Archives of Middlesex Hospital 2:127-137.
———. (1909a) The application of Mendelian rules to human inheritance. British Medical Journal 1:184, 372, 694.
———. (1909b) On the ancestral gametic correlation of a Mendelian population mating at random. Proceedings of the Royal Society 81B:225-229.
Pearson, K., E. Nettleship, and C.H. Usher. (1911-1913a) A Monograph on Albinism in Man. London: Dulau.
———. (1911-1913b) A Monograph on Albinism in Man, p. 490.
Pernet, G. (1904) Involvement of the eyes in a case of epidermolysis bullosa. Ophthalmoscope 2:308-309.
Peters, C.A. (1905) An interesting family history of epilepsy. Montreal Medical Journal 34:588-589.
Phillips, S. (1907-1908) Multiple telangiectases. Proceedings of the Royal Society of Medicine 1:64-65 Clinical.
Platt, R. (1929) Amaurotic family idiocy. British Medical Journal 1:177-178.
Pockley, E. (1915) Leber's disease. Australian Medical Journal 1:189-190.
Porter, J.H. (1907) Achondroplasia. British Medical Journal 1:12-14.
Poynton, F.J. (1906) A contribution to the study of amaurotic family idiocy. Brain 29:180-208.
———. (1908-1909) Amaurotic family idiocy. Proceedings of the Royal Society of Medicine 2:127-128 Clinical.
Poynton, F.J. and J.H. Parsons (1905) Amaurotic family idiocy. Transactions of the Ophthalmologic Society of the United Kingdom 25:312-314.
Prior, G.P. (1905) A case of angioneurotic edema. Australasian Medical Gazette 24:117.
Raffan, J. (1907) Case of neuromuscular paralysis (Charcot-Marie-Tooth). Scottish Medical and Surgical Journal 20:341-343.
Rankin, G. (1900) Pseudohypertrophic paralysis. Polyclinic 2:163.
———. (1902) Friedreich's ataxia. Lancet 1:150-153.
Reid, G.A. (1909) Review of Mendel's Principles of Heredity by William Bateson. Brain 32:93.
———. (1910a) The Principles of Heredity, 2nd ed. New York: Dutton, p. 360.
———. (1910b) The Principles of Heredity, p. 46.

———. (1910c) The Principles of Heredity, p. 54.
Reynolds, E.S. (1917) The cause of disease. Lancet 2:703-709.
Ribot, T. (1875) Heredity. New York: Appleton.
Riddoch, G. (1922-1923) Complete amaurosis, dementia and spastic paralysis in a Hebrew boy. Proceedings of the Royal Society of Medicine 16:29-30 Neurology.
Ridley, A. (1902) Glioma. Transactions of the Ophthalmologic Society of the United Kingdom 22:55.
Rischbieth, H. and A. Barrington (1910) Dwarfism. Treasury of Human Inheritance 1(XVa):355-554.
Roberts, J. (1964) Reginald Ruggles Gates. Biographical Memoirs of Fellows of the Royal Society 10:83-106.
Robinson, H.B. and W.H. Bowen (1908-1909) Inherited congenital claw foot. Proceedings of the Royal Society of Medicine 2:206-210 Clinical.
Rolleston, H.D. (1902) Persistent hereditary edema. Lancet 2:805-807.
Rolleston, H. (1927) The training of a physician. Practitioner 119:273-279.
———. (1928) Hereditary factors in some diseases of the hemopoietic system. Johns Hopkins Hospital Bulletin 43:61-80.
Rolleston, J.D. (1910-1911) Familial pigmentary dermo-fibromatosis. Proceedings of the Royal Society of Medicine 4:71-77 Clinical.
———. (1911) Inherited syphilis and blue sclerotics. Ophthalmoscope 9:321-324.
———. (1917) Persistent congenital edema of the legs (Milroy's disease). Review of Neurology and Psychiatry 15:480-482.
Rosett, J. (1922) A study of Thomsen's disease. Brain 45:1-30.
Rudolph, R.D. (1910-1911) Thomsen's disease. Canada Lancet 44:679-688.
Rushton, A.R., 2004. "Reginald Rugles Gates." Oxford Dictionary of National Biography, Oxford University Press, 2004, www.oxforddnb.com/view/article/33355. Accessed 7 October 2004.
Rutherfurd, W.J. (1919) Hereditary malformation of the extremities. Lancet 1:979-980.
Sandwirth, F.M. (1915) Four Gresham lectures on heredity. Clinical Journal 44:265-272, 273-280, 281-287, 294-296.
Savill, T.D. (1909-1910) Sequel of a case of scleroderma. Proceedings of the Royal Society of Medicine 3:33-35 Clinical.
Sawyer, E.H. (1910) A case of Huntington's chorea. Birmingham Medical Review 67:117-119.
Sawyer, J.E.H. (1907-1908) A peculiar deformity of the hands in four generations. Reports of the Society for the Study of Diseases in Children 8:393-394.
Sawyer, J. (1912-1913) A case of progressive lenticular degeneration. Brain 35:222.
Schiotz, I. (1920) The inheritance of colourblindness in man. British Journal of Ophthalmology 4:393-403.
Scourfield, D.J. (1905-1906) Mendelism and microscopy. Journal of the Quekett Microscopical Club 9:395-422.
Shannon, G.A. (1913) Notes on Huntington's chorea. Canadian Medical Association Journal 3:962-964.
Shaw, T.W. (1916) The transmission of some variations from a hereditary point of view. University of Durham Medical College Gazette 16:75-85.
Sinclair, W.W. (1905) Hereditary congenital night-blindness. Ophthalmic Review 24:255-258.
Smith, E.B. (1910) Amaurotic family idiocy. Ophthalmoscope 8:493-495.
Smith, P. (1910a) Heredity in relation to national welfare. Birmingham Medical Review 67:101-116.
———. (1910b) A note on the making of pedigree charts. Transactions of the Ophthalmologic Society of the United Kingdom 30:35-36.

———. (1910c) A pedigree of Doyne's discoid cataract. Transactions of the Ophthalmologic Society of the United Kingdom 30:37-42.

Snell, S. (1903) Numerous instances of night blindness (retinitis pigmentosa) occurring in five generations. Transactions of the Ophthalmologic Society of the United Kingdom 23:68-70.

———. (1904) Glioma occurring in two members of the same family. Transactions of the Ophthalmologic Society of the United Kingdom 24:230-237.

———. (1905) A further instance in which glioma occurred in more than one member of the same family. Transactions of the Ophthalmologic Society of the United Kingdom 25:261-266.

———. (1907a) Night blindness. Ophthalmic Review 26:93-94.

———. (1907b) Retinitis pigmentosa occurring in several members of a family. Transactions of the Ophthalmologic Society of the United Kingdom 27:217-219.

———. (1908) Coloboma of the iris of each eye occurring in five generations. Transactions of the Ophthalmologic Society of the United Kingdom 28:148-150.

Spillane, J.D. (1940) Familial pes cavus and absent tendon jerks. Brain 63:275-290.

Stephenson, S. (1915a) Blue sclerotics. Ophthalmoscope 13:278-281.

———. (1915b) Blue sclerotics. Transactions of the Ophthalmologic Society of the United Kingdom 35:274-276.

Steward, D.D.S. (1929) Notes on a pedigree of amaurotic family idiocy. British Medical Journal 1:101.

Stewart, D.S. (1929) Amaurotic family idiocy. British Medical Journal 1:479.

Stewart, H. (1922) Fragilitas ossium associated with blue sclerotics. British Medical Journal 2:498.

Stobie, W. (1924) The association of blue sclerotics and brittle bones and progressive deafness. Quarterly Journal of Medicine 17:274-287.

Sutherland, A.G. (1908-1909) Two cases of congenital adenoma of a family type. Proceedings of the Royal Society of Medicine 2:51 Clinical.

Sutherland, G.A. (1906) Case (?) of Von Recklinghausen's disease. Transactions of the Clinical Society of London 39:245-246.

Swanton, A.J. (1907) Hemophilia transmitted through the male. Lancet 2:1385-1386.

Sym, W.G. (1928) Familial glioma retinae. British Medical Journal 2:818.

Symonds, C.P. and M.E. Shaw (1926) Familial clawfoot and absent tendon jerks. Brain 49:387-403.

Taylor, J. and G. Holmes (1913a) Nervous symptoms associated with optic atrophy of the familial type. Transactions of the Ophthalmological Society of the United Kingdom 33:116-138.

———. (1913b) Two families with several members of each suffering with optic atrophy. Transactions of the Ophthalmologic Society of the United Kingdom 33:95-115.

Telling, W.H.M. and S.G. Scott (1905) A case of multiple neurofibromatosis. Lancet 1:921-923.

Torrance, H.W. (1922) Tay-Sachs disease. Glasgow Medical Journal 97:263-273.

Traquair, H.M. (1919) Hereditary glioma of the retina. British Journal of Ophthalmology 3:21-22.

Tubby, A.H. (1894) A case of "lobster claw deformity" of the feet and partial suppression of the fingers with remarkable hereditary history. Lancet 1:396-397.

Turner, J.G. (1906) Hereditary hypoplasia of enamel. Transactions of the Odontological Society of Great Britain 39:137-155.

Turner, J. (1912) Two cases of amaurotic idiocy or Tay-Sachs disease. British Journal of Children's Diseases 9:193-204.

Usher, C.H. (1906) Notes on a case of unilateral white eyelashes and tufts of hair. Transactions of the Ophthalmological Society of the United Kingdom 26:23-26.
———. (1914) On the inheritance of retinitis pigmentosa with notes of cases. Royal London Ophthalmic Hospital Reports 19:130-236.
———. (1924) A pedigree of congenital dislocation of lenses. Biometrika 16:273-282.
Warde, M. (1923) Hemophilia in the female. British Medical Journal 2:599-600.
Warrington, W.B. (1901) A family of three cases of the peroneal type of muscular atrophy. Lancet 2:1574-1577.
Watkins, D.J.G. (1904) A family tree. British Medical Journal 1:190.
Waugh, T.R. (1928) The inheritance of the blood groups. Canadian Medical Association Journal 18:64-66.
Webb, T.L. (1901) A case of hereditary brachydactyly. Journal of Anatomy 35:487-488.
Weber, F.B. (1916-1917) Cerebral degeneration and epileptiform fit with amaurosis. Proceedings of the Royal Society of Medicine 10:100-103 Children.
Weber, F.P. (1907) Multiple hereditary developmental angiomata. Lancet 2:160-162.
———. (1910) Family amaurotic idiocy. Ophthalmoscope 8:166-169.
Whitchurch Howell, H. (1924) Case of fragilitas ossium. Proceedings of the Royal Society of Medicine 17:21 Children.
Williamson, R.T. (1908-1909) Heredity in diabetes mellitus. Medical Chronicle (Manchester) 49:222-228.
Wilson, E.B. (1914) Croonian Lecture: The Bearing of Cytological Research on Heredity. Proceedings of the Royal Society 88B:333-352.
Wilson, J.A. (1914) The factor of heredity in myopia. British Medical Journal 2:393-395.
Wilson, J.J. (1905) Hemophilia. Practitioner 75:829-836.
Wilson, M.G. (1920) A case of hemophilia. Medical Press and Circular 109:134.
Wilson, S.A. (1912a) Progressive lenticular degeneration. Lancet 1:1115-1119.
Wilson, S.A.K. (1912b) Progressive lenticular degeneration. Brain 34:296-509.
Wise, W.D. (1920) A case of fragilitas ossium with blue sclerae. Medical Press and Circular 109:32.
Worster-Drought, C. and J.M. Allen (1929) Huntington's chorea. British Medical Journal 2:1149-1152.
Worth, C. (1906) Hereditary influence in myopia. Transactions of the Ophthalmologic Society of the United Kingdom 26:141-144.
Worton, A.S. (1913) Hereditary optic neuritis. Lancet 2:1112-1114.
Yealland, L. (1926) Huntington's chorea. Brain 49:580.
Yearsley, M. (1914-1915) The problem of deafness and its prevention. Eugenics Review 6:116-129.
Young, J. (1925) A new outlook on cancer. British Medical Journal 1:60-64.

Chapter Fourteen

Ashby, E. (1936) Genetics in the universities. Nature 138:972-973.
Barber, H. (1934) Familial acholuric jaundice. Guy's Hospital Reports 84:37-40.
Barnes, S. (1932) A myopathic family. Brain 55:1-46.
Bearn, A.G. (1993) Archibald Garrod and the Individuality of Man. Oxford: Clarendon, p. 131.
Bedichek, S. and J.B.S. Haldane (1937-1938) A search for autosomal recessive lethals in man. Annals of Eugenics 8:244-254.
Belisario, J.C. (1935) Two cases of xeroderma pigmentosum occurring in the same family. Medical Journal of Australia 2:148-150.

Bell, J. (1930-1931a) Some new pedigrees of hereditary disease A: Polydactylism and syndactylism B. Blue sclerotics and fragility of bone. Annals of Eugenics 4:41-48.
———. (1930-1931b) Three further cases of hereditary digital anomaly. Annals of Eugenics 4:233-237.
———. (1933) On the inheritance of migraine. Annals of Eugenics 5:311-325.
———. (1934) Huntington's chorea. Treasury of Human Inheritance 4(I):1-67.
———. (1935) On the peroneal type of progressive muscular atrophy. Treasury of Human Inheritance 4(II):69-140.
———. (1939) On hereditary ataxia and spastic paraplegia. Treasury of Human Inheritance 4(III):141-281.
Bell, J. and J.B.S. Haldane (1936) Linkage in man. Nature 138:759-760.
———. (1937) The linkage between the genes for colour blindness and hemophilia in man. Proceedings of the Royal Society 123B:119-150.
Biemond, A. and A.P. Daniels (1934) Familial periodic paralysis and its transition to spinal muscle atrophy. Brain 57:91-108.
Blakeslee, A.F. (1932) Genetics of sensory thresholds: taste for phenylthiocarbamide. Proceedings of the National Academy of Sciences 18:120-130.
Bloehm, T.F. (1936) Gaucher's disease. Quarterly Journal of Medicine 29:517-527.
Braid, F. and E.M. Hickman (1929) Metabolic study of an alkaptonuric infant. Archives of Disease in Childhood 4:389-398.
Brain, R.T. (1937) Familial ectodermal defect. Proceedings of the Royal Society of Medicine 31:69-70.
Bray, G.W. (1930) The hereditary factor in asthma and other allergies. British Medical Journal 1:384-388.
Bud, R., 2004. "Lancelot Thomas Hogben." Oxford Dictionary of National Biography, Oxford University Press. www.oxforddnb.com/view/article/31244
Accessed 7 October 2004.
Bulloch, W. (1928) Letter to K. Pearson. 13 February 1928 (P 647/5).
"Bureau of Human Heredity." (1936-1937) Eugenics Review 28:124, 297.
"Bureau of Human Heredity." (1938-1939) Eugenics Review 30:131.
Burns, J.L. (1933) Pregnancy with bilateral congenital cystic kidneys. Canadian Medical Association Journal 29:645-646.
Burrows, H.J. (1938) Developmental aberrations of terminal phalanges. British Journal of Radiology 11:165-176.
Cammidge, P.J. (1934) Heredity as a factor in diabetes mellitus. Lancet 1:393-394.
Caughey, J.E. (1933) Dystrophia myotonica. Proceedings of the Royal Society of Medicine 26:847-848.
Caughey, J.F. (1933) Cataract in dystrophia myotonica. Transactions of the Ophthalmologic Society of the United Kingdom 53:60-72.
"Charles John Bond, FRCS—Obituary." (1939) Eugenics Review 31:215-216.
Chrustschoff, G.K. (1935) Cytological observations on cultures of normal human blood. Journal of Genetics 31:243-261.
Clark, R.W. (1968) JBS: The Life and Work of J.B.S. Haldane. New York: Coward-McCann, p. 102.
"Clinical genetics." (1934) Medical Journal of Australia 1:756.

Clouston, H.R. (1939) The major forms of hereditary ectodermal dysplasias. Canadian Medical Association Journal 40:1-7.
Cockayne, E.A. (1931) Epicanthis and bilateral ptosis. Proceedings of the Royal Society of Medicine 24:847-848.
———. (1933) Inherited Abnormalities of the Skin and its Appendages. Oxford: Oxford University Press.
———. (1935a) Obesity, hypogenitalism, mental retardation, polydactyly and retinal pigmentation. Quarterly Journal of Medicine 28:93-120.
———. (1935b) A second piebald family from Suffolk. Biometrika 27:1-4.
———. (1936) Gargoylism. Proceedings of the Royal Society of Medicine 30:104-107.
———. (1938a) The genetics of transposition of the viscera. Quarterly Journal of Medicine 31:479-493.
———. (1938b) Recurrent bullous eruption of the feet. British Journal of Dermatology 50:358-363.
"Colour blindness and hemophilia." (1937) Lancet 1:611.
Cooke, A.M. (2004). "Lionel Sharples Penrose." Oxford Dictionary of National Biography, Oxford University Press. www.oxforddnb.com/view/article/31537 Accessed 7 October 2004..
Cooper, E.L. (1936) Progressive familial hypertrophic neuritis (Dejerine-Sottos). British Medical Journal 1:793-794.
Couch, H. (1938) Identical Dupuytren's contracture in identical twins. Canadian Medical Association Journal 39:225-226.
Cowen, S.O. (1936) Treatment of familial acholuric jaundice. British Medical Journal 1:690-692.
Crawford, B. (1936) Allergy in five generations. British Medical Journal 1:751-752.
Crew, F.A.E. and J.A. Fraser-Roberts (1933) Discussion on heredity as a factor in animal disease. Proceedings of the Royal Society of Medicine 26:377-380.
Critchley, M. and C.J.C. Earl (1932) Tuberose sclerosis and allied conditions. Brain 55:311-346.
Daniel, G.H. (1936-1937) A case of hereditary anarthrosis of the index finger. Annals of Eugenics 7:281-297.
Davis, E. (1939) Hereditary familial purpura simplex. Lancet 2:1110-1114.
Dawson of Penn, L. (1931) Hereditary icterus. British Medical Journal 1:921-928.
Debre, P. (1939) Familial hepatitis. Lancet 1:760-761.
de Silva, C.C. (1937) Ectodermal dysplasia. Journal of the Ceylon Branch of the British Medical Association 34:65-67.
———. (1939) Hereditary ectodermal dysplasia of anhidrotic type. Quarterly Journal of Medicine 32:97-113.
Dorrell, A. (1932) A case of familial optic atrophy. Royal Berkshire Hospital Report: 122-123.
Dukes, C. (1930) The hereditary factor in polyposis intestinalis. Cancer Review 5:241-256.
Ellis, R.W. (1940) Arachnodactyly and ectopia lentis in a father and daughter. Archives of Disease in Childhood 15:267-273.

Ellis, R.W.B. (1940) A syndrome characterized by ectodermal dysplasia, polydactyly, chondrodysplasia and congenital morbus cordis. Archives of Disease in Childhood 15:65-84.

Ellis, R.W. and W.W. Payne (1936) Glycogen disease. Quarterly Journal of Medicine 29:31-48.

Evans, C. (1930) Familial acholuric jaundice. St. Bart's Hospital Reports 38:25-28.

Evans, G. (1931) Familial incidence of cancer. British Medical Journal 1:157.

Fabing, H. (1934) Tuberous sclerosis with epilepsy in identical twins. Brain 57:227-238.

de F. Bauer, D. (1940) Genetical research in medical practice. Canadian Medical Association Journal 43:135-141.

Feldman, W.M. (1935) Transposition of the viscera. Proceedings of the Royal Society of Medicine 28:753-756.

———. (1941) Congenital transposition of the viscera. Proceedings of the Seventh Genetical Congress:85.

Feriman, D. (1941) The genetics of oxycephaly and acrocephalosyndactyly. Proceedings of the Seventh Genetical Congress:86.

Finney, D.J. (1940) The detection of linkage. Annals of Eugenics 10:171-214

———. (1941) An apparent linkage of the OAB blood groups with allergic disease. Proceedings of the Seventh Genetical Congress:209.

Fisher, R.A. (1911) Heredity. Minutes of the Cambridge University Eugenics Society.

———. (1918) The correlation between relatives and the supposition of Mendelian inheritance. Transactions of the Royal Society of Edinburgh 52:399-433.

———. (1934-1935a) Editorial. Annals of Eugenics 6:1.

———.(1934-1935ab) The detection of linkage in recessive abnormalities. Annals of Eugenics 6:339-351.

———. (1936-1937) Heterogeneity of linkage data for Friedreich's ataxia and the spontaneous antigens. Annals of Eugenics 7:17-21.

Fraser-Roberts, J.A. (1937) The place of genetics in the practice of medicine. Newcastle Medical Journal 17:115-134.

Garland, H.G. (1934) Hereditary scoliosis. British Medical Journal 1:328.

———. (1936) Progressive familial hypertrophic neuritis. British Medical Journal 1:909.

Garrod, A.E. (1933) Letter to E.A. Cockayne. 22 March 1933. Quoted in Bearn, A.G. (1993) Archibald Garrod and the Individuality of Man. Oxford: Clarendon, p. 145

Gates, R.R. (1933) A form of brachyphalangy in a cousin marriage. Lancet 1:194.

"Genetics and medicine." (1932) British Medical Journal 1:293-294.

Goodall, E. (1936) The need for keeping pedigrees. Lancet 2:168-169.

Gorer, P.A. (1937-1938) The genetic interpretation of studies on cancer in twins. Annals of Eugenics 8:219-232.

Gray, A.A. (1936) Otosclerosis. Glasgow Medical Journal 125:97-108.

Gruneberg, H. (1934) The inheritance of disease of the accessory nasal cavities. Journal of Genetics 29:367-374.

Gunther, M. and L.S. Penrose (1935) The genetics of epiloia. Journal of Genetics 31:413-430.

Haldane, J.B.S. (1932) Genetic evidence for a cytological abnormality in man. Journal of Genetics 26:341-344.

———. (1933) The genetics of cancer. Nature 132:265-267.

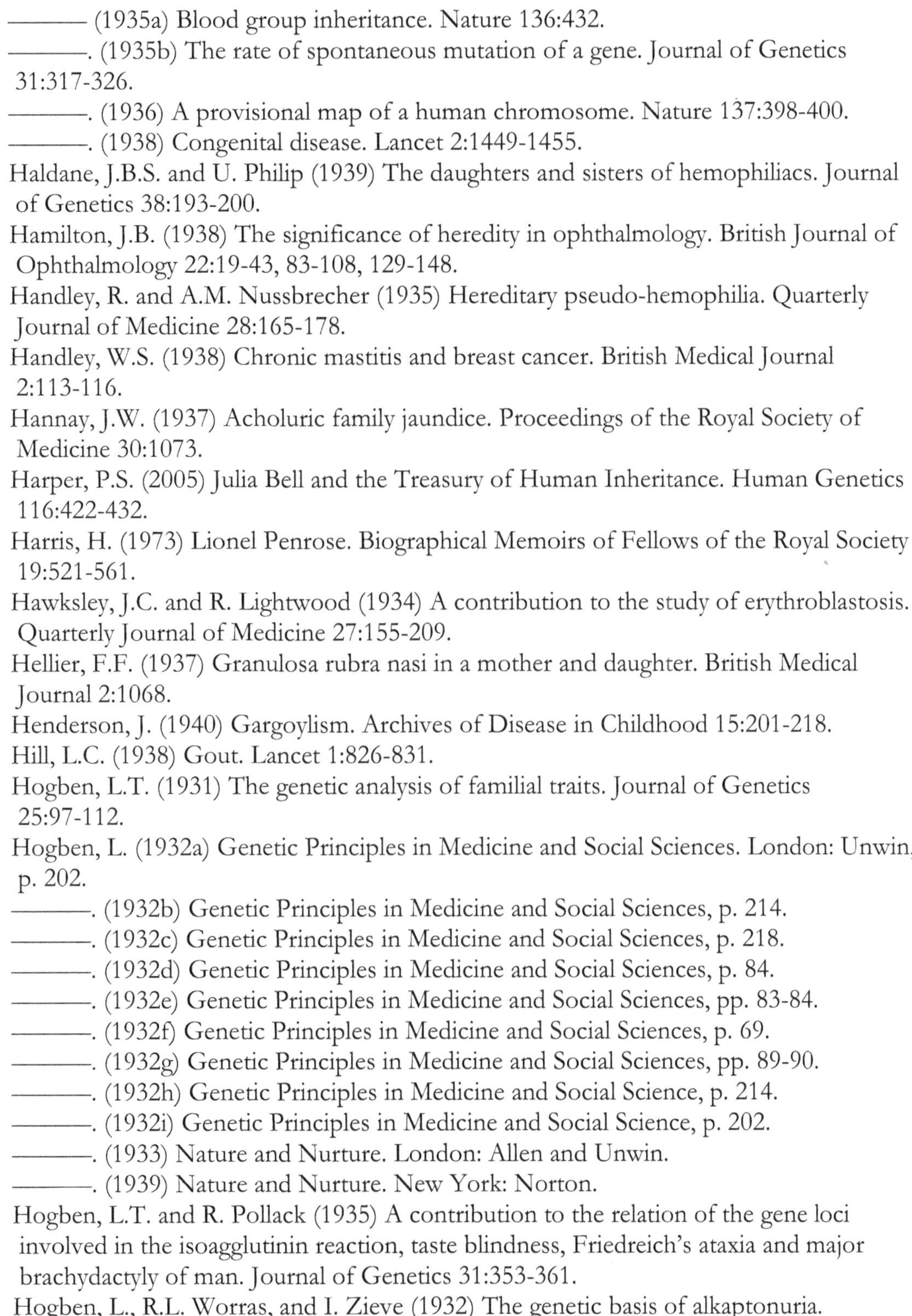

——— (1935a) Blood group inheritance. Nature 136:432.
———. (1935b) The rate of spontaneous mutation of a gene. Journal of Genetics 31:317-326.
———. (1936) A provisional map of a human chromosome. Nature 137:398-400.
———. (1938) Congenital disease. Lancet 2:1449-1455.
Haldane, J.B.S. and U. Philip (1939) The daughters and sisters of hemophiliacs. Journal of Genetics 38:193-200.
Hamilton, J.B. (1938) The significance of heredity in ophthalmology. British Journal of Ophthalmology 22:19-43, 83-108, 129-148.
Handley, R. and A.M. Nussbrecher (1935) Hereditary pseudo-hemophilia. Quarterly Journal of Medicine 28:165-178.
Handley, W.S. (1938) Chronic mastitis and breast cancer. British Medical Journal 2:113-116.
Hannay, J.W. (1937) Acholuric family jaundice. Proceedings of the Royal Society of Medicine 30:1073.
Harper, P.S. (2005) Julia Bell and the Treasury of Human Inheritance. Human Genetics 116:422-432.
Harris, H. (1973) Lionel Penrose. Biographical Memoirs of Fellows of the Royal Society 19:521-561.
Hawksley, J.C. and R. Lightwood (1934) A contribution to the study of erythroblastosis. Quarterly Journal of Medicine 27:155-209.
Hellier, F.F. (1937) Granulosa rubra nasi in a mother and daughter. British Medical Journal 2:1068.
Henderson, J. (1940) Gargoylism. Archives of Disease in Childhood 15:201-218.
Hill, L.C. (1938) Gout. Lancet 1:826-831.
Hogben, L.T. (1931) The genetic analysis of familial traits. Journal of Genetics 25:97-112.
Hogben, L. (1932a) Genetic Principles in Medicine and Social Sciences. London: Unwin, p. 202.
———. (1932b) Genetic Principles in Medicine and Social Sciences, p. 214.
———. (1932c) Genetic Principles in Medicine and Social Sciences, p. 218.
———. (1932d) Genetic Principles in Medicine and Social Sciences, p. 84.
———. (1932e) Genetic Principles in Medicine and Social Sciences, pp. 83-84.
———. (1932f) Genetic Principles in Medicine and Social Sciences, p. 69.
———. (1932g) Genetic Principles in Medicine and Social Sciences, pp. 89-90.
———. (1932h) Genetic Principles in Medicine and Social Science, p. 214.
———. (1932i) Genetic Principles in Medicine and Social Science, p. 202.
———. (1933) Nature and Nurture. London: Allen and Unwin.
———. (1939) Nature and Nurture. New York: Norton.
Hogben, L.T. and R. Pollack (1935) A contribution to the relation of the gene loci involved in the isoagglutinin reaction, taste blindness, Friedreich's ataxia and major brachydactyly of man. Journal of Genetics 31:353-361.
Hogben, L., R.L. Worras, and I. Zieve (1932) The genetic basis of alkaptonuria. Proceedings of the Royal Society of Edinburgh 52:264-295.
Harden, Lord. (1933) Eugenics and the doctor. British Medical Journal 2:1057-1060.

Horsfall, F.L. (1936) Congenital family clubbing of the fingers and toes. Canadian Medical Association Journal 34:145-149.
"Human genetics." (1939) Lancet 2:573, 663-664.
Hurst, L. (1940) Heredito-constitutional research in psychiatry. South African Medical Journal 14:384-390.
Ingram, J.T. and M.C. Oldfield (1937) Hereditary sebaceous cysts. British Medical Journal 1:960-963.
"John B Sanderson Haldane." (1970) Dictionary of National Biography 1961-1970:473-475.
Jones, G. (2004). "Julia Bell." Oxford Dictionary of National Biography, Oxford University Press. www.oxforddnb.com/view/articles/38514 Accessed 2 October 2004.
Jones, J.S. (1993) The Galton Laboratory—University College London. In M. Keynes (ed): Sir Francis Galton FRS—The Legacy of His Ideas. London: Macmillan, pp. 190-194.
Josephson, E. and M. Freiburger (1937) Carotene therapy for retinitis pigmentosa. Nature 139:155.
Joyce, J.C. (1933) Three cases of acholuric jaundice. Proceedings of the Royal Society of Medicine 26:366-368.
Kayne, G. (1933) Familial clubbing of fingers and toes. Proceedings of the Royal Society of Medicine 26:270-271.
Kemp, N.D.A. (2004). "Charles J. Bond." Oxford Dictionary of National Biography, Oxford University Press. www.oxforddnb.com/view/article/75292 Accessed 7 October 2004
Kemp, T. (1941) The human chromosomes. Proceedings of the Seventh Genetical Congress:152.
King, E.F. (1934) Three cases of arachnodactyly with ocular signs. Proceedings of the Royal Society of Medicine 27:298.
———. (1939) Leber's disease in twins. Proceedings of the Royal Society of Medicine 32:763-764.
Latham, A.M. and T.A. Munro (1937-1938) Familial myoclonus epilepsy associated with deaf mutism. Annals of Eugenics 8:166-175.
Law, W. (1934) The refractive error of twins. British Journal of Ophthalmology 19:99-107.
Lawrence, R.D. (1935) Hemochromatosis and heredity. Lancet 2:1055-1056.
Leak, W. (1934) Female bleeders. British Medical Journal 2:700.
Lockhart-Mummery, J.P. and C.E. Dukes (1939) Familial adenomatosis of colon and rectum. Lancet 2:586-589.
Loewenthal, L.J.A. and H.C. Trowell (1938) Xeroderma pigmentosum in African Negroes. British Journal of Dermatology 50:66-71.
Maas, O. (1937) Observations on dystrophia myotonica. Brain 60:498-524.
Macklin, M.T. (1929) Mongolian idiocy. American Journal of Medical Science 178:315-337.
———. (1932) Human tumours and their inheritance. Canadian Medical Association Journal 27:182-187.

———. (1933a) Heredity as an aid to modern therapy. Canadian Medical Association Journal 28:394-397.

———. (1933b) Inherited anomalies of metabolism. I. Diabetes mellitus. Journal of Heredity 24:349-356.

———. (1933c) The need of a course in medical genetics in the medical curriculum. Edinburgh Medical Journal 40:20-30.

———. (1934) The need of a course in medical genetics in the medical curriculum. In Scientific Papers of the Third International Congress of Eugenics. Baltimore: Williams and Wilkins, pp. 157-158.

———. (1935a) Education and research in the field of inheritance of disease. Canadian Medical Association Journal 32:80-82.

———. (1935b) Heredity in cancer. Edinburgh Medical Journal 42:49-67.

MacLachlan, T.K. (1932) Familial periodic paralysis. Brain 55:47-76.

Maddox, K. and M. Scott (1935) Concerning the role of heredity in diabetes mellitus. Medical Journal of Australia 1:7-13.

Maitland-Jones, A.G. (1936) Tay-Sachs disease. Proceedings of the Royal Society of Medicine 29:742-743.

Manson, J. (1935a) Hereditary myopathy. British Medical Journal 2:1256.

———. (1935b) Visceral transposition as a Mendelian recessive. British Medical Journal 2:38.

Mazumdar, P.M.H. (1992a) Eugenics, Human Genetics and Human Failings. London: Routledge, p. 170.

———. (1992b) Eugenics, Human Genetics and Human Failings, pp. 166-167.

———. (1992c) Eugenics, Human Genetics and Human Failings, pp. 237-239.

———. (1992d) Eugenics, Human Genetics and Human Failings, pp. 239-240.

———. (1992e) Eugenics, Human Genetics and Human Failings, p. 303.

———. (1992f) Eugenics, Human Genetics and Human Failings, p. 226.

———. (1992g) Eugenics, Human Genetics and Human Failings, p. 303.

McIlroy, J.H. (1930) Hereditary ptosis with epicanthus. Proceedings of the Royal Society of Medicine 23:285-288.

McQuarrie, M.D. (1935) Two pedigrees of hereditary blindness in man. Journal of Genetics 30:147-153.

Munro, T.A. (1941) The genetics of phenylketonuria. Proceedings of the Seventh Genetical Congress:208.

Munro, T.A., L.S. Penrose, and G.L. Taylor (1941) A study of the linkage relationship between the genes for phenylkenoturia and the ABR allelomorphs in man. Proceedings of the Seventh Genetical Congress:209.

Munro, T.B. (1937-1938) Hereditary sebaceous cysts. Journal of Genetics 35:61-72.

Murray-Lyon, R.M. (1935) Familial acholuric jaundice. British Medical Journal 1:50-52.

Norman, R.M. (1935) A case of juvenile amaurotic family idiocy. Journal of Neurology and Psychopathology 15:219-229.

Nussey, A.M. (1938-1939) A piebald family. Biometrika 30:65-67.

"Obituary of Julia Bell." (1979) Lancet 1:1152.

Ormond, A.W. (1930) The etiology of arachnodactyly. Guy's Hospital Reports 80:68-81.

Ottley, C. (1932) Osteopsathyrosis. Archives of Disease in Childhood 7:137-148.

———. (1934) Heredity and varicose veins. British Medical Journal 1:528.

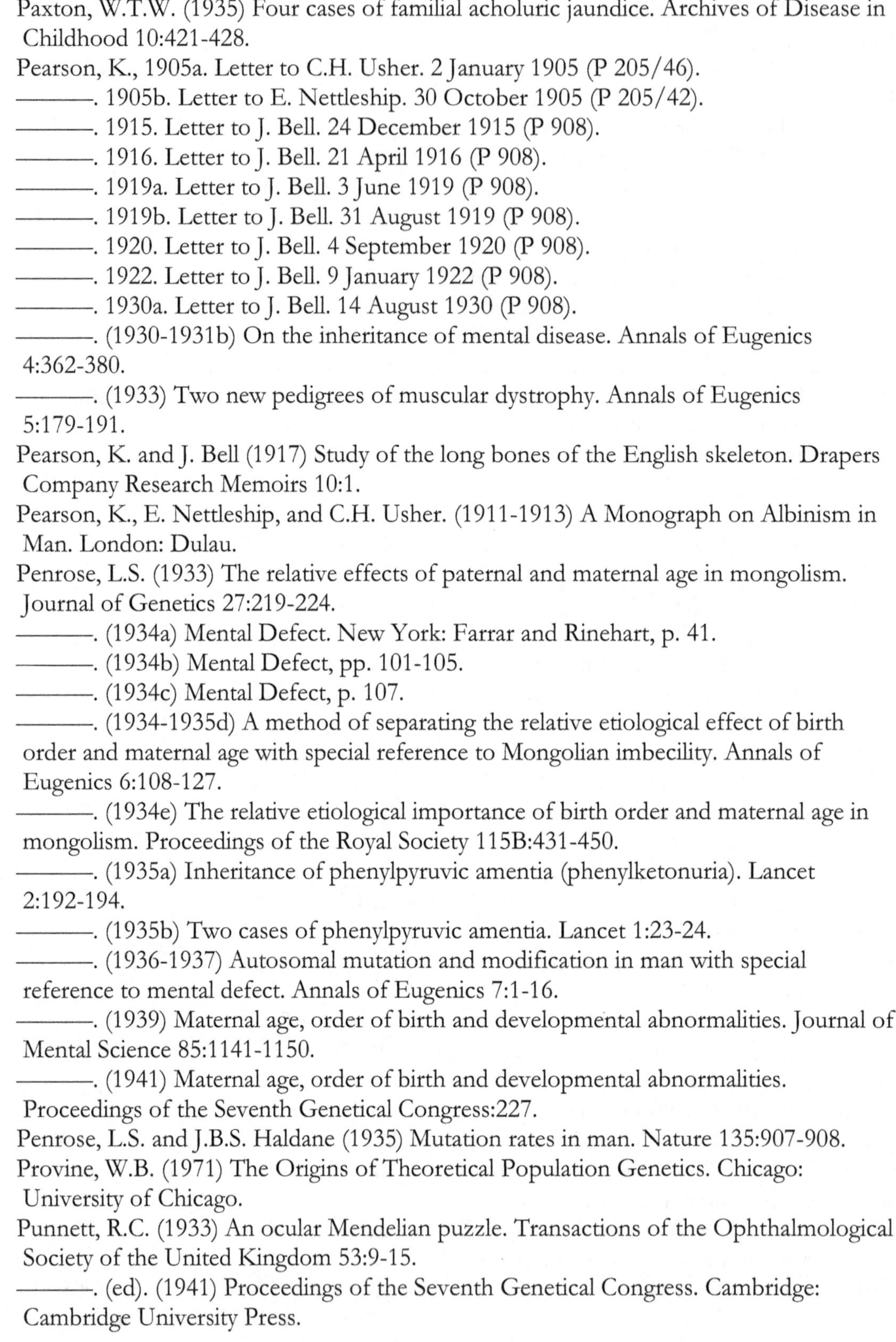

Paxton, W.T.W. (1935) Four cases of familial acholuric jaundice. Archives of Disease in Childhood 10:421-428.

Pearson, K., 1905a. Letter to C.H. Usher. 2 January 1905 (P 205/46).

———. 1905b. Letter to E. Nettleship. 30 October 1905 (P 205/42).

———. 1915. Letter to J. Bell. 24 December 1915 (P 908).

———. 1916. Letter to J. Bell. 21 April 1916 (P 908).

———. 1919a. Letter to J. Bell. 3 June 1919 (P 908).

———. 1919b. Letter to J. Bell. 31 August 1919 (P 908).

———. 1920. Letter to J. Bell. 4 September 1920 (P 908).

———. 1922. Letter to J. Bell. 9 January 1922 (P 908).

———. 1930a. Letter to J. Bell. 14 August 1930 (P 908).

———. (1930-1931b) On the inheritance of mental disease. Annals of Eugenics 4:362-380.

———. (1933) Two new pedigrees of muscular dystrophy. Annals of Eugenics 5:179-191.

Pearson, K. and J. Bell (1917) Study of the long bones of the English skeleton. Drapers Company Research Memoirs 10:1.

Pearson, K., E. Nettleship, and C.H. Usher. (1911-1913) A Monograph on Albinism in Man. London: Dulau.

Penrose, L.S. (1933) The relative effects of paternal and maternal age in mongolism. Journal of Genetics 27:219-224.

———. (1934a) Mental Defect. New York: Farrar and Rinehart, p. 41.

———. (1934b) Mental Defect, pp. 101-105.

———. (1934c) Mental Defect, p. 107.

———. (1934-1935d) A method of separating the relative etiological effect of birth order and maternal age with special reference to Mongolian imbecility. Annals of Eugenics 6:108-127.

———. (1934e) The relative etiological importance of birth order and maternal age in mongolism. Proceedings of the Royal Society 115B:431-450.

———. (1935a) Inheritance of phenylpyruvic amentia (phenylketonuria). Lancet 2:192-194.

———. (1935b) Two cases of phenylpyruvic amentia. Lancet 1:23-24.

———. (1936-1937) Autosomal mutation and modification in man with special reference to mental defect. Annals of Eugenics 7:1-16.

———. (1939) Maternal age, order of birth and developmental abnormalities. Journal of Mental Science 85:1141-1150.

———. (1941) Maternal age, order of birth and developmental abnormalities. Proceedings of the Seventh Genetical Congress:227.

Penrose, L.S. and J.B.S. Haldane (1935) Mutation rates in man. Nature 135:907-908.

Provine, W.B. (1971) The Origins of Theoretical Population Genetics. Chicago: University of Chicago.

Punnett, R.C. (1933) An ocular Mendelian puzzle. Transactions of the Ophthalmological Society of the United Kingdom 53:9-15.

———. (ed). (1941) Proceedings of the Seventh Genetical Congress. Cambridge: Cambridge University Press.

Race, R.R. (1942) On the inheritance and linkage relations of acholuric jaundice. Annals of Eugenics 11:365-384.

Race, R.R., G.L. Taylor, and J.M. Vaughan (1941) A genetic investigation of acholuric jaundice. Proceedings of the Seventh Genetical Congress:244.

Reason, C.H. (1933) Heredity and polycystic disease of the kidneys. Canadian Medical Association Journal 29:612-615.

Riddell, W.J.B. (1937) Hemophilia and colourblindness occurring in the same family. British Journal of Ophthalmology 21:113-116.

———. (1938) A hemophiliac and colour blind pedigree. Journal of Genetics 36:45-51.

———. (1939) Multiple factors in hereditary eye diseases. Transactions of the Ophthalmologic Society of the United Kingdom 59:275-291.

———. (1940) A pedigree of blue sclerotics, brittle bones and deafness with colour blindness. Annals of Eugenics 10:1-13.

Rolleston, H. (1928) Hereditary factors in some diseases of the hemopoietic system. Johns Hopkins Hospital Bulletin 43:61-80.

Ross, N. (1932) Congenital epicanthus and ptosis transmitted through four generations. British Medical Journal 1:378-379.

Rushton, M.A. (1934) Ectodermal dysplasia. Proceedings of the Royal Society of Medicine 27:725-727.

Russell, P.M.G. (1933) Mongolism in twins. Lancet 1:802-803.

Russell, W.R. (1931) Hereditary aspects of Leber's optic atrophy. Transactions of the Ophthalmologic Society of the United Kingdom 51:187-202.

Russell, W.R. and H.G. Garland (1930) Progressive hypertrophic polyneuritis. Brain 53:376-384.

Rutherfurd, W.J. (1933) Hereditary knock-knee with recurrent dislocation of the patella and aplasia of nails of fingers and toes. British Journal of Children's Disease 30:34-38.

———. (1934) Hereditary scoliosis. British Medical Journal 2:87.

Salaman, R.N. (1941) Breeding for immunity to blight and other diseases of the potato. Proceedings of the Seventh Genetical Congress:261.

Savin, L.H. (1935) Atypical retinitis pigmentosa associated with obesity, polydactyly, hypogenitalism and mental retardation (the Lawrence-Moon-Biedl syndrome). British Journal of Ophthalmology 19:597-600.

Seaton, D.R. (1938) Familial clubbing of the fingers and toes. British Medical Journal 1:614-615.

Sheldon, W. (1938) Hypertrophic pyloric stenosis. Lancet 1:1048-1049.

Sinnott, E.W. and L.C. Dunn (1932) Principles of Genetics. New York: McGraw-Hill.

Slome, D. (1933) The genetic basis of amaurotic family idiocy. Journal of Genetics 27:363-376.

Smith, A.B. (1939) Unilateral hereditary deafness. Lancet 2:1172-1173.

"Something better." (1939) Lancet 2:655.

Sorsby, A. (1934) Three groups of unusual fundus disturbances. Proceedings of the Royal Society of Medicine 27:694-700.

———. (1935) Congenital coloboma of the macula together with the account of the familial occurrence of bilateral macular coloboma in association with apical dystrophyy of the hands and feet. British Journal of Ophthalmology 19:65-90.

———. (1939) Obesity, hypogenitalism, mental retardation, polydacytlism, and retinal pigmentation. Quarterly Journal of Medicine 32:51-68.
Souter, W.C. (1933) Two cases of cataract extraction in myotonia atrophica. Transactions of the Ophthalmologic Society of the United Kingdom 53:73-85.
Spencer, H.G. (2004). "Ronald Aylmer Fisher." Oxford Dictionary of National Biography, Oxford University Press. www.oxforddnb.com/view/article/33146. Accessed 7 October 2004
Stallard, H.B. (1938) A case on intraocular nevus (Von Recklinghausen's disease) of the left optic nerve head. British Journal of Ophthalmology 22:11-18.
Stewart, R.M. (1925) The problem of the mongol. Proceedings of the Royal Society of Medicine 19:11-25 Psychiatry.
Stuart, A.M. (1937) Three cases exhibiting Ehler-Danlos syndrome. Proceedings of the Royal Society of Medicine 30:984-985.
Susman, M.P. (1934) Rudimentary patellae, other skeletal defects and dystrophy of the nails. Medical Journal of Australia 1:685-686.
Templeton, H.J. (1936) Hereditary dystrophy of the nails. British Journal of Dermatology 48:248-249.
Thomas, J.C. and E.J.C. Hewitt (1939) Blood groups and mental disease. Journal of Mental Science 85:667-688.
Thompson, A.H. and C.T. Willoughby Cushell (1935) A pedigree of congenital optic atrophy. Proceedings of the Royal Society of Medicine 28:1415-1425.
Thompson, R.H.S. and G.P. Wright (1937) Studies on the chemistry of Gaucher's disease. Guy's Hospital Reports 87:30-45.
Usher, C.H. (1930-1931) Two pedigrees of retinitis pigmentosa. Annals of Eugenics 4:215-231.
———. (1932) Hereditary esotropia. Biometrika 24:1-20.
———. (1933) Heredity and eye disease. Transactions of the Ophthalmologic Society of the United Kingdom 53:16-29.
———. (1935a) Bowman Lecture—On a few Hereditary Eye Affections. Transactions of the Ophthalmologic Society of the United Kingdom 55:164-245.
———. (1935b) Pedigrees of hereditary epicanthus. Biometrika 27:5-25.
Van der Hoeve, J. (1932) Eye symptoms in phakomatoses. Transactions of the Ophthalmologic Society of the United Kingdom 52:380-401.
Van Duyse, A. (1933) Heredity and eye disease. Transactions of the Ophthalmological Society of the United Kingdom 53:29-42.
Watson, E.M. (1934) Diabetes mellitus in twins. Canadian Medical Association Journal 31:61-63.
Weber, F.P. (1931) A hemolytic jaundice family. International Clinics 3 Series 41:148-156.
———. (1933) Familial asthenic type of thorax. Lancet 2:1472-1473.
Wells, G.P. (1978) Lancelot T. Hogben. Biographical Memoirs of Fellows of the Royal Society 24:183-221.
Wiener, A., I. Zieve, and J.H. Fries (1936-1937) The inheritance of allergic disease. Annals of Eugenics 7:141-162.
Wigley, J.E.M. (1938) Ehler-Danlos syndrome. Proceedings of the Royal Society of Medicine 31:257.

Wilson, J.A. (1932) Twins and eye defects. British Journal of Ophthalmology 16:421-423.
Wilson, R. (1936) Congenital blindness: ?bilateral pseudoglioma. Proceedings of the Royal Society of Medicine 29:1433-1434.
Witts, L.J. (1932a) The constitutional factor in diseases of the blood. Practitioner 129:450-454.
———. (1932b) The heredity of hemorrhagic diatheses. Guy's Hospital Reports 82:465-474.
———. (1937) The hemorrhagic states. British Medical Journal 2:689-692.
Wordley, E. (1932) Epistaxis without telangiectasia. Lancet 2:1331.
Worster-Drought, C. (1932) Unusual form of familial myopathy. Proceedings of the Royal Society of Medicine 25:1540-1542.
———. (1940) A form of familial presenile dementia with spastic paralysis. Brain 63:237-245.
Worster-Drought, L. and W.H. McMenery (1933) Presenile familial dementia with spastic paralysis. Journal of Neurology and Psychopathology 15:27-34.
Yacoub, K. (1938) Tay-Sachs disease in Egypt. Journal of the Egyptian Medical Association 21:377-387.
Yates, F. (1970) Ronald A Fisher. Dictionary of National Biography 1961-1970:361-362.
Zieve, I., A. Wiener, and J.H. Fries (1936-1937) On the linkage relations of the genes for allergic disease and the genes determining the blood groups MN types and eye colour in man. Annals of Eugenics 7:163-178.

Chapter Fifteen

Gates, R.R. (1929) Heredity in Man. London: Constable.
———. (1946) Human Genetics. New York: Macmillan.
Greenblatt, S.H. (2003) Harvey Cushing's paradigmatic contributions to neurosurgery and the evolution of his thoughts about specialization. Bulletin of the History of Medicine 77:789-822.
Haldane, J.B.S. (1942) New Paths in Genetics. New York: Harper.
Hukk, D.L. (1988) Science as a Process. Chicago: University of Chicago Press.
Krantz, D.L. and L. Wiggins (1973) Personal and impersonal channels of recruitment in the growth theory. Human Development 16:133-156.
Levenson, T. (2003a) Einstein in Berlin. New York: Bantam, p. 44.
———. (2003b) Einstein in Berlin, pp. 44-45.
———. (2003c) Einstein in Berlin, pp. 215-216.
———. (2003d) Einstein in Berlin, pp. 25-26.
———. (2003e) Einstein in Berlin, p. 352.
———. (2003f) Einstein in Berlin, pp. 352-353.
Meyer, A.W. (1936) An Analysis of De Generatione Animalium of William Harvey. Stanford, CA: Stanford University Press, p. 25.
Pearson, K. (1909) On the ancestral gametic correlation of a Mendelian population mating at random. Proceedings of the Royal Society 81B:225-229.
———. (1911) The Grammar of Science, 3rd ed. London: Black, p. 9.

Pearson, K., E. Nettleship, and C.H. Usher. (1913) A Monograph on Albinism in Man, Vol. 2. London: Dulau, p. 490.
Rushton, A.R. (1994) Genetics and Medicine in the United States 1800-1922. Baltimore: Johns Hopkins University Press, p. 153.
Youngson, A.J. (1979) The Scientific Revolution of Victorian Medicine. London: Helm.

Index

Index